Essentials of
Long-Term Care Insurance

Financial Advisor Series

C. Bruce Worsham, Editor

Future titles to be published in the Series

<u>*Sales Skills Techniques*</u>

Techniques for Marketing Financial Services Products

Techniques for Advising Financial Services Clients

Techniques for Building a Financial Services Career

<u>*Product Essentials*</u>

Essentials of Annuities

Essentials of Business Insurance

Essentials of Disability Income Insurance

Essentials of Life Insurance Products

Essentials of Life Insurance Law

Essentials of Employee Benefits

<u>*Planning Foundations*</u>

Foundations of Senior Planning

Foundations of Estate Planning

Foundations of Retirement Planning

Foundations of Financial Planning: An Overview

Foundations of Financial Planning: The Environment

Another American College book about long-term care insurance:

Meeting the Financial Needs of Long-Term Care
Burton T. Beam, Jr., and Thomas P. O'Hare
© 2003

Financial Advisor Series: Product Essentials

Essentials of
Long-Term Care Insurance

Richard A. Dulisse
Kirk S. Okumura
Glenn E. Stevick, Jr.
C. Bruce Worsham

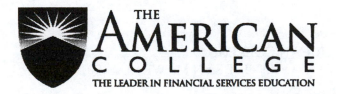

THE
AMERICAN
COLLEGE
THE LEADER IN FINANCIAL SERVICES EDUCATION

ISBN 1-57996-071-5

To Dr. Gary K. Stone on the occasion of his retirement from The American College. His ownership of a long term care insurance policy was a motivating force behind our writing this book. We pray that he will forever remain healthy and never have to avail himself of his policy's benefits.

RAD
KSO
GES
CBW

Contents

1. Getting Started

2. Identifying and Approaching Prospects

3. Long Term Care Caregivers, Settings, and Financing Alternatives

4. Meeting with the Prospect

Preface

The mission of this book is to develop your professionalism as a financial advisor counseling prospects and clients about the need for long-term care insurance (LTCI). We intend to do this by teaching you the *product essentials* of LTCI, by enhancing your marketing and *sales skills techniques,* and by stressing the importance of *planning foundations* in shaping your performance as a successful advisor. It is our hope that this book has the right blend of sales skills techniques, product essentials, and planning foundations to accomplish this mission.

While much of the text material will be new to you, some will, no doubt, refresh knowledge you acquired in the past. In either case, all of the text material is both valuable and necessary if you aspire to be successful in the LTCI marketplace. The benefits you gain from studying the text material will be directly proportional to the effort you expend. So read each chapter carefully and answer both the essay and multiple choice review questions for the chapter (preferably before looking in the back of the book for the answers); to do less would be to deprive yourself of a unique opportunity to become familiar with LTCI and to learn more about selling it.

The book includes numerous pedagogical features designed to help you focus your study of LTCI. Among the features found in each chapter of the book are

- an overview and learning objectives
- a chapter outline, examples, quotes, and lists
- key terms and concepts
- review questions (essay format)
- self-test questions (multiple choice format)

Features located in the back of the book are

- a glossary
- an answers to questions section
- an index

Finally, all of the individuals noted on the acknowledgments page made this a better book, and we are grateful. However, in spite of the help of all of these fine folks, some errors have undoubtedly been successful in eluding our eyes. For these we are solely responsible. At the same time, however, we accept full credit for giving those of you who find these errors the exhilarating intellectual experience produced by such discovery. Nevertheless, each of the authors acknowledges that any errors discovered are the fault of one of the other authors.

Richard A. Dulisse
Kirk S. Okumura
Glenn E. Stevick, Jr.
C. Bruce Worsham

Acknowledgments

This book was written by Richard A. Dulisse, Kirk S. Okumura, Glenn E. Stevick, Jr., and myself, C. Bruce Worsham, all from The American College.

The College would like to acknowledge Burton T. Beam, Jr., associate professor of insurance at The American College, and Thomas P. O'Hare, adjunct professor of insurance at The American College and authors of The American College textbook, *Meeting the Financial Needs of Long-Term Care*, for allowing the authors to borrow liberally from their book. Also, the College wishes to thank Samuel H. Weese, president and CEO of The American College, and Gary K. Stone, executive vice president of The American College, for initiating the development of this book, and for providing continued support and encouragement in writing this book.

For their valuable contribution to the development of this book, appreciation is extended to Todd Denton for editing the manuscript and Pat Berenson, Susan Doherty, Charlene McNulty, Evelyn Rice, and Jane Hassinger for production assistance.

Very special thanks to Alyse Blumberg, Rick DiLaurenzo, Hollie Gandy, and Ginny Thompson, who gave a great deal of their time and expertise to advise on the writing of this book. Also, special thanks to Robert A. Arzt for providing guidance and encouragement to keep the project moving.

The College would also like to thank the following individuals for their substantial contributions to this book:

Paul Barbin	Earl Gordon
Bob Barrett	John Gray
Irv Beitler	Ron Hagan
Ed Boyce	Jeff Hughes
Lucia Bryson	Maryanne Ibach
Shalyn Clark	Lori Ann Jones
Barry Cook	Craig Lafferty
Kathryn Cover	Anna Marie Lombardi
Charles Day	Bill Lombardo
John Ebner	Tom O'Connell
Darren Featherstone	Larry K. Oxenberg
Rebecca Freeman	Mark Papa
Jason Goetze	Dennis Poulous
Joel Goodhart	Tom Schreiner

Mark Seidenberg   Robert Whitaker
John Seigler   Larry Wright
Gregory Smith   Tom Young
Jeff Swenson

To all of these individuals, without whom this book would not have been possible, the College expresses its sincere appreciation and gratitude.

C. Bruce Worsham
Associate Vice President and Editor
Financial Advisor Series
The American College

About the Authors

Richard A. Dulisse, MSM, MSFS, LUTCF, CLU, ChFC, RHU, REBC, is an author/editor at The American College. His responsibilities at the College include writing and preparing text materials for the LUTC *Retirement Planning* and *Planning for Seniors* courses. He also writes articles for *Advisor Today,* the national magazine distributed to members of NAIFA.

Before joining the College, Mr. Dulisse worked in the life insurance industry from 1979 through 2001. His experience includes 5 years as a life agent—initially with Metropolitan Life and then with New York Life. At New York Life, he also served as a sales manager before becoming a training manager in 1985. As a training manager, he helped implement the company's training curriculum to teach agents product knowledge and selling skills.

Mr. Dulisse earned a BSoc.S degree, cum laude, from The Pennsylvania State University. He also holds both the MSM and the MSFS degrees awarded by the College.

Kirk S. Okumura is an author/editor at The American College. His responsibilities at the College include writing and preparing text materials for the LUTC *Exploring Personal Markets* and *Employee Benefits* courses. He also writes articles for *Advisor Today,* the national magazine distributed to members of NAIFA.

Before joining the College, Mr. Okumura worked for State Farm Insurance as a supervisor in a regional life/health office and as a trainer in the Pennsylvania regional office's agency training area.

Mr. Okumura earned a BS degree from The Pennsylavnia State University.

Glenn E. Stevick, Jr., MA, CLU, ChFC, is an author/editor at The American College. His responsibilities at the College include writing and preparing text materials for the LUTC *Meeting Client Needs* and *Business Continuity* courses. He also writes articles for *Advisor Today,* the national magazine distributed to members of NAIFA.

Before joining the College, Mr. Stevick worked for New York Life as a training supervisor for 15 years in its South Jersey office. He also served as an agent with New York Life for more than 2 years. Prior to his insurance industry experience, Mr. Stevick taught psychology at the college level and worked in various educational and mental health programs.

Mr. Stevick earned his BA degree from Villanova University and his MA degree from Duquesne University.

C. Bruce Worsham, MA, JD, LLM, CLU, is an associate vice president and director of educational development at The American College. He has been with the College since 1969 and his current responsibilities include supervising the development of LUTC course materials and editor of the Financial Advisor Series of books. He also is the examination consultant for the Academy of Life Underwriting's FALU professional designation program for home office underwriters.

Prior to assuming his current duties at the College, Mr. Worsham was in charge of the College's professional designation programs (i.e., CLU, ChFC, RHU, and REBC) as director of the Huebner School. In addition, he was responsible for the College's CFP™ Certification Curriculum for students interested in earning a CFP™ designation.

Mr. Worsham earned his BS degree from the University of California at Berkeley and an MA degree from the Wharton School at the University of Pennsylvania, where he held a Huebner Foundation fellowship. He also received his JD degree, cum laude, from Widener University School of Law and an LLM degree from Villanova University School of Law.

Special Notes to Advisors

Text Materials Disclaimer

This publication is designed to provide accurate and authoritative information about the subject covered. While every precaution has been taken in the preparation of this material to insure that it is both accurate and up-to-date, it is still possible that some errors eluded detection. Moreover, some material may become inaccurate and/or outdated either because it is time sensitive or because new legislation will make it so. Still other material may be viewed as inaccurate because your company's products and procedures are different from those described in the book. Therefore, the authors and The American College assume no liability for damages resulting from the use of the information contained in this book. The American College is not engaged in rendering legal, accounting, or other professional advice. If legal or other expert advice is required, the services of an appropriate professional should be sought.

Caution Regarding Use of Illustrations

The illustrations, sales ideas and approaches in this book are not to be used with the public unless you have obtained approval from your company. Your company's general support of The American College's programs for training and educational purposes does not constitute blanket approval of the sales ideas and approaches presented in this book, unless so communicated in writing by your company.

Use of the Term Financial Advisor or Just Advisor

Use of the term "Financial Advisor" as it appears in this book is intended as the generic reference to professional members of our reading audience. It is used interchangeably with the term "Advisor" so as to avoid unnecessary redundancy. Financial Advisor takes the place of the following terms:

Account Executive	Life Insurance Agent
Agent	Life Underwriter
Associate	Planner
Brokers (stock or insurance)	Practitioner
Financial Consultant	Producer
Financial Planner	Property & Casualty Agent
Financial Planning Professional	Registered Investment Advisor
Financial Services Professional	Registered Representative
Health Underwriter	Senior Advisor
Insurance Professional	

Answers to the Questions in the Book

The answers to all essay and multiple choice questions in this book are based on the text materials as written.

About the Financial Advisor Series

The mission of The American College is to raise the level of professionalism of its students and, by extension, the financial services industry as a whole. As an educational product of the College, the Financial Advisor Series shares in this mission. Since knowledge is the key to professionalism, a thorough and comprehensive reading of each book in the Series will help the practitioner advisor to better service his or her clients. A task made all the more difficult because the typical client is becoming ever more financially sophisticated with each passing day and demands that his or her financial advisor be knowledgeable about the latest products and planning methodologies. By providing practitioner advisors in the financial services industry with up-to-date authoritative information about various marketing and sales techniques, product knowledge, and planning considerations, the books of the Financial Advisor Series will enable many practitioner advisors to continue their studies so as to develop and maintain a high level of professional competence.

When all books in the Financial Advisor Series are completed, the Series will encompass 15 titles spread across three separate subseries, each with a special focus. The first subseries, *Sales Skills Techniques,* will focus on enhancing the practitioner advisor's marketing and sales skills, but will also cover some product knowledge and planning considerations. The second subseries, *Product Essentials,* will focus on product knowledge, but will also delve into marketing and sales skills as well as planning considerations in many of its books. The third subseries, *Planning Foundations,* will focus on various planning considerations and processes that form the foundation for a successful career as a financial services professional. When appropriate, product knowledge and sales and marketing skills will also be touched upon in many of its books.

When all 15 titles in the Series are completed, they will be divided among the 3 subseries as follows:

Sales Skills Techniques
- *Techniques for Marketing Financial Services Products*
- *Techniques for Advising Financial Services Clients*
- *Techniques for Building a Financial Services Career*

Product Essentials
- *Essentials of Annuities*

- *Essentials of Long-Term Care Insurance*
- *Essentials of Business Insurance*
- *Essentials of Disability Income Insurance*
- *Essentials of Life Insurance Products*
- *Essentials of Life Insurance Law*
- *Essentials of Employee Benefits*

Planning Foundations

- *Foundations of Senior Planning*
- *Foundations of Estate Planning*
- *Foundations of Retirement Planning*
- *Foundations of Financial Planning: An Overview*
- *Foundations of Financial Planning: The Environment*

This book, *Essentials of Long-Term Care Insurance,* is the inaugural book in the Series. Other books in the Series will be forthcoming over the ensuing months and years.

Overview of the Book

Essentials of Long-Term Care Insurance is designed around a 10-step selling process (or sales cycle) that is covered in more depth in other American College publications. Chapter 1 reviews the 10-step selling process, defines long-term care (LTC), and discusses the exploding need and interest in purchasing long-term care insurance (LTCI).

From there, the book discusses the markets for LTCI and effective prospecting, preapproach, and approach strategies that will help you get started in exploring LTCI sales opportunities. Next, the book focuses on the sales interview and what must be done to discover the prospect's needs, to design solutions to meet those needs, to present them in an effective manner, and how to handle any of your prospect's concerns and objections. This will give you a good foundation for identifying prospects and working with them to explore the LTC need.

In addition, the book provides an in-depth look at LTC services, settings, and different financing alternatives. The LTCI product and optional riders are covered thoroughly, reflecting the impact that HIPAA (Health Insurance Portability and Accountability Act) has had on new LTCI products and their marketing in general. Understanding these technical aspects of LTCI is critical to designing and presenting customized solutions to your prospects. Although the book focuses on LTCI, it also reviews some of the combination products that are available, such as a universal life/LTCI hybrid policy.

The final chapters in the book look at some of the distinctive issues associated with underwriting and delivering a LTCI policy. They examine the servicing and claim handling aspects of the LTCI product that distinguish it from life insurance. Also, the book discusses how LTCI is an integral part of a prospect's retirement, estate, and overall financial plan. In chapter 8, the book concludes with discussions on marketing LTCI to business owners, ethics, professionalism, and building a profitable practice in the LTCI market.

Essentials of
Long-Term Care Insurance

1

Getting Started

Overview and Learning Objectives

Chapter 1 reviews the 10-step selling process covered in other American College publications. In addition, it provides a brief overview of long-term care (LTC), the needs and opportunities for long-term care insurance (LTCI), and three major market segments for the LTCI product. By reading this chapter and answering the questions, you should be able to:

1-1. Identify the 10 steps of the selling process.

1-2. Explain the principles of client-focused selling.

1-3. Define LTC.

1-4. Describe the relationship among the components of the LTC crisis.

1-5. Identify who will need LTCI based on financial and emotional motivations.

1-6. List the three age-based market segments.

Chapter Outline

The Selling Process

Welcome to the *Essentials of Long-Term Care Insurance*, a book designed to teach you how to market and sell long-term care insurance (LTCI). It assumes you have general marketing and selling skills for insurance products.

In this book, LTCI is discussed within the framework of the universally recognized components of what is generically referred to as the selling process or "sales cycle." In this regard, it is appropriate to provide an overview (and for some of you a review) of the selling philosophy and selling process that provides the underlying framework for our discussion of LTCI.

> **Anything worth doing is worth doing well.**

Selling Philosophy

A selling process is based on a selling philosophy. Over the years, many authors have written about selling the "right" way. In doing so, they have used many terms to describe the "right" way: relationship, client-centered, counselor, consultative, needs-based, values-based—the list goes on. Each is based on the same basic principles of communication: asking good questions and listening carefully to people. The end goal is the same: to cultivate a long-term, mutually beneficial relationship with a client. For our purposes we will refer to this selling philosophy as client-focused selling.

Client-focused selling stresses that a financial advisor's **(see page xv for an explanation of the meaning of the term "financial advisor" or just "advisor" as used in this book)** job is to help people achieve their objectives by providing solutions to their insurance and financial needs in an open, honest, ethical and forthright manner. The process focuses on helping people achieve their goals by removing obstacles and presenting strategies that lead to success. It is founded on the premise that people want to feel that they bought a product they need, will help them, and has personal value. People like to buy; they do not like to be sold.

Compare such ends and means with the "commando" approach of high-pressure, exaggerated pitches, arm-twisting, and manipulative closing techniques. The main objective of such a process is to get the sale at all costs. It is transaction-oriented and results in an adversarial advisor-client relationship, pitting the advisor against the client. Transactional selling is an endless series of one-shot deals and poor service, if any at all. The transaction-selling mantras, "the sale begins when the prospect says no" and "close early and often" reflect this combative relationship. The financial advisor must outthink, outmaneuver, and outtalk the prospect to make the sale.

On the other hand, the client-focused selling approach is a win-win situation. A sale should not be a victory for the advisor alone, but for everyone involved. People deserve to work with a reliable, trustworthy professional who has their best interest in mind. When they are able to do so, they view their financial advisor as a trusted professional. Consequently, the advisor will receive repeat business, referrals, and increased persistency. Client-focused selling will elevate the sales experience for both the advisor and the client, as well as the status of and respect for the insurance and financial services industry. In the LTCI marketplace, there is no other way to proceed.

10-Step Selling Process or "Sales Cycle"

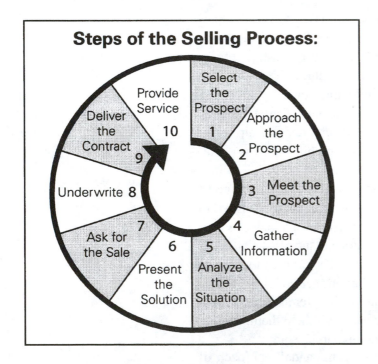

Steps of the Selling Process:

This book divides the selling process into 10 steps. Think of the selling process as a blueprint for building clients. Following the selling process enables you to organize your marketing and selling efforts so you can develop a systematic approach rather than leave them to chance. Systems enable you to duplicate success and equally important, to analyze failure.

1. Select the Prospect—Effective selling begins with getting in front of the right prospect. Not only do you want to look for prospects who have a high probability of needing, wanting, and affording your products; you should also be aware that

LTCI requires a higher emphasis on the insurable aspect of a qualified prospect. As always, when prospecting outside your current client base, you will want to find people who will value your expertise and become a source of repeat business and referrals. A systematic approach can help you find target markets of potential clients and enable you to market efficiently and effectively.

2. Approach the Prospect—This step involves getting appointments and can be done either by telephone or face to face. If you are cultivating relationships, you will generate more referral-based business. With the negative feelings people have toward telemarketers, cold calling is becoming more difficult and, consequently, referrals have become much more critical.

3. Meet the Prospect—This is where you establish rapport, explain your business purpose, ask some thought-provoking questions, and listen, listen, and listen. The importance of listening cannot be overstated; it is essential when building any relationship. Gain the prospect's agreement to let you proceed with the information-gathering process by distinguishing yourself from the competition.

4. Gather Information—When you think of the word interview, you think of someone asking questions of someone else. That is exactly what you want to do with your prospect. Questions help you uncover the prospect's needs, goals, priorities, and attitudes. It is good to discover as much about the prospect's financial and attitudinal landscape as you can.

The key skills in the interviewing process are:

> **Focus on Listening**
>
> Don't be anxious to make a sale. Focus on listening to people and their needs. LTCI is a needs-based sale, so explain the need. If the prospects don't know they have a need, you have to educate them. They will only buy what they think they need.

- Questioning. Ask open-ended questions to probe for needs, goals, prioritizing and attitudes. Ask confirming questions to clarify.
- Listening. Actively listen, rephrase, and reflect to ensure that you and the prospect are on the same page.
- Uncovering. Provide information or ask open-ended questions designed to help the prospect see the reality of the situation. Be fair and honest, not manipulative.

- Taking notes. Jot down numbers, goals, needs, priorities, and feelings.
- Summarizing. Review what the prospect has told you and confirm that you have clearly understood him or her.
- Acting. Agree on a proposed next action.

5. Analyze the Situation—Once you have a good idea of the needs, goals, priorities, and attitudes of the prospect, analyze the concepts and products you have that might best fit the prospect's situation; organize these into a plan — no matter how basic or sophisticated, it is an insurance plan. If your product does not fit correctly, send the prospect where they can get what they need. Because you focus on the long-term relationship, the prospect may not do business with you today, but he or she will remember that you were honest even when it meant you did not write the business. People want to do business with those they trust!

> **Selling made easier:**
> **Ask good questions**
> **and learn to listen.**

6. Present Solutions—Position your product based on the information gathered in the interview. Cover only relevant features and benefits, not every feature and benefit. Confirm throughout the presentation that the prospect is in agreement so you can address any questions or concerns that arise. Immediately deal with any miscommunication or misunderstanding.

7. Implement the Solution—Help the prospect acquire the financial products and services required to put the plan into action. Ask if the prospect has further questions or concerns. If so, address them immediately. Then propose the next steps.

8. Underwrite—Complete the application, perform all field underwriting requirements that are needed, and submit the case to the company. Advise the prospect of the time frame and any responsibility he or she may have (such as having a medical exam). Use this opportunity to proactively discuss situations that might result in a rating.

9. Deliver the Contract—At delivery, review the benefits you are providing and how they resolve the applicant's problem. Reinforce the concept of an insurance plan and the need for monitoring the situation to ensure that the client remains properly insured as time passes and life changes. You can do this by offering a periodic review, annually or at some other agreed-upon time frame.

10. Service the Plan—This may be the most important step in preserving your hard work and expanding on it. Through service you enhance and cement your relationship with each new client, make additional sales, and set the stage to obtain quality referrals to new prospects. In contrast to life insurance sales, you will have ongoing contact with your clients and their families during the claim period.

Summary

No matter what insurance or financial service product you sell, the basic selling (or planning, if you prefer) process is universal. Following the selling process ensures that you duplicate success and enables you to diagnose failure because you have clearly defined what you want to accomplish at each step and how you will do it.

The Need
and Opportunity

The headline of a March 21, 2002 news release from the U.S. Senate's Special Committee on Aging bears the title, "Sen. Breaux Warns of National Long-Term Care Crisis." Senator Breaux's use of the word *crisis* in association with LTC is something with which many Americans are beginning to identify. The country's collective awareness is growing and many people approaching retirement would at least like to prevent the LTC crisis from personally affecting them. Unfortunately, the awareness of the need does not make the solution self-evident. People need your professional advice and, sometimes, a little motivation to buy the LTCI policy that will meet their needs.

The purpose of this section is to provide enough information for you to picture the opportunity that exists for financial advisors who sell LTCI. It begins with an overview of LTC and is followed by a discussion of the factors involved with the impending LTC crisis, namely

- the increasing need for LTC services
- the decreasing ability of families to provide care
- the high cost of care
- the lack of viable options to pay for care

The section ends with a brief overview of the possible markets for prospects.

What Is LTC?

The definition of LTC seems to have grown more complex over the years. Because of the public misconception of LTC, it is important to emphasize that LTC is not simply nursing home care. It is much more than that. LTC can best be defined as the broad range of medical, custodial, and other care services provided over an extended period of

> **Long-term care is more than just nursing home care!**

time in various care settings due to a chronic illness, physical disability, or cognitive impairment. Examining this definition closely will help you to understand and explain LTC to your prospects and clients.

Medical, Custodial, and Other Care Services

LTC can require any one or a combination of the following types of services: medical, custodial, and other.

Medical—Medical care services imply that the supervision of a physician is required to direct the care provided by skilled, licensed health care professionals, such as registered nurses, licensed practical nurses, and therapists. This could be 24-hour around-the-clock care, which is commonly referred to as *skilled care*, or it could be less frequent, which is commonly referred to as *intermediate care.*

Custodial—Custodial care (or personal care) services include assistance with the activities of daily living (ADLs) or instrumental activities of daily living (IADLs). ADLs are those activities geared toward the care of bodily needs that enables an individual to live independently. They include bathing, dressing, toileting, eating, transferring, and continence.

On the other hand, IADLs deal more with one's overall ability to function cognitively. IADLs include ancillary activities such as preparing meals, shopping, cleaning, managing money, taking medications, and so forth.

Custodial care can usually be provided without professional medical skills or training. Family members often provide custodial care at home.

Other Care Services—The realm of services provided under the auspices of LTC has broadened beyond physical and medical needs. One example is social care, aimed at preventing the loneliness and isolation that a person requiring LTC often experiences. Also included are the services that are required in order to adapt the home to the care recipient's needs. Examples of adaptations would include

---

Financial Advisor's Perspective

One advisor related the story of how her best friend's husband kept putting off buying a LTC policy. He eventually had a stroke, and is now uninsurable. The advisor visited the couple and summarized her feelings in this way: "When I came back from seeing my friend, I wanted to get on top of my office building with a bullhorn and scream to everyone in town, 'Don't be stupid; get your LTCI.' But I realized I couldn't get the word out like that. So I've chosen to do it one family at a time. And it's a very slow process. I get frustrated that I cannot do it faster."

- bathroom balance bars
- widened doorways
- improved lighting
- nonslip flooring
- phones with amplification capability and larger buttons

Provided over an Extended Period of Time

Generally speaking, LTC is associated with chronic illnesses and disabilities. This means that it excludes *acute care* services. Acute care can be thought of as an emergency intervention or treatment typically brief and severe in nature. The reasonable assumption is that after the person has been successfully treated he or she will recover back to his or her previously healthy condition. Acute care is provided by a hospital and many times will involve an intensive care unit and, obviously, requires professional medical attention. Examples of conditions requiring acute care include a broken hip, pneumonia, or a heart attack.

Various Care Settings

Unfortunately, LTC was once synonymous with nursing home care only. But the care setting for LTC has evolved as technology, services, and market demands have dictated. Now care can be provided in a variety of care settings, including

- skilled-nursing facilities, such as a LTC facility or a nursing home
- residential communities, such as an assisted living facility
- community-based facilities, such as an adult day care center
- the home of the person receiving care

Some levels of care do require staying in a specified facility, such as a skilled-nursing facility. For example, skilled care that requires medically necessary, 24-hour physician-directed care must be provided in a skilled-nursing facility. However, intermediate care could be provided in a skilled-nursing facility or in the recipient's home.

Impairment and Illness

Cognitive impairments, physical disabilities, and chronic illnesses associated with aging (Alzheimer's disease, arthritis, and the general effects aging has on mobility) are the reasons people typically need LTC. But many people require LTC services because of a disability caused by an accident or a stroke—something that could happen to anyone at any age.

The Increasing Need for LTC Services

Whether or not Senator Breaux and his congressional colleagues are using the word *crisis* for political reasons, the fact is that the need for LTC will only increase for the foreseeable future, very likely dramatically. Let us examine the most prominent factors: the relationship between LTC and aging and the changing demographics.

The Relationship Between LTC and Aging

Regardless of the fact that many people under the age of 65 require assistance with daily living due to physical or cognitive disabilities, the greatest single predictor of the need for LTC is advancing age. This is due to the gradual and inevitable decline in physical and mental abilities that usually occurs as one ages. Consider the following often-quoted statistics:

- Approximately 20 percent of Americans older than 65 need assistance with every day activities. The number increases to almost 50 percent for those older than 85.[1]
- Those who attain age 85 are four times as likely to enter a nursing home than those who have attained age 65.[2]
- About 90 percent of all nursing home residents are aged 65 or older.[3]
- Over 51 percent of all nursing home residents over age 65 are aged 85 or older.[4]

The direct correlation between aging and the need for LTC is the central ingredient for the LTC crisis. This is a fact that medical advances have done very little to change.

Changing Demographics

In light of the direct correlation between aging and the need for LTC, consider the following demographic changes.

Increased Longevity—People are living longer because advances in medicine, nutrition, and so forth have developed preventions, cures, and treatments for diseases and conditions that were once fatal. Consider that the average life expectancy in 1900 was 47 years; in 2000 it reached 76.9 years. Perhaps more significantly, people who survive to age 65 can expect to live to age 83; in 1900 they could expect to live only to age 68. Unfortunately, while medical advances mean people will live longer, such advances have not done as much to improve the quality of life during these extra years.

Thus, there are more people reaching advanced ages in which dependency on others is more prevalent. As lifespans increase, the length of time people will need LTC due to such dependency will almost certainly increase as well.

Nursing Home Resident Demographics (By Percentages)	
Age at Interview	**Percentage of Residents**
Under 65 years	9.7
65 years and older	90.3
65-74	12.0
75-84	31.8
85 +	46.5

Source: Jones, A. The National Nursing Home Survey: 1999 Summary. *National Center for Health Statistics. Vital Health Stat 13(152), 2002.*

Baby Boomers—The baby boom generation with retirement years between 2011 and 2030 will swell the population in these categories significantly. A few statistics using the population projections in Figure 1-1 make the case.

- In the year 2000, there were approximately 35 million people over age 65, constituting 13 percent of the country's population of 275.3 million; by 2030, when the last of the baby boom generation (those born between 1946 and 1964) turns age 65, there will be 70 million seniors constituting 20 percent of the population (351.1 million).
- Individuals aged 85 and older constitute the fastest growing segment of the senior population and are expected to increase from 4.3 million or 1.6 percent of the population in 2000 to almost 9 million by 2030, when they will represent over 2.5 percent of the population.
- By 2050, when the full effect of the baby boom retirees is felt, the age 85-and-over category will exceed 19 million and comprise almost 5 percent of the population (403.7 million).

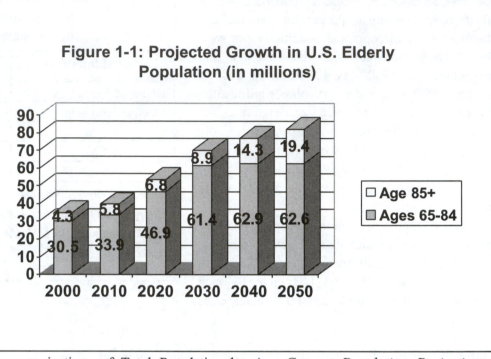

Figure 1-1: Projected Growth in U.S. Elderly Population (in millions)

	2000	2010	2020	2030	2040	2050
Age 85+	4.3	5.8	6.8	8.9	14.3	19.4
Ages 65-84	30.5	33.9	46.9	61.4	62.9	62.6

Source: projections of Total Population by Age Groups, *Population Projections, Population Division,* U.S. Census Bureau, Washington, DC, December 1999–January 2000, NP-T3A-F.

Increased longevity already means that more people will reach ages that will require LTC. The baby boom phenomenon will further accentuate this due to the sheer numbers of those associated with this demographic group. The bottom line is that more people will require LTC in the not-so-distant future, and require it for a longer period of time.

The Decreasing Ability of Families to Provide Care

How is society positioned to handle this increasing need? Currently, family members provide a great deal of LTC for their elderly relatives, often at considerable personal sacrifice. Immediate family members, other relatives, and friends render approximately 70 percent of LTC in the home. This care would cost over $200 billion per year if provided by paid caregivers. In addition, these caregivers spend billions of dollars of their own money in the process of providing care. This does not take into account the billions of dollars in lost wages and opportunities that caregivers forfeit because they are no longer able to work outside the home.

Regardless of the cost, informal caregivers will continue as a principal source of LTC because families prefer to care for their elderly relatives. However, it is becoming more difficult for families to provide that care at the very time the need for LTC is increasing. Limits arise from demographic, social, and economic factors that can be categorized under the headings of availability and capacity.

Availability

Compared to previous generations, family members are simply less available today to meet the needs of their elderly parents and relatives because of the increased participation of women in the paid workforce, lower birth rates, and the geographic dispersion of families.

Increased Participation of Women in the Paid Workforce—Women have been and continue to be the major providers of LTC services in the home. However, their availability has become restricted because of their increased participation in the paid work force. Due to economic necessity, the desire for a higher standard of living, and/or the pursuit of their own careers, a majority of women have made their careers a priority. Regardless of the motivation, the hours spent at work are unavailable for caregiving and often exclude assistance to a parent who needs continuous care, thereby requiring the need for professional care at home or in a nursing home. But many women (and men) with jobs outside the home still provide care to elderly parents. Indeed, about 64 percent of family caregivers are employed, many (54 percent) full-time.

Lower Birth Rates—Unlike the baby boom generation, today's average family is smaller and there are fewer large families. Because of the cost of living, standard of living concerns, and marriages later in life, people are having fewer children. In addition, there are more childless families and more people are remaining single. As a result, today's aging

---

A Buyer's Perspective

"I don't want my family milked dry because of the care that I may need. Why would I want to do that to my family when there is a simple solution? And LTCI is a simple solution. It's not a complicated thing at all.

---

parents have fewer children to look to for their care than in previous generations.

Geographic Dispersion of Families—Family members are dispersed geographically to a greater extent than in previous generations. Sons and daughters, brothers and sisters often leave the area in which they grew up when they marry or they relocate to take advantage of employment and career opportunities. To the extent they are dispersed geographically, family members are unavailable to care for elderly parents or other relatives.

Capacity

A caregiver's capabilities, a family's situation, and the condition of the family member being cared for limit the capacity of family members to provide LTC. These capacity limitations frequently arise from multiple priorities, increased longevity, divorce, and the required necessary medical technology.

Multiple Priorities—Even when family members are available, they often face multiple priorities that restrict their ability to provide care. The caregiver may have a spouse or children who also have a claim on the caregiver's available time and attention. Financial priorities may also conflict if the family caregiver must pay for a portion of a parent's LTC expenses while meeting his or her own financial obligations for retirement and child education.

Increased Longevity—Longevity makes it difficult to predict the availability of family support. An extended life span leaves a greater proportion of older people requiring support from a younger but aging generation. Thus, family members are increasingly at an advanced age when they find themselves responsible for their spouses or their 80- to 90-year-old parents. At this period in their lives, they could easily be unable to provide the extent of care required by the age and condition of their loved one and because of their own declining capabilities. A retiree's limited financial and other resources can easily be insufficient to support a disabled spouse or parent, especially if medical care or other expensive services are needed.

High Divorce Rates—Divorce has the effect of restricting the capacity to provide informal care in several ways. Not surprisingly, a person is more likely to care for the parents of a spouse than those of his or her ex-spouse. Aged divorced persons, especially fathers, are less likely to receive care from their adult children. Stepparents are only half as likely to receive care from their stepchildren as are parents of natural children. Single parent families, often created by divorce, have lower incomes on average than dual-parent families and are often below the poverty level. They are, consequently, less able to assume the burdens of or contribute to the care of a parent or other relative.

Required Necessary Medical Technology—The level of assistance a family provides for an elderly relative at the initial stages of a chronic condition may be nothing more than occasional visits to check on or observe routine activities and provide assistance when needed. Inevitably, the initial level almost always escalates to the point of required continuous care with major responsibilities for a broad range of needs. At some point hereafter, available medical technology to improve nutrition, provide therapy, and prevent infection may be required even if the care setting has remained in the caregiver's or recipient's home. While the family member may continue to provide custodial care, the use of the medical technology may require professional assistance one or more days a week.

High Cost of Care

The out-of-pocket payments for LTC by people who must pay their care from personal resources can be astronomical. Currently, average annual nursing home costs are approximately $52,195 for a semi-private room ($61,320 for a private room) and can range much higher.[5] The average nursing home stay is 2.5 years.[6] Two visits a day by a home health aid to help with bathing and dressing and household chores can cost $2,500 a month ($30,000 annually).[7] By 2030, the annual cost of nursing home care is expected to rise to $200,000 with comparable increases in home care charges (see figure 1.2—Projected Annual Cost of LTC).[8]

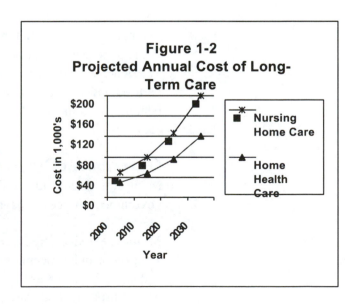

Figure 1-2
Projected Annual Cost of Long-Term Care

These estimates are based on a 4.73 percent increase each year. While that might seem high, it actually might be quite low. With the numbers of people requiring LTC projected to double by 2030 and the shrinking number of health care workers, costs could rise even higher and faster.[9]

Few Viable Options

The rising costs would not be as much of a problem if there were viable ways to pay for the needed care. Now we will look at three major classifications of sources: personal resources, government programs, and LTCI. We will cover each of these alternatives in depth in later chapters. What is important to note here is how well any of these options can handle the LTC problem.

Personal Resources

Personal resources (out of pocket) include income, savings, and assets that comprise one's personal or family wealth. The single question most relevant to personal resources is whether they can pay for all LTC expenses often incurred at unanticipated times and for an extended or indefinite period at the levels mentioned previously. Statistics indicate that 50 to 75 percent of all couples are impoverished within one year after one of them enters a nursing home. Only 15 percent of Americans can afford to pay for more than a 3-year nursing home stay at today's rates.[10] Even if personal wealth is sufficient to meet expenses for a specific episode of LTC, the adequacy of the remaining resources to maintain a spouse's or family's desired standard of living and leave an estate to be passed on to heirs must also be considered.

Benefits from traditional forms of life and health insurance may also be used under certain circumstances to meet LTC needs. However, these benefits are limited in both the amount and the situations in which they are available.

Government Programs

Medicare, Medicaid, and veterans' benefits are frequently cited government sources of payment for LTC services.

Medicare—Medicare is a medical expense insurance program for people aged 65 or older, people with disabilities under age 65, and people with end-stage renal disease (permanent kidney failure that requires dialysis or a transplant). Medicare provides coverage for acute hospital, surgical, and physician care but pays only limited benefits for the expenses of LTC. These benefits do not extend to custodial care unless this care is needed along with the medical or rehabilitative treatment (post-acute skilled care) provided in skilled-nursing facilities or at home. Unfortunately, Medicare's limited coverage of post-acute care services in a skilled-nursing facility and payment of home care services often gives the mistaken impression that Medicare provides payment for custodial LTC services required by the elderly with chronic conditions.

Medicaid—Medicaid is a federal-state funded entitlement program that is designed to provide medical assistance for individuals and families with low incomes and resources. Unfortunately, it has also become the de facto program for funding LTC for the middle class as well. This is why Medicaid is the largest source of payment for LTC services, covering 43 percent of all LTC services provided. It is also why a cottage industry of Medicaid attorneys and specialists has emerged to assist middle class clients in hiding assets in order to qualify for Medicaid's standards. But what can Medicaid provide?

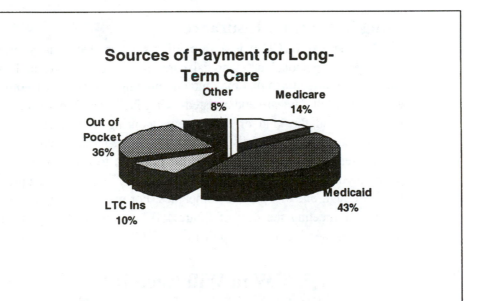

Sources of Payment for Long-Term Care

Other 8%
Medicare 14%
Out of Pocket 36%
Medicaid 43%
LTC Ins 10%

Source: How Will You Pay for Long-Term Care if You Need It? Office of Personnel Management for the Government. *http://www.opm.gov/insure/ltc/posters/pay_for_ltc.htm*. Citing: Department of Health and Human Services, HCFA, Office of the Actuary, National Health Statistics Group, Personal Health Care Expenditures, 2001

Already Medicaid is straining under a burden it was not designed to bear. It is one of the reasons that Medicaid does not pay a LTC facility full market value for a bed. Thus, many LTC facilities only carry limited numbers of Medicaid beds. The result is a waiting list for those potential residents who will pay via Medicaid. Factor in the scores of baby boomers on the edge of needing such care and as the Center for Long-Term Care Financing report puts it: "…Medicaid will not withstand the tidal wave of aging baby boomers."[11]

Veterans' Benefits—The Veterans' Administration (VA) may provide limited nursing home benefits for veterans in one of its own facilities or private nursing homes. Service-connected disabilities and illnesses or low income are eligibility requirements for admission to VA nursing homes. This care is always further conditioned on available space. Use of private nursing homes is possible upon discharge from a VA facility, but is normally not provided in excess of 6 months, unless service-related care is required. Direct admission to a private nursing home is almost always limited to someone receiving care for a service-related condition.

Long-Term Care Insurance

Finally, there is LTCI. It is a form of insurance that usually provides coverage for personal or custodial care, intermediate care, and skilled care in various settings that may include nursing homes and at-home care as well as adult day care and assisted-living facilities. Benefits often vary by setting and the kind of care received during a specified period of covered care (typically daily). In addition, benefits are paid either as a reimbursement of expenses incurred, usually up to a maximum, or as a payment of a defined amount. Approximately 5 million people have LTCI through one of over 120 companies. For many people, it is the best option for meeting the cost of future LTC expenses. And you will do them a great service if you help them buy a LTCI policy.

Who Will Need It?

In this section we will identify some issues related to prospect needs and then review some market segments. The information discussed here will help you get started in identifying some prospects. The marketing and prospecting topics are developed further in chapter 2.

Financial and Emotional Needs

An often-quoted statistic indicates that over 40 percent of all 65-year-olds will spend some time in a nursing home. The older one gets, the greater the probability he or she will need LTC. However, needing LTC does not directly correspond to needing LTCI. Some will not have enough assets to warrant LTCI and others will not have a strong enough emotional reason to buy it. As with other insurance products, the LTCI "need" has two aspects: a financial one, and to a greater degree, an emotional one. Specifically, the need depends greatly on how the prospect perceives the financial and emotional aspects of LTC.

Financial—The financial reason for purchasing LTCI is to protect a person's assets. But not everyone has viable assets to protect. The NAIC in its publication, *A Shopper's Guide to Long-Term Care Insurance*, specifies suitability guidelines of $30,000 in assets (not including primary residence) and that LTCI premiums not exceed 7 percent of monthly income.

Who Can Afford LTCI?	
Ages	**Percent**
35–39	73
40–44	71
45–49	81
50–54	75
55–59	63
60–64	47
65 +	31
Total	62

Source: American Council of Life Insurance.
Note: Affordability is defined as spending no more than 2 percent of income for ages 35-44, 3 percent for ages 45-54, 4 percent for ages 55-59, 5 percent for ages 60–64, and 10 percent for ages 65+

The baseline for suitability is not too difficult for many people to meet at younger ages. For example, if the average LTCI premium with inflation protection for someone aged 50 is $800 per year, a person with an annual income of $11,500 and $30,000 in assets (excluding primary residence) would meet the suitability guidelines. In contrast, if the average premium at age 65 is $1,900 per year, the annual income guideline increases dramatically to $27,150, a more difficult standard to meet. Your company's guidelines may be more stringent (higher requirements), in which case use your company's guidelines instead.

To help you identify the specific income and net worth levels you wish to target, here are some guidelines that the United Seniors Health Cooperative, a nonprofit organization dedicated to educating seniors on health issues, suggests that consumers use. The prospects should

- have assets of at least $75,000 (excluding home and automobile).
- have annual retirement income of at least $25,000–$35,000 if single, or $35,000–$50,000 if married. (These are national averages and may be higher or lower depending upon costs in your community.)
- be able to pay LTCI premiums without adversely affecting lifestyle.
- be able to absorb possible increases in LTCI premiums without financial difficulty.[12]

You will want to derive your own guidelines based on your natural and target markets as well as your own personal convictions.

Buyer's Perspective on LTCI

Authors' Note: The following excerpt from the June 27, 2002 article, Navigating the Maze of Long-term Health Insurance, *found at* http://www.cnn.com/2002/HEALTH/06/27/long.term.health.ap/index.html. Reprinted with permission of The Associated Press.

Marian and Rubin Ferziger:
For Marian Ferziger, a 57-year-old New York accountant, the decision to buy her own long-term care policy came after her mother-in-law applied for one in her 80s and was turned down.

"It turned out she had a health problem that hadn't been diagnosed," she said. "It was found during the (qualifying) physical. She's doing fine, but she was turned down for coverage."

Ferziger and her husband, lawyer Rubin Ferziger, 53, figured that because they were in good health, they should consider getting their own coverage. They had a broker show them a number of policies. They also used the insurance planner available from Weiss Ratings Incorporated, a Palm Beach Gardens, Florida firm that evaluates policies and the companies that offer them.

"I feel better having it," Marian said. "If I get sick, I don't want to eat up all of our assets so Rubin has nothing. The reverse is true, too."

Emotional—Buying LTCI is more than a financial decision; it is an emotional one as well. Therefore, it is necessary to examine the motives behind the purchase. These are the real reasons people buy LTCI and by understanding them, you will have a great deal of success in selling LTCI and helping people protect themselves from a potential financial catastrophe. People need LTCI because:

- *They desire independence.* For some buyers, the purchase of LTCI means they do not have to depend on anyone else for their care; they want to be self-reliant. In other words, it is about dignity and pride. They do not want their children or spouse assisting them with personal care issues because it would be embarrassing and possibly degrading. Even more so, they do not want to depend on public assistance to pay for their care.

- *They do not want to burden family and/or friends.* Similarly, some may not want to burden their loved ones with having to provide care for them. We have already seen the financial burden that is involved with LTC. It can leave a caregiving spouse impoverished. In addition, providing such care can have physical and emotional consequences as well. For example, Alzheimer's victims are sometimes abusive to their caregivers.

This only adds to the emotional stress of watching a loved one deteriorate to a point where he or she cannot recognize family and friends.

- *They desire a choice of providers and settings.* With the news reports of elder abuse in nursing homes[13] and the often poor reputations of Medicaid homes, many buyers want to have the flexibility of choosing a setting other than a nursing home. They typically would prefer to "age in place" by receiving the necessary assistance in their own homes. When their care requires a skilled-nursing facility, they would like to be able to choose the facility. In both situations, choice means better care and greater flexibility—two things Medicaid cannot provide.

- *They want to protect assets.* This reason for buying LTCI has two different manifestations. For those with moderate assets, the motive is to prevent bankruptcy. Given that the number one reason for bankruptcy among seniors in America is paying for LTC, this is a real concern. For those with a sizable net worth,

---

Reasons Given for Buying LTCI

1. I do not want to burden my loved ones with taking care of me when I get old.
2. I want to stay in my own home.
3. I want to make sure I get the best care I can afford.
4. I want to leave an inheritance for my children.
5. I want to be able to afford medical care when I get older.
6. I do not want my spouse to become impoverished.
7. I am afraid I might not be able to qualify to purchase it later in life should my health fail.
8. I do not want to depend on public assistance (Medicaid).
9. Government assistance will not be able to cover LTC in the future.

the motive is more about leaving a legacy for their children than preventing LTC expenses from causing bankruptcy.

Markets

You have probably been in the financial services industry long enough to know that success comes from finding groups of prospects with common needs and characteristics, a process known as *segmenting*. The ultimate goal is to find a segment that is large enough so you do not run out of prospects and that has a communication system that will facilitate the process of identifying prospects. Such a segment is known as a *target market.*

Because of the relationship between needing LTC and age, we will first segment the markets for LTCI in terms of age: under age 50, ages 50 to 65, and over age 65. Following is a brief overview of these market segments to give you a better feel for and understanding of why segmenting is important.

Under Age 50—Typically, people under age 50 do not feel the need for buying LTCI as keenly as those who are older than age 50. This segment is a little more resistant because there are many other needs that are more important. For example, many are still worried about saving enough for their children's education and protecting their incomes from death and disability. Nonetheless, you will find two distinct opportunities in this market for selling LTCI. The first and most obvious opportunity is that you can sell these people a policy to cover themselves. The second and less obvious opportunity for you is to convince this under-age-50 group to motivate their aging parents or other relatives to buy LTCI, or in some cases, actually purchase a policy for these aging loved ones.

Ages 50 to 65—While many in this market segment who are parents may still have other financial concerns (such as saving for children's educations and the life and disability insurance mentioned in the under-age-50 segment), a transition of priorities takes place with a greater emphasis now being placed on their retirement needs. Premiums are still very affordable for those in this segment and the need is appreciated more, especially for those who are watching their own parents cope with aging. This is the bread and butter market segment and will be for several years to come due to the fact that baby boomers (born 1946-1964) comprise a growing percentage of this market.

Over age 65—The premium rates for LTCI begin to increase rapidly for prospects over age 65, not to mention the fact that a smaller percentage of the people in this market segment actually qualify because many have age-related illnesses and medical conditions. Because of the high premiums and smaller percentage of people qualifying healthwise, this market segment requires more stringent prequal-ification than the other two markets. In spite of these facts, however, the average age for LTCI buyers is age 67, indicating that most of the buyers currently come from this market segment.

<hr>

Getting Started

The following is one financial advisor's suggestion to other advisors who are getting started in the LTCI business:

1. Buy the product for yourself. You cannot sell something you have not bought yourself.
2. Sell the product to your staff or assistants.
3. Know your product.
4. Ask everyone to buy it.
5. Do not assume that someone does not need it or is not interested in it.

<hr>

Summary

A popular paradigm describes how the Chinese word *crisis* is expressed by combining the two concepts *danger* and *opportunity for change*. In other words, in Chinese thought, a crisis is a danger that is impregnated with an opportunity for change. The LTC crisis truly represents a danger for an aging population. For financial advisors who sell LTCI, the LTC crisis presents a real opportunity to change what could otherwise be a bleak future.

The market penetration of LTCI is currently less than 8 percent. This means many of your clients and prospects are not ready to face the coming LTC crisis. Therefore, you have an opportunity to beneficially change the future of many of your clients and prospects who would otherwise find their financial fortunes swept away by the need to pay for LTC.

NOTES

1. American Council of Life Insurance. *Long-Term Care Insurance: What Long-Term Care Insurance Can Do For You/Tips on Buying Long-Term Care Insurance,* page 1, taken from *www.acli.com/public/consumer/longterm/ltc.htm* on May 12, 2002
2. Lewin, V.H.I. *Brookings-ICF Long-Term Care Model: Model Assumptions.* Prepared for the Office of the Assistant Secretary for

Planning and Evaluation, U.S. Department of Health and Human Services, 1992.

3. Jones, A. *The National Nursing Home Survey: 1999 Summary*. National Center for Heatlh Statistics. Vital Health Stat 13 (152), 2002.

4. Sahyoun, Nadine, et. al. *The Changing Profile of Nursing Home Residents 1985-1997*, page 2, published for the Centers for Disease Control and Prevention.

5. MetLife Mature Market Institute. *MetLife market Survey on Nursing Home and Home Health Care Costs 2002*. April 2002, Westport, CT: Metropolitan Life Insurance Company, page 4.

6. Jones, A. page 30.

7. American Council of Life Insurance, *Long-Term Care Insurance: What Long-Term Care Insurance Can Do for You/Tips on Buying Long-Term Care Insurance,* taken from American Council of Life Insurance Web site at *web2.acli.com/public/consumer/longterm/ltc.htm.*

8. American Council of Life Insurance, *Can Aging Baby Boomers Avoid the Nursing Home?* March 2000, Washington, DC, page 15.

9. Mulvey, Janemarie and Li, Annelise. *Long-Term Care Financing: Options for the Future*. Benefits Quarterly, Second Quarter 2002, page 7.

10. The John Hancock/National Council on Aging 1997 *Long Term Care Survey,* prepared by Matthew Greenwald and Associates, Washington, DC, Report of Findings, page 15.

11. Ibid.

12. United Seniors Health Cooperative. *Long Term Care Insurance: Making the Right Decision*. *http://www.unitedseniorshealth.org/html/long_term_care_insurance.htm*

13. *Abuse of Residents Is a Major Problem in U.S. Nursing Homes*. Prepared for Rep. Henry A. Waxman, July 30, 2001. This congressional report estimates that one in three U.S. nursing homes was cited for an abuse violation during the 2-year period from January 1, 1999 to January 1, 2001

Case History
Why I Sell LTCI

Authors' Note: The following case history summarizes the responses of several finanical advisors to the question, "Why do you sell LTCI?"

"It's Personal"

For many of the advisors we interviewed, selling LTCI is nothing short of a personal crusade against the devastating effects of a catastrophe waiting to happen. The reason for their missionary zeal is a personal experience and here are three of them:

Advisor 1—"I am motivated by the fact that my mother needed LTC but was ineligible for LTCI. I personally had to care for her and went into debt to do it. In addition, I had a college friend who, at age 34, had a bad accident and is now paralyzed from the waist down. He needs LTC but he cannot qualify to buy LTCI."

Advisor 2—"Even though my mother suffered from Alzheimer's and was bedridden, the last thing we wanted was to place her in a nursing home. At first, my 86-year-old father tried to care for her at home by himself, but lifting her and moving her around proved too much for him. Consequently, we turned to the wide range of home health care services to assist us in caring for my mother. Her care toward the end of her life was costing $9,800 per month. I could see that it was not something my dad and I could afford for very long.

I also have a dear friend from high school whose husband had a stroke at age 54. This was a situation where I had talked to them many times about LTCI before the stroke but was unable to close the sale. These two experiences have made a lasting impression on me. Seeing the need for LTCI has made me realize that I owe it to my clients to sell this product."

Advisor 3—"I have a personal motivation. My grandmother is 91 years old and has been incapacitated for almost 15 years. My grandfather was her primary caregiver until he passed away 2 years ago at the age of 95. When he died, my grandmother went to live with my sister. That was when we realized how hard my grandfather's job must have been. With everyone else in the family working or involved with their families, we needed the services of a home health care provider in order to keep her at my sister's home. This experience has really given me an appreciation of what other families go through in similar situations. It has also educated me about the cost of LTC. I am now motivated to help people buy this product."

"It's Profitable"

Some advisors shared their thoughts on the profitability of selling LTCI. They believe that helping people protect themselves from the devastation of LTC costs is not only the right thing to do, but it also has financial benefits as well. Here are the thoughts of three advisors.

Advisor 1—"I can see from a purely business standpoint that there is a lot of money to be made selling LTCI with very little service work involved. For my company, the claim process involves getting the insured's physician to certify that he or she needs care. I write a letter to the physician telling him or her that the insured has been moved to an LTC facility and that I need a physician's statement certifying the need. The physician sends me the certification letter and we submit it with a claim form to the claim's office. That's all there is to it."

Advisor 2—"I got into the LTCI market because I saw the demographics of a graying America. Every year there will be more people needing this coverage, especially with the first wave of baby boomers rapidly approaching age 65. Furthermore, 43 percent of all people aged 65 and older will spend time in a LTC facility at some point in their lifetimes. This means that baby boomers are watching their own parents either pay for LTC or obtain financial assistance from Medicaid, raising their awareness of the emotional and financial costs involved.

LTCI is the fastest growing market opportunity in the industry."

Advisor 3—"It's a very lucrative market. Advisors can make good money selling LTCI and feel good that they have done the right thing for their clients."

"What about You?"

The finanical advisors quoted above have seen firsthand the tremendous impact LTC can have on family and friends. Because of their experiences, they want to help people avoid similar hardships and are passionate in doing so. In the process, they also realize that selling LTCI is a lucrative business.

It has been said that success and satisfaction happen when your passion intersects opportunity. Passion alone has created many starving artists. Opportunity alone has created many greedy CEO's. If you enter the LTCI market both to help people and make money, you will likely be both satisfied and successful.

What about you? What is your story? Why do *you* want to sell LTCI?

Chapter One Review

Key Terms and Concepts are explained in the Glossary. Answers to the Review Questions and Self-Test Questions are found in the back of the book in the Answers to Questions section.

Key Terms and Concepts

selling process

prospect

long-term care (LTC)

custodial care

activities of daily living (ADLs)

instrumental activities of daily living
(IADLs)

other care services

social care

care setting

long-term care insurance (LTCI)

cognitive impairment

Alzheimer's disease

financial and emotional needs

Review Questions

1-1.   Name and briefly explain each of the 10 steps in the selling process.

1-2.   What are the four major factors involved with the impending LTC crisis?

1-3.   Briefly define LTC.

1-4.   List several emotional reasons why people buy LTCI.

1-5.   List the three age-based market segments described in the text.

Self-Test Questions

Instructions: Read chapter 1 first, then answer the following questions to test your knowledge. There are 10 questions; for questions 1 through 4, match the statement with the step in the 10-step selling process to which it relates; for questions 5 through 10, circle the correct answer. When finished with the test, check your answers with the answer key in the back of the book.

Match each statement below with the step in the 10-step selling process to which it relates.

1-1.   Fact-finding occurs in this step.   _____

1-2.   The objective of this step is to get an appointment.   _____

1-3.   This step is where you create a plan that best meets the needs, goals, priorities, and attitudes of the prospect.   _____

1-4.   This step is where you establish rapport, explain your business purpose, and ask some thought-provoking questions.   _____

   (a)   select the prospect
   (b)   analyze the situation
   (c)   gather information
   (d)   meet the prospect
   (e)   approach the prospect
   (f)   present solutions

1-5.   Which of the following factors is the greatest predictor of the need for LTC services?

   (a)   a geographically dispersed family
   (b)   a person's advancing age
   (c)   a divorce
   (d)   a lack of income and assets

1-6. Approximately what percent of residents in nursing homes are under the age of 65?

(a) 10 percent
(b) 20 percent
(c) 30 percent
(d) 40 percent

1-7. Activities of daily living (ADLs) include which of the following?

I. shopping
II. preparing meals

(a) I only
(b) II only
(c) Both I and II
(d) Neither I nor II

1-8. Aspects of client-focused selling are described by which of the following?

I. Client-focused selling relies on asking good questions and listening carefully.
II. The goal of client-focused selling is long-term mutually beneficial relationships.

(a) I only
(b) II only
(c) Both I and II
(d) Neither I nor II

1-9. All of the following are demographic changes that have made it more difficult for families to provide care for relatives **EXCEPT** the

(a) increased participation of women in the paid workforce
(b) large number of priorities that face family members
(c) geographic dispersion of family members
(d) increased size of the average family

1-10. All of the following are emotional reasons why people buy LTCI **EXCEPT** to

    (a)   take advantage of Medicaid
    (b)   not burden family and/or friends
    (c)   maintain independence
    (d)   protect assets

2

Identifying and Approaching Prospects

Overview and Learning Objectives

Chapter 2 begins with a focus on identifying markets and approaching prospects. It examines the three market segments identified in chapter 1 plus other marketing concepts. It also provides an in-depth look at seminars, which are one of the more popular prospecting methods for selling LTCI. By reading this chapter and answering the questions, you should be able to:

2-1.   Describe a qualified prospect for LTCI.

2-2.   Describe the common characteristics and needs for each of the three age-based market segments.

2-3.   Describe five market segments (in addition to the three age-based segments) identified in this book.

2-4.   Explain the most commonly used methods for prospecting, preapproaching, and approaching a prospect for LTCI.

2-5.   Identify the main benefits and aspects of conducting a successful seminar.

Chapter Outline

Marketing and Prospecting

This section of the chapter discusses the application of conventional target-marketing and prospecting concepts to identify and approach prospects for long-term care insurance (LTCI). We will examine the characteristics of a qualified prospect for LTCI, then describe some different ways to segment and target your markets in order to find groups of qualified prospects. Finally, we will duscuss how to identify individual prospects for LTCI and review the preapproach and approach strategies used to create interest and set appointments with them. A review of these concepts will help you put together your plan for marketing LTCI.

Qualified Prospects

The process of selling any insurance or financial product begins with creating a profile of the typical person who will believe in you and buy your products and services. In other words, you need to define the characteristics of qualified prospects.

Generically, *qualified prospects* are people who

- need and value your products and services
- can afford to pay for your products and services
- are insurable
- can be approached by you on a favorable basis

Let us apply this definition to create a profile of a qualified LTCI prospect.

Need and Value

Who needs LTCI? Although people in their 80's have a greater probability of needing long-term care (LTC) than do people in their 30's, strokes, accidents, and disease can occur at any age. With nursing home

---

LTCI: Not Just for the Elderly

Here is one advisor's thoughts about marketing and prospecting for LTCI: "Talk to everyone. I talk to anyone between the ages of 37 and 80. If they are not interested, I ask if they would mind if I spoke with their parents or other relatives. For younger prospects, I tell them that LTCI is not just for the elderly. Forty percent of all LTC recipients are under the age of 65."

---

care costing on average $52,195 per year in 2002, a couple of years of such care would seriously jeopardize the financial well-being of many individuals and families. Furthermore, if a person's money runs out he or she will need to obtain assistance from Medicaid. Such assistance will most likely mean a reduction in the quality of care for the LTC recipient. Clearly, possible LTC expenses create a financial need for many people.

However, no matter how logical the financial reason for buying LTCI, the prospect must have a strong enough emotional reason to buy it. He or she must value LTCI more than other competing wants, needs, and desires. In other words, it makes sense for a prospect to not want LTC expenses to impoverish his or her family, but does the prospect *feel* that it is worth the premium he or she must pay for LTCI?

Emotional needs are not easily observable. The best way to uncover them is to ask prospects about their experiences with family members and friends who have needed nursing home or LTC. One seasoned financial advisor uses a series of questions to explore a prospect's feelings toward LTCI:

- Do you know anyone who has needed nursing home or LTC?
- How was the situation handled?
- How would you want the situation handled if you were facing such a need?

There are some characteristics that may indicate that a prospect will value LTCI. We suggest you compile your own list of characteristics, starting with these few examples. Look for people who:

- are implementing a retirement plan or seriously considering one. People who have bought LTCI consider it to be a major component of their retirement plan.
- own other insurance products such as life or disability insurance. People who own these types of insurance products demonstrate they value the concept of risk transfer.
- work for an employer that offers group LTCI. In general, people who work for employers who offer LTCI have a greater

familiarity with the issues surrounding LTC than does the general public.

Can Afford the Premiums

One of the biggest obstacles to the LTCI sale is price. Note that price and value are interrelated. For example, a middle-aged couple may say that the premiums for LTCI are too much. You discover, however, that they own a vacation home. What this couple is really saying is that they value LTCI less than their other needs, wants, and desires. In contrast, an older couple living on a fixed income may really want LTCI but truly not be able to afford to pay the premiums.

We discussed affordability indirectly in chapter 1. If you have not done so already, identify the income and net worth ranges you will target in order to avoid affordability issues. Describe any characteristics you will look for that may indicate a prospect's ability to pay premiums. For example, you might look for the prospect who:

- owns a home
- owns a business
- has supplemental policies in place, such as a personal articles floater policy on an engagement ring
- has high liability limits on property and casualty insurance
- owns a personal liability umbrella policy

Are Insurable

There are many people who want LTCI and can afford to pay the premiums but who are uninsurable because of poor health. The worst thing for everyone involved is for a prospect to be declined for health reasons. When declinations occur, both the prospect and the financial advisor feel bad. In addition, the advisor fears the damage this might cause to his or her business relationship with the prospect. For this reason, many successful advisors recommend prequalifying the prospect over the phone. We will discuss prequalifying later when we cover the topic of approaching the prospect. As a proactive step, financial advisors should target markets where most of the people are healthy enough to

---

A Buyer's Perspective

Roger is a professor at a small college. He purchased LTCI when he was age 59. Here are his reasons for buying the policy:

"My aunt and uncle needed LTC and did not have LTCI. From that experience I was able to see the financial and emotional drain that such a situation can have on a family. This impacted my decision to buy LTCI because I don't want to leave my wife and children in a lurch. I don't like having their security affected by my problems. Furthermore, I also wanted to leave my wife and children an inheritance. It is important to me that I do not use up resources that I would use for that purpose. I guess you could say that I want to feel that my family is secure, and that's why I bought LTCI."

qualify for LTCI. For example, instead of an advisor targeting prospects over the age of 70, he or she could target prospects aged 50 to 65. Younger prospects tend to be healthier than older ones.

Can Be Approached by You On a Favorable Basis

The first three aspects of qualified prospects focuses solely on the characteristics of the prospects. In contrast, this last aspect considers the financial advisor's characteristic and how well they match those of his or her prospects. For example, an advisor in her 30's may not be successful approaching prospects in their 50's to talk to them about LTCI because these prospects may perceive her as too young and inexperienced. However, for an advisor in her 50's such prospects would more than likely be in her natural market because she probably will be perceived as more experienced.

While the financial advisor in his or her 50's would seem to have the advantage, that may not necessarily be the case. It all depends on how well each advisor establishes rapport with prospects and develops his or her reputation.

Rapport—The importance of rapport underscores the value of starting your marketing and prospecting efforts in your natural markets. Your natural markets include people you know and people to whom you have access for reasons other than direct personal acquaintance. Examples include your existing client base, people you know from a former occupation or employer, professionals with whom you have a natural ability to work, and so forth.

Rapport, however, is equally important when working with cold leads. For example, if you are making a cold call on the telephone, you need to be able to project a warm and professional image. Your words and voice mannerisms are critical because the prospect cannot pick up on any of your non-verbal cues.

Reputation—Many of your prospects will be people whom you have not met before. Some of these prospects will know about you because of your reputation. Thus, the first order of business is to make sure that you have a good reputation, especially in your target markets. Then you will need to find ways to have your reputation precede you, which will cause prospects to be more responsive to your approaches. We will cover this topic in more detail a little later in this chapter when we discuss preapproaches.

Identifying Market Segments

Having determined the profile of a qualified prospect, the next step is to find groups of qualified prospects, or *market segments*. We will begin by reviewing the age-based market segments overviewed in chapter 1. Age-based segments are an appropriate place to start because the older the prospect, the greater the level of his or her awareness of the need for LTCI. Age currently plays a more important role in the marketing and selling of LTCI than any other insurance product except Medicare supplement policies.

Once we have established the common characteristics and needs of the age-based market segments, we will then look at some other useful ways to segment the LTCI market.

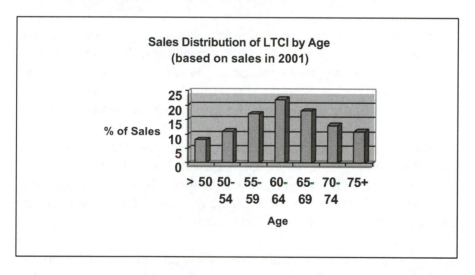

Source: Based on data from Broker World, July 2002, page 154.

Age-Based Market Segments

From the definition of a qualified prospect, it is easy to conclude that an effective way for you to segment the LTCI market is by age. Intuitively you will have greater success with prospects in the age range where they typically need LTC, can afford to pay LTCI premiums, are insurable, and can be approached on a favorable basis. Fortunately, this age range can be easily identified: Statistics show that currently most LTCI sales fall into two categories: ages 50 to 64, and ages 65 and older.

Because of the general acceptance of age 65 as the traditional or normal retirement age (even though for Social Security purposes, this will eventually increase to age 67), we have slightly modified the age ranges used with the statistics. Under our methodology, the age groups are separated into three market segments:

1. prospects who see retirement as a distant goal (those under age 50)
2. prospects who see retirement as a more immediate concern (those ages 50 to 65)
3. prospects who are enjoying retirement or semi-retirement (those over age 65)

(Throughout this discussion of market segments, you will see boxed material on various generations, as commonly used by demographers. One word of caution: These generations do not exactly match up with our age-based market segments. For example, Baby Boomers can be found in both the under age 50 and the ages 50 to 65 market segments.)

Under Age 50—As mentioned in chapter 1, the prospects in the under age 50 market segment can be approached in two different ways. The first way involves them buying LTCI for themselves. The second way involves them buying or facilitating the buying of LTCI for their parents or other relatives for whom they feel responsible.

LTCI for the Prospect—Traditionally, prospects in the under-age-50 market segment have been much less receptive than prospects from the other two market segments to purchasing LTCI for themselves. Probably the most universal reason for this reluctance to buy LTCI is that people in this market segment consider other needs and wants to be more important. Examples include saving for a house, saving for retirement, buying a new car, saving for a child's education, and securing life and/or disability income insurance. There is only so much income to spend.

Another reason for the lack of receptivity to buying LTCI is that prospects in the under-age-50 market segment perceive LTCI to be a need for people much closer to retirement or actually in retirement. They may feel that they still have plenty of time to plan. In fact, many of these prospects feel that they will never need LTC.

This is not to say that you should not approach prospects from this market segment. Obviously, people with the discretionary income to pay for LTCI premiums may be good prospects. Their income notwithstanding, however, you should look for prospects who:

- know a friend or family member who has needed LTC
- are in their 40s
- have no dependent children at home
- are single or divorced with no dependents
- have high liability limits on their property and casualty insurance
- own a personal liability umbrella policy

One of the major needs for prospects in the under-age-50 market is for them to purchase LTCI now, while they can qualify. Nobody can predict how his or her health may change. Prospects who have a family history of longevity and/or a hereditary disease such as Alzheimer's may respond to this need. In addition, prospects who understand the benefits of guaranteeing future insurability, such as those who have a guaranteed insurability option on their life and/or disability insurance policies, may feel strongly about this need.

> **Affinity Marketing**
>
> One advisor's marketing strategy:
> "The best way to reach the under age 50 market is through affinity marketing. Set up alliances with credit unions and other organizations that will allow you to market to their members."

A second need common to prospects in the under-age-50 market is asset protection in the context of retirement and/or estate planning. The whole goal of retirement planning is to build a nest egg that will last. One of the major risks facing everyone is outliving one's resources. This risk dramatically increases when you factor in the possibility of needing LTC. Prospects with whom you have actually done retirement planning make good prospects for LTCI discussion. The same holds true for prospects with whom you have done estate planning to maximize the value of the estate. When the possibility to pay for LTC is considered, even moderately large estates can suffer a severe shrinkage from LTC costs. LTCI should always be a part of any discussions about retirement and/or estate planning.

LTCI for the Prospect's Parents or Relatives—Even though many people in the under-age-50 market may not be receptive to purchasing LTCI for themselves, this market can nonetheless provide you with prospects. This is because adult children often feel morally obligated to ensure that their parents are provided for should they require LTC. This obligation quite frequently translates into a need for LTCI for several reasons.

First, while adult children traditionally have been the caregivers for elderly parents, they typically are not able to provide skilled LTC requiring a physician or a nurse.

Second, adult children are often unable to care for their elderly parents because of the financial burdens of raising their own children,

---

Generation X

Demographers often divide the population into age-based segments known as generations. The process is not an exact science so you will find that dates for when a generation begins and ends vary slightly from source to source.

The basis for a demographic generation is the theory that the general population's psyche and behavior are shaped by significant life experiences, such as the way people are raised, national and world events, wars, the social and economic climate of the times, and so forth. While each prospect will need to be treated as an individual, generalizations allow you to be aware of the different types of attitudes you may encounter from members of each of these generations so that you can recognize them quickly and make adjustments.

People born between 1965 and 1980 have been labeled as Generation X, or Xers for short. They were shaped by events like Watergate, the energy and gas crisis, the Iran hostage crisis, the space shuttle Challenger disaster, the Pan Am Flight 103 incident, the Exxon Valdez oil spill, and the fall of the Berlin Wall. Some of the resulting characteristics these Xers share are:

- Risk-takers—they are ambitious and push the boundaries. Entrepreneurial opportunities appeal to them.
- Work/life balance—their reaction to their latchkey childhood has been to seek a balance between work and home life. An increasing number stay home voluntarily to raise children.
- Skeptical—they can spot a fake quickly. They expect and will pay more for quality.
- Self-oriented—they want to know what is in it for them.
- Practical—they want something that works; they want a plan with specific steps and a well-defined result.

Generation X has also been tabbed as the Baby Bust generation. In direct contrast to the Baby Boom generation, fewer babies were born during the Baby Bust generation. This means that Xers' parents had fewer children. Given the earlier discussion on the driving forces of the LTC crisis, while Xers may not be as open to discussing LTC and LTCI for themselves, they may be interested in helping their parents purchase LTCI. In addition, because of their self-orientation and practical nature, Xers may be concerned about their inheritance—another motivation for them to want their parents to have LTCI.

and/or the impact that being a caregiver would have on their lifestyles and their relationship with their parents. In either of these situations, the children still want their parents to receive the best care possible. They also want to ensure that if one of the parents is not receiving LTC, his or her lifestyle will not deteriorate.

Third, studies show that caregiving takes its toll on the caregiver both physically and emotionally. It also negatively impacts the caregiver's career and earning capacity.

Fourth, adult children should consider how they feel about watching their inheritance dwindle to nothing. One successful financial advisor noted that when he confronts children with this possible scenario, they view LTCI as the protector of their inheritance and are often willing to pay the premiums.

Selling to the Under Age 50 Market

The under age 50 market may not be your target market, but you should take advantage of the opportunities for selling LTCI to this market. Specifically:

1. Offer the coverage to everyone because stroke, disease, and accidents know no age limitations.
2. Educate prospects about the risks for needing LTC and the associated high costs. The information can result in a sale or plant the seeds for a future sale.
3. Educate prospects on the impact that LTC can have upon them if their parents should need it. This will help you gain access to their parents through a referral. A simple question works: "How do you and your parents plan on handling LTC should they need it?"

Have a transition ready. For example:

"Mr. and/or Ms. Prospect, I understand that you feel that you cannot afford LTCI right now. Do you understand the importance of having LTCI?" (Yes)

"Great, when you feel that you can afford this coverage come and see me. And by the way, do your parents live in-state?" (Yes)

"Have they purchased their LTCI policies yet? Because guess who is going to take care of them if they have not—probably you. Do you mind if I call on them?"

Because of facts like these, many people in this market will either buy or encourage the purchase of LTCI for their parents. The market trends seem to support this. Consider that a large insurance company has created a LTCI policy that allows up to four extended family members to be covered by the same policy. This policy was developed based on feedback from nationwide focus groups revealing that while many adult children are concerned about their parents' LTC needs, they do not know how to start a conversation on the subject.[1] However, they generally will be more receptive to talking about their parents' LTC needs if they:

- demonstrate a sense of responsibility for the care of a parent or parents
- live a long distance from their parents
- have no or few surviving siblings
- are dual-income families
- have young children

In addition, while the above discussion is focused on parents, there are situations where a person may feel obligated to care for another relative such as a grandparent, aunt, uncle, and so on. Keep this fact in mind as you talk with prospects in the under-age-50 market.

Ages 50 to 65—This market segment will be the bread and butter market for LTCI for the next several years for a variety of reasons.

First, recall that the baby boomers represent a bulge in the population. Many demographers refer to the baby boom phenomenon as a "rat in a snake." Over the next several years, the Baby Boomer population bulge will dominate the ages-50-to-65 market segment, making it the market segment with the most prospects by sheer numbers alone.

Second, people in this market segment typically are at their peak income levels and LTCI premiums are relatively low for the younger ages in the segment. Thus, prospects in the ages-50-to-65 market segment typically have the means to afford LTCI premiums. A related factor is that prospects in this segment are generally healthier than those in the over-65 market segment. Therefore, the chances of qualifying to buy LTCI are much better at the younger ages.

Third, the public generally views LTC as a retirement planning issue and ages 50 to 65 are when planning for retirement becomes a front-burner issue.

Finally, prospects in this market segment have a greater likelihood of experiencing a parent or other elderly relative needing LTC. Financial advisors consistently report that when all other factors are equal, people who have had this type of experience are more receptive to buying LTCI.

The needs of prospects in this market segment are many. One of the more significant needs is that they do not want to burden their children and/or spouse with having to care for them. They do not want to be a financial, physical, or emotional burden on their relatives. People who have experienced caring for an elderly loved one will be more likely to feel this way because they have firsthand knowledge of just how taxing caregiving can be.

Another important need is to preserve independence. When a person has a self-reliant attitude, they want to avoid having to depend on government welfare programs and and/or a spouse or child. There also may be a sense of dignity involved. Having a child take care of personal custodial needs might be embarrassing and demeaning for some. You will find this independent, self-reliant attitude among the middle class, especially those who have worked hard to accrue a nest egg for retirement. They are the people who have planned for their retirement and take great pride in having done so. Again, as previously indicated, LTC and the purchase of LTCI should be a part of any retirement planning discussion.

A third need is to have choices. For example, people typically desire to have a choice of settings for any LTC they might need. For most people, this generally means in their own home or in an independent living community. Most people also want to be able to obtain the best care they can afford. LTCI allows them to not only choose the setting for the care they might receive, but it also enables them to cover the potentially staggering costs of LTC in exchange for paying a specified periodic premium. Since people aged 50 to 65 are for the most part employed and the premium rates for LTCI are still reasonable for people in this age range, LTCI coverage is affordable for most.

Finally, prospects in this market segment have the need to purchase LTCI while they are still insurable. As they age, they typically become more aware of the effects of aging and the potential costs

> **Ask Everyone!**
>
> An advisor reflects on his LTCI marketing practices:
>
> "At first I was trying to contact people age 65 and older because most of the statistics showed that these people were most receptive. However, I found that the premiums were so high that these older people could not afford to buy LTCI. I also discovered that 20 to 30 percent of these people were declined for medical reasons. Now I only write business in the ages-50-to-65 market and have experienced a lot more success."

How to Talk to Parents: "The Conversation"

Authors' note: The following excerpt is from an article by Beth Witrogen McLeod, a journalist, speaker, and consultant on caregiving, spirituality, and wellness at midlife. Ms. McLeod is the author of the book, "Caregiving: The Spiritual Journey of Love, Loss, and Renewal" (Wiley, 2000). The entire article can be found at http://www.dhs.cahwnet.gov/cpltc/Articles/TheConversation.pdf.

It may be the most frustrating concern among Baby Boomers today: how to get parents to talk about long-term care needs—before a crisis hits.

A recent American Association of Retired Persons (AARP) survey found that two-thirds of adult children have never had this conversation because they don't know what information their parents need or where to find it. Talking to parents about private, uncomfortable matters is never easy. From long-term care insurance to end-of-life wishes, this conversation is loaded not only with concerns about maintaining independence, but also with unexamined family dynamics, sibling rivalries, and communication problems.

How do you know when a parent needs help? How do you bring up the subject? When you start having these concerns, it is time for "the conversation."

The best way to start this process is to learn about home- and community-based programs. This can be done by calling the local Area Agency on Aging (AAA) and by searching Internet caregiving and aging sites.

The next step is communication: Set up a family meeting in person, by e-mail, in private Web chat rooms, or through telephone conferencing. Everyone should be involved: parents, adult children and their spouses, grandchildren, and concerned relatives or neighbors.

Because it is not always easy to bring up these topics, approaches might include:

- Saying you are beginning your own family's estate planning and need their advice.
- Sharing your emotional concerns directly.
- Assuring you do not want to take over their affairs, but are concerned that needs will be met, especially if a crisis occurs.
- Giving them a list of questions and scheduling time to talk later.
- Admitting you are worried about their driving, for example, and offering to find alternate arrangements.

The meeting should focus on facts and issues, not on negative emotions or past conflicts. Each person should be allowed time to share concerns and suggest solutions. Then family members can agree to specific actions, such as what help is needed and who will provide it. Even siblings located far away can handle bills, make phone calls, or do Internet research. And remember that just because your parents have different views does not mean they are invalid.

Here are questions to explore at the meeting:

- What are your parents' perceptions about current needs and biggest worries?
- What are your parents' health conditions today? Future prospects?
- Is their home still accessible, or does it need modifications for disabilities and hazards? Is a move warranted?
- Do they need help with daily chores, meals, bathing, errands?
- Can they still drive safely?
- What are your parents' current and future financial needs? Do they need planning assistance?
- Have they executed the necessary legal papers (wills, trusts, powers of attorney), and are they up to date?
- Do they have adequate health insurance and long-term care insurance?
- What are their wishes for end-of-life care?

The Baby Boomers

Demographers have labeled people born from 1946 to 1964 as the Baby Boom generation, reflecting their impact upon the population. They comprise 76 million of the 281 million people in the United States (27 percent of the population). Picture a snake that has just swallowed a rat and you have a picture of the demographic phenomenon known as the baby boom.

The Baby Boom generation was impacted by events such as the Vietnam War, the Cuban Missile Crisis, the assassinations of President Kennedy and the Reverend Martin Luther King, and the music event known as Woodstock. The resulting common characteristics of Baby Boomers are

- *Spenders*—although Baby Boomers have more money than preceding generations in the middle years, they tend to spend it. It is not that they do not save at all, but they save less percentage-wise.
- *Inheriters*—it is anticipated that they will be collecting over $9 trillion in inheritances between 1990 and 2030.
- *Image-conscious*—Boomers are very image-conscious; perception matters a great deal to them. Cosmetic surgery, designer clothing, careers, and luxury cars are examples of their near-obsession with image.
- *Youth-oriented*—they want to retain their youth. Health, fitness, and laser eye surgery exemplify the Boomer desire to remain young forever.

The Baby Boomers will enter retirement with money saved from their working years and inheritances. They will be able to afford premiums for LTCI. Their preoccupation with image makes LTCI an appealing product because it is designed to help them preserve their dignity and independence. In addition, Boomers are keenly aware of the stigma attached to nursing homes and thus choice of settings for their LTC, if needed, is important to them. Finally, the importance of careers and their standard of living make Boomers appreciate the value of LTCI for their parents.

of LTC. As a result, some of them will be more receptive to buying LTCI, realizing that if they do not act now while they still qualify, their health might deteriorate and foreclose the possibility of obtaining coverage.

People in the ages-50-to-65 market that might make good prospects are those

- with no dependent children in the household (so-called "empty nesters")
- with few children and/or children that are geographically dispersed
- who have saved for retirement

The Silent Generation

Demographers have labeled people born from 1925 to 1945 as the silent generation.

This generation was impacted by events such as the Great Depression, World War II, and the Korean War. The lives of the Silents were shaped by their parents' desire to protect them from the perceived dangers of the time. Common characteristics of the Silents are:

- *Private*—they do not like the limelight and making waves.
- *Cautious*—growing up as children of people who had gone through the Great Depression, they were taught not to take risks.
- *Self-reliant*—although they may not take risks, they still want to be independent and self-reliant. They saw firsthand the effects of a mass failure of banks and businesses. They do not want to trust others for their security.
- *Hard-working*—they equate success with hard work. In Horatio Alger fashion, they believe in the ability to overcome obstacles with hard work. The recovery from the depression and World War II may have had an impact on that belief.
- *Frugal*—during the Great Depression, parents of the Silents saved every dime and instilled this value in their children. This frugality has translated into the unprecedented wealth that they carry into their elderly years.

From these characteristics, you can see that the youngest of the Silents are a good target market for LTCI. More than any generation that preceded them, they have the money to spend on LTCI. Their self-reliance motivates them to purchase it. They do not want to depend on their families or the government to take care of them. In addition, the Silents' desire to leave as much wealth as they can to their heirs is another factor motivating them to purchase LTCI. They do not want the rapidly escalating expenses of LTC to erode the fruits of their labor and prevent them from passing it on to their heirs. These characteristics make them receptive to purchasing LTCI.

Be aware that many people in this market segment face pressure to save both for retirement and for their children's post-secondary educations. In this regard, they face the same challenges as their under-age-50 counterparts. The difference is that they probably have a higher income and thus a greater ability to pay for LTCI.

Over Age 65—Since the advent of LTCI, the over-age-65 market segment has generated the majority of sales. However, studies show that the current trend is toward more sales for the younger market. Because of age-related illnesses and conditions, people in the over-age-65 market experience a higher percentage of coverage declinations than people in the other two market segments. Nevertheless, there are still many healthy prospects in this market segment that can afford to pay the higher premiums required because of their advanced ages.

Prospects in the over-age-65 market segment generally have the same needs as those in the ages-50-to-65 market segment, except that prospects over age 65 are definitely more sensitive to healthcare issues, especially those related to Medicare and LTC. In addition, because the majority of people in the over-age-65 segment are no longer employed, they have a heightened fear that their monthly income and assets are not going to pay for everything. They fear that a lack of money will force them to depend on relatives, friends, or public assistance and limit their access to the quality LTC they want.

Because of their age and retirement status, prospects from the over-age-65 market are much more concerned about protecting and conserving their assets than are younger prospects. As retirees, the over-age-65 prospects are generally not able to add to their retirement nest egg. Consequently, they readily relate to the risks involved in outliving their assets.

Because this market segment is largely comprised of retirees, they have more spare time. Thus they are more deliberate in their decision-making and very receptive to seminars. One topic that makes for a great seminar is Medicare. If you sell Medicare supplement insurance, a seminar could serve a dual purpose because the topic of Medicare can be utilized effectively to also sell LTCI, too.

Other Market Segments

There are many ways to segment a market and each way may shed new light on how best to approach your prospects more effectively. Segmenting your markets in different ways provides you with fresh perspectives of your prospects, leading to new approach and presentation techniques that could help them better understand the LTC need. Here are some examples.

Couples Versus Singles—Couples and singles buy LTCI for different reasons. For couples, the desire to protect their standard of living is paramount. Should one partner need LTC, the other partner could face impoverishment even though Medicaid qualification standards are less stringent in these situations. Can a couple sustain a $60,000 per year expense for one of them to be in a nursing home? How would such an expenditure impact the healthy partner?

Some couples may insist that the healthy partner would be the caregiver for the other partner. In their mind, LTC would then be affordable. Do they know just how expensive LTC can be? Have they considered the emotional and physical strain upon the caregiving partner? How would they handle the situation if they discover that the demands of caregiving are too rigorous? How important is it to ensure that the partner needing LTC had the best care they can afford? With LTCI the best care can be purchased with discounted dollars. And, for many companies, a couple can take advantage of a spousal or partner discount.

A challenging situation occurs when one of the partners is uninsurable because couples often decide not to buy LTCI for the other partner who is healthy as well. An experienced advisor who struggled early on with this problem recommends that you prepare the couple ahead of time if you sense that a declination is possible. For example, you could say to the prospect, "If we find out that you cannot get coverage because of some insurability factor, let's not overlook your spouse. Let's get that coverage. Then we can look at other carriers or perhaps try to qualify you later."

At first glance, single people may appear to need LTCI less than couples. After all, they do not have a spouse to worry about should they need to use their entire retirement savings to pay for LTC. Interestingly, the absence of a partner may actually increase their sensitivity to LTCI because they are more aware that there is no one there to care for them should they need it. Who

---

Talking to Couples about LTCI

Here is one financial advisor's approach to couples about LTCI:

"Did you know that one out of every two people will need LTC? Perhaps you have already seen it in your family because your mother had to take care of your father, or vice-versa."

To the woman: "If he had a stroke today, could you lift him?"

To the man: "Would you want her to?"

"Let's talk about LTCI."

---

will care for them? What quality of care do they want and how much will it cost? Is it possible for them to outlive their assets paying for LTC? Being alone causes a whole different set of concerns to arise. Furthermore, single people with children may want to preserve an inheritance for them.

Women—LTC has been branded a women's issue (for example, see the government's "Women and Aging Letter" found on the Administration on Aging's Web site at www.aoa.gov/elderpage/walltc.html). Consider the following statistics from the California Partnership for Long-Term Care (CPLTC) Web site.

- Women live longer than men by an average of 7 years.
- Women comprise 60 percent of the population that is age 65 and older.
- Women tend to marry men older than themselves. Seven out of 10 "baby boom" women will outlive their husbands.
- Women are nearly twice as likely to spend time in a nursing home.
- Women are nearly twice as likely to live in poverty.
- Women comprise about 75 percent of the 7 million informal caregivers in the United States.[2]

Also consider the following statistics from the U.S. Department of Labor Pension and Welfare Benefits Administration:

- About three-fourths of nursing home residents are women.
- Two-thirds of home care consumers are women.
- The average woman could spend 17 years caring for a child and 18 years caring for a parent.
- Among those who reach 85 or older, 75 percent are women.
- At age 85 or older, women account for four out of five individuals receiving help for two or more disabling conditions.[3]

These statistics have prompted the branding and subsequent promotion of LTC as a women's issue. They are why there are events like a bipartisan Mother's Day rally to lobby for better tax incentives for LTCI. They are why more print and web articles about LTCI are being published for forums that target women. Take advantage of all this free publicity touting LTCI for women.

> **"Women are on the Titanic. The iceberg of caregiving is only a few miles away" —Phyllis Shelton, President of LTC Consultants**

Women and LTCI

The statistics point to LTC being a women's issue. Intuitively, women recognize this fact. The following comments from three successful advisors support this notion:

Advisor 1: "I am finding single women are the most receptive to buying LTCI, especially those in their 50s. They are alone and afraid."

Advisor 2: "Traditionally, women have been the caregivers for their children and parents. Because of this, they are more realistic about the emotional and financial stresses of providing LTC for someone. When working with couples, I have found that the women motivate the men to buy LTCI because most men think, 'My wife will take care of me.'"

Advisor 3: "Just as a general observation, I have found that women make the decisions on LTCI. It is the men who still believe that they are invulnerable, that nothing is going to happen to them. A wife intuitively knows that her husband is going to need LTC first and that she's going to end up taking care of him."

In targeting women, there are some interesting facts to note. First, women, because of their longevity, have a greater exposure to LTC than men. Their longevity means that they have a much greater probability of needing care for themselves and of providing care for their husband. This situation contributes to the disproportionate numbers of elderly women living in poverty. Whether dealing with a single or married woman, find out how she plans to insure against this possibility.

Second, unless the caregiving trends change, women have a much higher probability of caring for an elderly parent or relative than do men. How will such caregiving impact them physically, emotionally, and financially? What salary will they forego? What career opportunities will they sacrifice?

Third, women and men tend to buy LTCI for different reasons. Women typically purchase LTCI because they do not want to be a burden to their loved ones—probably because they have personally experienced the demands of caregiving. In contrast, men typically purchase LTCI to preserve assets.

Business owners—Because of the Health Insurance Portability and Accountability Act (HIPAA) passed in 1996, a business owner has possible tax deduction incentives for purchasing LTCI. While there is a tax advantage for any small business owner to purchase LTCI, the owner of a close C corporation benefits the most. The opportunities in the business market are covered in greater detail in chapter 8.

Wealthy—The biggest mistake financial advisors make when dealing with wealthy prospects is to assume that they want to self-insure, overlooking the underlying emotional nature of the LTCI sale. A prospect's motives for buying LTCI do not change just because he or she has a lot of money.

A point often made is that most wealthy people still purchase automobile and homeowner's insurance even though they could self-insure. What this reflects is that many wealthy people prefer to transfer risks because they do not want to pay for losses, dollar-for-dollar, out of their own pocket. The reasons for such feelings are many. For instance, they may feel that paying for LTC is not a good use of their hard-earned money and that their money should be inherited by their children or grandchildren, or gifted to a foundation or charity. As always, it is a question of what prospects value most when prioritizing the possible uses of their money.

In addition, to self-insure would mean setting aside a large sum of money (since it is not known when care would be needed or, if needed, for how long) that they could not use for other purposes without jeopardizing its role as an insurance fund for LTC expenses. An open-ended risk does not sit well with even those who have means.

As with any prospect, exploring values, goals, and dreams is an effective way to uncover possible needs for LTCI. With wealthy prospects, it is no different. They may still desire to protect their children from having to provide any type of care for them. They may still be concerned about receiving the best possible care in the desired setting. For these reasons, approach them with an open mind. Do not assume anything.

Other Cultures—As more of a footnote, be aware of the differences that you may encounter when working with prospects from differing ethnic and cultural backgrounds. For example, in Asian and Latino communities, children are expected to care for their aging parents. While this objection may seem insurmountable, it may turn out to be an unexpected motivation for buying LTCI. In these situations approach the adult children of the prospects. As these children express their sense of responsibility for the care of their aging parents you can ask questions that will help them see how buying LTCI does not conflict with their values. Instead, buying LTCI can reflect their values and can make honoring them possible. It also can ensure that the parents receive quality care in any setting

> **Working with Wealthy Prospects**
>
> One advisor gives his input on working with wealthy prospects:
>
> "When I encounter higher-net-worth prospects ($2 to 4 million), I work through the self-insuring theory. It depends on the prospect's age and the cost of the LTCI, but quite often the total possible expenses make it not worth it to self-insure. They are smart enough to see that. In addition, I point out that market downturns do happen and can wreak havoc upon a plan to self-insure."

desired, including in the home of one of the adult children. Ask the adult children a series of motivating questions like the following:

- What type of care do you want your parents to have?
- Where do you want your parents to receive it?
- What if your parents need medically necessary care? How much would it cost? Can they and/or you afford it?
- What plans do you have to handle such contingencies?

In many situations where the adult children feel responsible for the care of their parents, they will also be willing and able to pay the premiums.

Targeting a Market

Market segmentation is a powerful marketing strategy that allows you to customize your approach and presentations based on the common needs and characteristics of the prospects in the segmented market. If you can find a market segment that has a communication or network system, then you have a target market. The communication system can be formal such as a newsletter or regular meeting, or it can be informal, such as word-of-mouth within a tightly-knit ethnic community. Either way, the communication system or network provides the means by which your reputation as a professional advisor can precede you. In other words, before you personally meet with any prospects in a target market, they will know about your abilities as a financial advisor.

Targeting Markets for LTCI—Because of the nature of LTC, LTCI can be marketed successfully using age-based market segments as "makeshift" target markets (age-based market segments are very broad and lack a communication system and for that reason do not technically qualify as a target market). Many successful advisor do this by targeting narrow but specific age ranges. For example, one successful advisor targets prospects ages 55 to 65 because most of them are probably empty nesters who are focused on retirement.

An extension of the age-based target market theme is when advisors target people in a specific, but narrow, age range who are also members of an association, service organization or club. The ideal situation occurs when the majority of the membership is in the chosen age range. For example, if an advisor wants to target prospects age 50 to 65, he or she may consider targeting a service organization (such as the Rotary,

Jaycees, Kiwanis, and so forth) or club (such as a VFW, Elks, or a country club) in the community that has a sizeable membership of people in the desired age range. Besides age range and membership, other common characteristics of the prospect group, such as a narrow income range, could help in establishing a new target market. If you use this method for targeting a market, you will need to develop a list of desirable characteristics that you want the prospects to possess to guide you in the process of establishing the new target market.

For many advisors, LTCI is just one of several insurance and financial products they sell, so they position it in a manner consistent with their current target market's view of them as advisors. For instance, if an advisor works as an estate planner for businessowners making $100,000-$500,000 per year, he or she will want to position LTCI as an estate preservation tool. Likewise, if an advisor's target market is teachers in a large city, he or she will want to position LTCI as a strategy for safeguarding their retirement nest egg. Similarly, financial advisors selling property and casualty insurance will want to position LTCI as a piece of their prospect's overall insurance and financial plan.

Target markets enable you to focus on the unique needs of your prospects. Such focusing will foster not only your reputation within the target market as an expert in LTCI or in insurance and financial products in general, but it will also allow you to better understand your prospect's needs. With this knowledge, you will soon discover the efficiencies of tailoring a marketing strategy for a large number of prospects with common characteristics and needs.

> **Target Markets**
>
> One advisor found that his direct mail campaign discovered a target market that he was unaware of. As it turned out, a sizeable number of the prospects who responded were professional caregivers who work with LTC recipients. These professionals make excellent prospects because they understand the financial and emotional plight of many of the uninsured LTC recipients. In similar fashion the following market segments could make excellent target markets or centers of influence for you.
>
> - Medical personnel—nurses, doctors, and therapists
> - Eldercare attorneys
> - LTC providers—nursing home administrators and home health care workers
> - Social workers

Prospecting

Once you have identified a few target markets or market segments, the next task is to select prospecting methods that will effectively create a stream of prospects from these markets. In this section, we will review some general prospecting and preapproach strategies that you can use to

---

identify and precondition prospects for approaching them about LTCI. What works will depend on your specific market, as well as your personality and skills.

Prospecting Methods

There are many different prospecting methods. We will provide a brief overview of some of the more popular ones that successful advisors have used to sell LTCI.

Referrals—Successful advisors have found referrals, or recommendations, to be a very efficient and effective means of generating an endless list of prospects. Referrals are people to whom you are introduced by someone who knows and values your work. In their highest form, referrals are unsolicited and the prospects come to you because of the enthusiastic recommendations that satisfied clients make to them. Until your practice evolves to this level, you will have to ask for referrals.

It is advisable to pave the way for referrals early on in the selling process, preferably during the initial meeting. Create the expectation of receiving referrals if the prospect appreciates what you do for them. For example:

"Mr. and/or Ms. Prospect, as we work together, if you find what we are talking about to be important and valuable, then give me the opportunity to meet with people you know and care about so that I may help them, too."

Then, when you ask for referrals it will not surprise the prospects. The best time to ask is when the prospect indicates an appreciation for you and/or LTCI. It could be as simple as, "I'm so glad you showed me that. I always thought Medicare would pay for LTC." Obviously, if the prospects purchase LTCI policies from you, they have demonstrated an appreciation for the product. However, even if the prospects do not buy policies, ask them about the value of the process. If they have a favorable opinion of you and the process, ask for the referrals.

> "Ms. Prospect, I know you have decided that you do not need LTCI. May I ask what, if anything, in this process you found to be of value? [Wait for a response.]   "That's great. I am glad I could help you clarify the issues of Medicare and Medicaid. May I ask who you know who might also benefit from this type of advice?"

Of course, if your prospects have parents who may be eligible for LTCI, you can specifically ask for their names.

> "Mr. Prospect, although I disagree with your waiting to buy LTCI, I respect your decision. I am glad, however, that you see the need for LTCI. LTC is a catastrophe waiting to happen. I was wondering, do your parents have LTCI yet? Do they live in this state? Would it be okay if I met with them?"

When you ask for general referrals (that is, when you do not specifically ask for the name of the prospect's parents) try to help the prospect identify people you would like to meet. Describe the kind of person who would make a good prospect by providing details such as:

- Age range
- Income range
- Occupation types
- Living situation (for example, older single females or childless couples)
- Health (that they are healthy)

As always, remember to follow-up on referrals by providing an update to the referrer to let him or her know how the meeting went.

Children Referring Their Parents

When I get resistance because a prospect feels it is not his or her time to buy LTCI, I pivot to another product. Once I have completed any sale that results, I transition to LTCI for their parents:

"Do your parents live in this state, or are they out of state? Where are they located? I would like to talk to them. The reason I need to see them is to protect your income and lifestyle. If anything happens to your parents and they do not have LTCI, either you or they will pay the costs for LTC. It makes more sense for you to write a $193 check each month to ABC Insurance than to write a $3,953 check each month to the Shifting Sands Nursing Home. Would it be all right if I call your parents?"

Center of Influence (COI)—By definition a *center of influence* is an influential person who knows you favorably and agrees to introduce or recommend you to others. A client may become an effective center for you, just as a center may become a client, but this is not necessary to the relationship you need to establish.

In general, you will find that COIs

- are active in a community or sphere of influence
- are sought out for advice by the community or within their sphere of influence
- seek to communicate with others
- are givers, not takers

Good COIs know the people in your target markets regardless of their occupation or profession. However, some occupations and professions deal directly with your target markets and finding COIs in these occupations and professions could prove very profitable. Examples include:

- eldercare attorneys
- CPAs
- fee-based financial planners
- advisors who sell non-competing lines of insurance (for example a property and casualty agent)
- health care providers
- clergy
- senior activity center coordinators
- members of a golf club
- members of a volunteer organization

Once you have identified some possible COIs, you will need to set up meetings with them. Write and practice a script if you do not know them very well.

One strategy for you is to approach the COI by explaining how the meeting will benefit him or her. For example you might approach a non-competing advisor by saying, "Pat, you have a great reputation in the community and I would feel comfortable referring clients to you. I would like to get together with you to brainstorm ways we can help each other build successful practices. Would breakfast sometime next week work for you or would a lunch be better? My treat."

In contrast, you could approach a community leader by explaining how the meeting will benefit the community. You may say, "Kim, you really command the respect of the seniors in this community. One of the critical questions many seniors are asking is 'How do I pay for LTC?' Unfortunately, many people are making decisions about LTC based on inaccurate information. I would like to discuss this issue with you, along with ways you could help the seniors in this community make well-informed decisions. I am not going to try to sell you anything; I only want to show you how I can help you help the community. Would next Wednesday be a good day to meet, or would another day work better for you?"

Your meeting with a COI is as important as a sales appointment. Therefore, plan your presentation. Keep it brief and consistent with your approach. For example, if you are meeting with a community leader, the goal of your presentation is to show the COI just how he or she can help others by referring them to you. Your approach to accomplish this objective may include the following steps:

- Share the impact that the LTC crisis will have on people needing it and upon society in general.
- Illustrate the impact with any personal stories.
- Demonstrate how LTCI can prevent this disaster for many people and reserve Medicaid for those who truly need it.
- Provide the COI with some practical actions that he or she can take to help.

You will probably want to ask the COI for names of qualified prospects. If so, have a brief written description of how to identify qualified prospects. Although referrals are important, you may find other ways the COI can help you. For example, if the COI is a leader for a senior community service organization, you can approach him or her about doing an educational presentation for the rest of the organization. Be creative.

Networking—*Networking* is the process of continuous communication and the sharing of ideas and prospects with others whose work does not compete with yours. In turn, their clients might also be shared with you and become your clients.

Most networking groups have the same general rules. Membership is limited to one person from each type of sales background, whether insurance, real estate, stock brokerage, or some other sales profession. Each person attending the meeting is required to bring a prescribed number of names. For example, the real estate agent member of the group just sold a house located in an over-55 community that she represents exclusively. She gives you the name of that person as a prospect who may be interested in LTCI. On the other hand, your client has expressed a desire to live in an independent living or retirement community and thus would be a good prospect to share with the real estate agent.

If you can find an existing networking group in your community, it might be worthwhile to investigate joining it to provide you with a steady stream of prospects.

Seminars—Some advisors have found that seminars are an extremely effective way to prospect, especially in the senior market. Seminars enable advisors to accomplish two key objectives. First, seminars are a means to present LTCI to several prospects at one time, resulting in less time needed to conduct one-on-one interviews. Second, seminars cast financial advisors as the experts, especially if they play a significant role in the presentation. Many successful advisors in the LTCI market use seminars as their main prospecting tool. We will discuss the hows and whys of seminars in the next section of this chapter.

Cold Calling—Many advisors avoid cold calling because they do not want to be seen as telemarketers. However, many experienced advisors still use this prospecting tool with excellent results. The key to cold calling is the list of prospects. Advisors who have success with cold calling use lists to select prospects who likely would have an interest in LTCI—for example, a list of AARP members. Some companies provide lists to their advisors through market segmentation programs; check with your company to see if one is available. Otherwise you will want to buy one from a reputable vendor.

When dealing with a vendor, exercise caution. Here are some points to keep in mind:

- Select lists that reflect your target markets.
- Check to see how recently the data was collected.
- Make sure that the list has current phone numbers.
- Verify the source of the leads.

- Make sure that the list has been "scrubbed." This means that any "do not call" and undeliverable names have been eliminated.
- Check to see if duplicate entries or incomplete names have been deleted.

One final thought on cold calling lists: Keep good records so you can evaluate the quality of the leads and compare different vendors until you find the one that gives you the best return on your investment.

Preapproach

The purpose of a preapproach is to create awareness of who you are and interest in your products. You want to precondition your prospects to meet with you when you call them. They will be less apt to do so if they have no idea who you are and what you can do for them.

How do you feel when you receive a cold call? If you react like most people do, you are suspicious and defensive and do not listen to what the caller says. You are too busy thinking, "Who is this, how did he get my number, and how can I get rid of him?" Compare this scenario to receiving a call from a CPA you met briefly at a wedding or who sent you a postcard introducing herself as "a CPA for insurance advisors, helping them to maximize their tax breaks." Are you listening? Use the preapproach to make your prospect curious—this can be done in many different ways. We will discuss some of the more standard preapproaches. The ones you use will depend on your target market, your prospecting methods, and your creativity.

Direct Mail—Direct mail is one of the more common preapproaches because it is an easy and relatively inexpensive way to precondition prospects to be receptive when you call them. It allows people to see your message who otherwise might not be looking for your name in the telephone book or see your billboard advertisement. Furthermore, you can use direct mail to customize your message to different target markets. For example, you may send prospects ages 45 to 65 a

> ### Using Direct Mail with a Giveaway
>
> One advisor's company offers a giveaway that requires interested prospects to mail a tear-off response card back to the advisor, providing their names, addresses, and telephone numbers. Then the advisor contacts them to set up a time to drop off a copy of the promised material. Here is the advisor's script:
>
> "Hello, Prospect, my name is Jeff. I'm calling for XYZ Company. I'm following up on the information about LTC that you requested. I'm not a telemarketer; I'm an advisor with the company and I have been for years. I would like to stop by and give you this information. I am going to be in your area on Tuesday and Wednesday of this week. All I want to do is give you the information you requested, and take a couple minutes of your time to talk to you about LTC and answer any questions you might have. Would the morning be good for you, or would the afternoon be better?"

postcard that talks about LTCI as a major component of a retirement plan. For prospects under age 45, you may instead send a postcard that talks about the LTC needs of their parents.

Your company may have a direct mail program that requires you to supply the list of prospects you want to approach, select the particular letter you wish to send, and to choose a giveaway offer if desired. Although the giveaway offer could be a remembrance item such as an atlas or a coffee mug, a better choice would be a booklet, book, or video on LTC.

As mentioned when we discussed cold calling, many companies also offer market segmentation programs that allow advisors to create a list of prospects who meet specific criteria. Examples of often-used criteria include marital status, age range, income level, zip code, home ownership, phone number available, and so on. Consider a reputable vendor if you are dissatisfied with your company's options or if your company does not offer this service. Some vendors also have customizable direct mail pieces that they will send for you. Whether you use a direct mail piece from a vendor or one of your own, remember to have them approved by your company's compliance area before you send them out.

Here are some additional tips for a direct mail campaign.

- If you are working with a list of prospects you have generated through referrals, centers of influence, and casual meetings, make sure the names are spelled correctly.
- Before you purchase a list, check the undeliverable rate. Also check to see if the vendor uses a 5- or 9-digit zip code (5 digits have a greater chance of being undeliverable).
- Select a letter that matches the type of prospects on your list. Be conscious of both the content and the layout. For example, some companies use larger fonts for seniors.
- The letter should be short. The main paragraph that creates interest should be no more than three or four sentences; otherwise people will not read it.
- Try using postcards. Many people do not open "junk mail" but they will take time to read a postcard.
- Use stamps rather than metered mail (no stamp). Metered mail to most people is perceived as "junk mail."
- Try the "wave" mail technique, which involves sending several pieces of mail to the prospect over a period of time. For example,

you may send three or four mailing pieces over a 3 or 4-week period, or perhaps over a 12-month period. Direct mail results show that people often respond between the third and sixth time they have seen a letter or an idea.

- Follow-up direct mail with a phone call; it gives you an excuse to call. In the "wave" mail technique, wait and call after the prospects have received a few mailings from you. The mailings will help the prospects feel that they know who you are and as a result they will be more receptive to your call.
- Track your leads to monitor the effectiveness of your direct mail and other preapproach efforts.

Building Prestige—Prestige, or reputation, is your personal public relations campaign. It is your standing or esteem in the eyes of others; it is the position or influence you command in people's minds. A good reputation increases the probability of approaching prospects on a favorable basis. Therefore, take great care in building and maintaining it. In general, make professionalism a priority. For example:

- Dress professionally but not showy.
- Keep your car and office clean and organized.
- Build your knowledge of LTC and LTCI. Consider earning an industry-recognized designation.
- Be approachable and personable.

Furthermore, implement a strategy that will publicize your reputation, especially to your target markets. You want as many people in your target market to know you as the expert on LTCI. For example, if you target the senior market, sponsoring a little league team would not be part of your strategy. However, teaching a personal finance class at the local senior center would be an excellent prestige-building activity. Here are some other prestige-building ideas.

- Advertise on local radio stations. Select shows and stations that appeal to your target market. For example, Saturday with Sinatra would be a good radio show on which to advertise if you are targeting prospects over the age of 55.
- Advertise in local papers.

- Make yourself available to the local media. Alert journalists that you are knowledgeable about LTC issues and would be willing to provide expert information and quotes.
- Give back to your community in ways that both you and your target market value.
- Leave LTCI brochures (with your contact information on them) in places people from your target markets frequently get free information—for example, doctors' offices, train stations, and credit unions.
- Educate key advisors, such as attorneys and CPA's, who work with your target markets.
- Work with a local paper to publish achievements such as receiving your LUTCF, CLU, ChFC or CFP™ certifications.
- Join a local organization that addresses the impact LTC has or will have on the community.

10-Second Commercial—Socializing provides an excellent way to create awareness and interest in what you do. One opportunity is to have well-thought, customized responses to the question, "What do you do for a living?" Have a short response that is relevant and interesting to the person to whom you are talking. A response like, "I sell LTCI" tells the person how you make money; it also tells the person specifically what you can do for him or her. However, it is not interesting or attention grabbing.

Contrast such a response with the following example: If you were talking to a 55-year old married man, you could say, "Do you know what conservationists do?" (Answer: They preserve the environment.) "Well, I do something similar with retirement nest eggs. I help couples, like you and your wife, put plans into place that preserve their retirement savings from the costs of LTC. Do the two of you have a plan like that?"

Using a Preapproach with Referrals

An excellent preapproach strategy is to ask clients to introduce you to the referred lead. If the client cannot arrange a face-to-face meeting or telephone call, then ask the client if he or she would be willing to write a note of recommendation for you on his or her personal letterhead or stationery. One advisor recommends carrying around samples of what to say in case the client does not know what to say. The note should be short and simple such as:

Dear John,

Kelly shared with me some great strategies about protecting my retirement nest egg. She could help you, too.

- Mark

Then you send the note with your personal letter introducing yourself and the services you provide, and letting the referred lead know that you will be calling him or her. Send the letter in a hand-addressed envelope with a regular postage stamp. This will ensure it is opened and read.

The conversation should be different if you are talking to a 65-year old retiree. You might say, "Are you familiar with Medicare and Medicaid? (Answer: Yes, or No.) I help people like you maximize their health coverages by coordinating these government health programs with insurance like Medicare supplement and LTCI. Would that interest you?"

Here are some tips for creating a commercial:

- Ask a "positioning" question that is relevant to a prospect's need for your services. The question positions your response to be a solution to a problem or question that they might be asking.
- Follow up with your 10-second commercial, stating your value in terms of the results you achieve for your clients.
- Be creative and make it interesting, but follow your company guidelines. You may be restricted in the way you describe your work. Because of today's compliance issues, exercise caution and do not misrepresent the products you sell.
- End with a question that measures the prospect's interest.
- Have a business card with you to give the prospect if you feel it is appropriate.

The key is to customize your commercial to the prospects and refer to a need that they might have. By doing so, you are not only creating awareness about your products and services, you are creating interest—and interest will get you an appointment.

Résumé—Some financial advisors use a résumé as one of their preapproach methods. The résumé is a one-page self-promotional piece that introduces the advisor. Some advisors create their own résumés and then reproduce them using a local printing company. Other advisors use a vendor to design and print them. The goal is to impress potential clients, so do not let price be the only consideration.

The self-promotional piece includes information such as:

- Name and contact information
- Short biography
- Credentials (designations, experience, and so forth)
- Services
- Products

All of this is printed on high quality paper; some advisors use a glossy finish. Some advisors send résumés to referred leads along with a cover letter that tells them to expect a phone call. It is also an appropriate handout to give new prospects as part of your introduction when you meet them for the first time. Make the résumé a part of your sales presentation binder.

As always, your résumé needs to meet your company's compliance standards.

Approach

Generally, advisors use the telephone to approach prospects for sales appointments. This section will review some of the basics of effective telephone approaches and include a discussion on prequalifying prospects during the appointment-setting call. However, since many advisors view LTCI as one of several products they use to meet a client's financial and insurance needs, this section also looks at pivoting to LTCI after selling another product.

Telephone Approach

The Objective—Your objective is to introduce yourself to the prospect and set the appointment. Obviously, you will not need to introduce yourself to an existing client, but you will want to re-establish rapport if you have not spoken to him or her for some time.

Sometimes a prospect or client may ask you a question related to the product. One you probably hear often is, "How much does it cost?" Some advisors cannot resist the temptation to answer these questions

---

Multi-line Advisor to Existing Clients

Multi-line advisors have access to a slew of qualified prospects through their existing client base. LTCI may be a new product for the company or simply a product the advisor had not previously marketed. Either way, here is an approach that will work:

"Hello, this is your insurance advisor, Kelly Smith. How are you today? I wanted to let you know that I can now meet your LTC needs through LTCI. I thought this might be something that would interest you. Let's get together to review how LTCI can help you maintain your retirement savings and lifestyle. Would some time this week work for you or would next week be better?"

Essentials of Long-Term Care Insurance

over the telephone. Resist it. Save such answers for the interview; you simply want to get the appointment.

System—You may already have a system for setting appointments. If you do not, now is a good time to make one. A system ensures that appointment setting is done effectively. It is critical especially if you delegate the task of setting appointments to an assistant. A system provides you or your assistant with clear expectations and a game plan that will increase confidence and improve results. Here are some points to consider as you create or modify your system:

- *Use a telephone script*—Write and practice your telephone script. Your script should reflect the needs and characteristics of your target markets. In addition, the script will vary depending on the source of the prospect and the preapproach, if one was used. For example, if you approach a referred lead, you would want to mention the referrer's name.

- *Coordinate logistics*—Plan a specific time to make your calls. Have a goal for the number of appointments you will make based on your sales, commission, and/or fee goals. Maintain a prospect list of names, telephone numbers, and addresses (to confirm where the appointment will be).

- *Follow the laws*—Follow federal and state laws concerning telemarketing. For example, keep and observe a do-not-call list and abide by the call curfews set by your state.

- *Use good telephone techniques*—Smile, project your voice, and enunciate your words. These are just a few of the many suggested techniques.

- *Track your results*—Record keeping enables you to evaluate your prospect list and your target markets. Without adequate records, you may miss a target market because you are relying on "feel" to measure results rather than objective numbers.

Follow-up to a Mailing

"Hello, this is Tom Smith from DEF Company. I recently mailed you a letter pertaining to one of the hottest issues in the financial and insurance industry today. It's LTCI. I would like to get together with you and just explain what LTCI is and how it works. Is an afternoon good for you or do evenings work better?"

"Hello, this is John Doe from XYZ Insurance. Recently I sent you some information on LTCI. Really what we ought to do is set up a time to visit about it. It may or may not be appropriate for you but come in and visit with me or you won't know. It's certainly worth your time to learn some of the facts about LTCI. Would next Tuesday work for you, or would Thursday be better?"

- *Confirm the appointment*—Send a letter, post-card, and/or call the prospect to confirm the appointment to prevent being stood up.

Writing a Script—Many advisors balk at the words *telephone script*. They feel a script will restrict them or cause them to sound mechanical. Actually, the opposite is true. Scripts help you feel more comfortable and enable you to project a more confident phone personality. They free you to focus on the prospect and listen for clues to gauge his or her level of interest. In addition, they help you repeat success and diagnose failure.

A good script is short and creates interest. For example:

> "Good afternoon, Prospect, this is Joe Advisor from ABC Financial. I will only take a moment of your time. I work with people like you who are thinking more and more about retirement. I help them understand the challenges they could face during their retirement years and how they can prepare for them by carefully planning now. I would like to meet with you to review some strategies involving insurance products that can help you protect your standard of living throughout your retirement. Would some time during the day work for you, or are evenings better?"

If you do not have a script, here are some of the basic elements of a good script. As always, remember to follow company guidelines and get any necessary compliance approval.

A Greeting—You want to make a good first impression.

- Open your conversation with something upbeat like, "Good morning/Good afternoon."
- Identify yourself and the company you represent.
- Consider adding a phrase such as "I will only take a moment of your time." This demonstrates that you are sensitive to their busy schedule.

Create Interest—Remember, you are trying to motivate prospects to see you.

- Tell why you are calling.

- Give a unique benefit statement that describes the results you create for people like the prospect (your target market).

Ask for the Appointment—This is why you are calling.

- Explain the purpose of the meeting in terms of the results you hope to achieve for them.
- Personalize these results.
- Avoid using the word appointment. Use meet, see, or get together.

A Closing—As they say in gymnastics, "stick the dismount."

- Give or get directions depending on where you will meet for the appointment.
- Reconfirm the appointment and affirm your desire to meet the prospect.

Asking Prequalifying Questions—Many successful advisors prequalify prospects once they have agreed to an appointment. Others wait to prequalify during the initial interview. When you prequalify, your prospects will depend on your type of practice and your personal views on this matter. For example, if you have multiple products, prequalification before the initial interview is not as crucial because you have other products to satisfy other needs the prospects may have. Even so, having prequalification information before you hold the sales interview could save you from raising the prospect's hopes only to dash them when you find out he or she is uninsurable. Such a scenario is not only bad for the prospect it could damage your relationship with him or her. Thus, prequalifying before the initial interview will allow you to prepare a smooth transition to other needs and products and avoid this situation altogether.

If you decide to prequalify before the initial interview, the next step is to decide what information you need to know and build a script. What questions you ask will depend on your philosophy of prequalification. For instance, one advisor prequalifies for age only. His philosophy is that although LTCI is his main product, it is not his only product. He can pivot to a discussion of the prospect's possible need for an annuity or life insurance. Even so, he cannot help anyone over the age of 85. If he detects that the person might be over age 85, he will ask them, "How young are you? You sound like you are 65."

Other advisors prequalify for health as well. The transition from getting the appointment to asking the prequalifying questions needs to be smooth—that is why a script is important. One commonly used transition is: "I know your time is valuable. In order to save some time, it would help for me to know some basic information about your health and medical history. I am going to ask a few general questions, will that be okay with you?" Once you have transitioned to asking the prequalifying questions, keep them short and general. Here are a few different questions successful advisors ask:

- How is your health?
- What medications are you taking?
- What surgeries have you had?
- Can you tell me a little about your medical history?
- Are there any medical problems you manage daily?

Still, other advisors ask more than just health questions. Some will ask questions to identify other people who will influence the prospect's decision, such as children or a CPA. If these advisors find that there are other people involved in the decision-making process, they will ask for them to be present at the interview. Here are a few of the questions they ask:

- Do you have any children? How many? Where do they live?
- Do you rely on anyone to help you make decisions about finances and insurance? If so, who?

Finally, have a short close scripted that you can use to let the person down if you know he or she will not qualify. This takes the utmost care and sensitivity. You do not want them to feel bad. An example script might be: "Prospect, I am really sorry but it looks like from the health information you gave me, we will not be able to help you at this time. I highly recommend that you consider seeing an attorney or another advisor who specializes in alternative strategies for meeting LTC needs. I can recommend a few attorneys if you would like."

For more information on prequalifying during the initial interview, see the section in chapter 4 titled, "Qualifying Prospects." It covers some techniques for prequalifying during an initial interview that can be used over the telephone, too.

Pivot Approach

If you walk into a computer store to purchase a computer, a good salesperson will ask questions to understand your needs. For example, she will

probably ask you how you plan to use it. Your answer will help her suggest the right system. In the beginning her focus is upon finding you the right computer. Throughout the process she gathers information about your total needs and, when you finally decide on your system, she will begin to ask about other computer equipment like a printer or a monitor upgrade.

The conversation might sound something like this: "You have made a great choice. I really think the Orange 2000XP is going to meet your needs. Since you are going to use it for graphic design, I was wondering what type of graphics printer you plan to use with it?"

This is an example of a good pivot or transition. It uses previously shared information as the context for asking a question relevant to another product. Pivoting can occur from any type of product sale. Most likely, you will discuss LTCI as a part of a retirement or estate planning discussion. But if you are a property and casualty advisor or an advisor who is working the income replacement market, you will have the opportunity to pivot as well.

How and when to pivot are going to depend on factors such as what type of product the prospect bought from you (or did not buy from you), your personality, and so forth. Try to use something from the previous discussion to lead into the LTCI approach. Furthermore, pivot when there is closure to the previous discussion. For instance, one of the best times to pivot is when you deliver a policy. After you have reviewed the policy and other important information, you could say:

"Prospect, you have made a great choice to buy this life insurance policy. You are really thinking and planning ahead. Since you seem to be the planning type, I was wondering, have you thought about your plans for the time when you or your parents may need ongoing care? What do you know about LTC? Have you ever been in a situation where a neighbor, friend, or family member has needed LTC?"

If your prospect responds affirmatively to the last question, ask him or her to tell you about it. Then you can simply ask for the appointment. For example: "That is a compelling story. Stories like that are the reason I want to make sure you are aware of the issues and solutions to the rising costs of LTC. Can we get together next week or another time convenient for you to discuss this?"

If your prospect has not had an experience where someone he or she knows has needed LTC, then tell him or her about your experience (if you have had one) or share a story from the newspaper. Keep it brief and then ask for the appointment.

Summary

Successful selling begins with effective marketing. Defining target markets for a product enables you to create efficient and effective preapproach and approach strategies that are customized to appeal to the needs of your prospects. As you begin marketing LTCI, treat it as any other product you sell and take the time to define your target markets and strategy, including details like your telephone and pivot scripts. The execution of a well-thought plan will enable you to take advantage of the marketing opportunities in LTCI sales.

Notes

1. See page 10.
2. *http://www.dhs.cahwnet.gov/cpltc/html/consumer.html*. July 1, 2002
3. *http://www.dol.gov/dol/pwba/public/adcoun/report2.htm*. June 18, 2001

Seminars

Seminars are a form of mass marketing. Although classified in this text as a prospecting method, seminars do more than help you identify prospects. They create awareness and interest in your products and services, and serve to establish and build your reputation as an expert in LTCI. In these ways, seminars function as a preapproach as well.

Think of seminars as live infomercials that educate people about the LTC need and motivate them to want to know how LTCI can help them. Because of the educational and motivational aspects of seminars, they are an extremely effective way to obtain appointments. Not surprisingly, in one study insurance advisors who were classified as "high earners" ranked seminars as the third most effective marketing tool for reaching targeted prospects, just behind referrals or centers of influence and the effective use of newsletters and brochures.

The general success of seminars and, specifically, the success that advisors have had using them to sell LTCI are why the text provides an in-depth look at this prospecting method. This section will discuss the advantages of seminars, some planning considerations, presentation tips, and the most important aspect—follow-up.

Advantages

Seminars are a popular prospecting method for LTCI because they appeal to the demographics most interested in LTCI: people age 50 and over. But there are other reasons why you should consider using this prospecting method.

Use Time Efficiently

Seminars enable you to present yourself and your products to a larger number of prospects at one time. This will inevitably shorten the amount of time you will need to spend discussing the topics covered in the seminar when you meet with the prospects individually. For example, if the

---

Time Is Money

One successful advisor gives his reason for prospecting using seminars: "I prospect almost exclusively through seminars even though they require a lot of effort and expense. I justify them because I view the seminar as the initial interview that establishes the need for LTCI in the minds of a group of prospects. So, if I have 20 people in the seminar, I am able to do at least 10 initial interviews (this assumes I have a group of married couples) in the time it would take me to do one. As they say, 'time is money.'"

---

seminar covers Medicare and Medicaid and disqualifies them as sources for funding LTC, you will probably not need to cover this in your one-on-one interview with each prospect.

Meet Prospects in a Nonthreatening Way

In a sales interview, you ask prospects many questions, some of which are very personal. Many prospects are reluctant to give their financial and health information to someone they do not know too well. Seminars help such prospects to warm up to you because they do not have to share any information. They can listen to your presentation of the issues without feeling vulnerable, allowing them to learn more about LTC and LTCI. Most importantly, they can learn more about you and see your professionalism and expertise. This gives prospects the confidence and trust so they will want to meet with you.

Maximize Public Speaking Ability

If you are someone who enjoys presenting and teaching, seminars are a way to leverage these abilities. Some advisors are natural-born public speakers, making this form of marketing extremely enjoyable and effective.

If you have an aversion to public speaking, you can still take advantage of seminars by arranging for other advisors, agents, company specialists, and experts to speak. A great format is to share the presentation with them, giving them the bulk of the speaking time. When working with new prospects and not current clients, taking an active role in the presentation will enable new prospects to gain some sense of your professionalism and expertise.

If you pair up with another advisor, you will need to agree on some form of compensation such as a split in the commission. If you both invite prospects, you could offer to pay for the cost of the seminar since he or she is doing the majority of the speaking.

Prequalify Prospects

To some extent, seminars prequalify prospects. Although you initiate the seminar by inviting the prospects, they confirm their interest by attending and represent a much better prospect pool than a cold call list. If you can bring together the right people, ask the right probing questions, present the right solutions, and project yourself as the professional source for insurance and financial planning, your seminar will be tremendously successful.

Planning a Seminar

Arrangements, program content, and follow-up are critical to the success of a seminar. If a seminar is not well planned, you risk losing credibility with the people who attend. Therefore, developing a well-thought-out plan is essential.

It is helpful to have a written game plan, a step-by-step description of what you need to do and when you need to do it. A checklist lets you see at a glance where you are and what remains to be done. Developing a seminar checklist requires a good bit of thought, and should answer the five "W" questions:

- who?
- what?
- when?
- where?
- why?

Your Objective

The first step in the planning process is to set your goal or objective. Before you do anything else, ask yourself what the seminar will accomplish. Your goal should be specific, attainable, and measurable. For example, you may set a goal of making 10 appointments with seminar attendees. Or your goal may be to provide an informational seminar for 15 of your best clients.

The goal you set is important because it will impact other decisions. If your goal is to make 10 appointments with seminar attendees, you must get more than 10 people to attend your seminar.

> **Seminar Objectives**
>
> Says one experienced advisor, "I want to accomplish three objectives during the seminar: create an awareness of the need for LTCI, show the alternatives, and anticipate objections. If I am successful, then the one-on-one interview is nothing more than a closing interview."

The Audience

Seminars involve target marketing. The people you invite should have a common interest or need. This allows you to focus on the specific needs of the audience. For example, you could present a seminar that covers Medicare, Medicaid, and LTCI, which would appeal to prospects over age 65. Whereas a seminar that focused on LTCI as it relates to planning for retirement would appeal more to prospects under age 65.

Sometimes the audience is determined by the purpose of the seminar. For example, if your purpose were to create centers of influence, your audience would be made up of other professionals who work with prospects in your target market. You would probably invite professionals such as attorneys, CPA's, and fee-based financial planners and advisors. If your objective were to improve retention in your multi-line book of business, you would invite a market segment from your current client-base. Finally, you may want to expand your client base. In that case, you would invite new prospects (not current clients) from a specific market segment or target market. The point is that you need to make a list of invitees who have some common characteristics and needs.

To determine how many people to invite, begin by setting a goal for the number of attendees you wish to have. Initially, aiming for 15 to 20 prospects is reasonable. If 15 to 20 prospects attend, you can justify costs. At the same time, the group is small enough to allow interaction between the speaker and attendees. You will learn from experience how many people to invite to have the desired number of attendees. A good rule of thumb is to invite 10 people for each desired attendee. The ratio of invitees to attendees will improve as your seminars become better known.

Once you have created a list of invitees, your next step is to design a way to invite them to your seminar. Individual invitation letters are the most effective way. However, newspaper ads may be effective for attracting new prospects. Regardless of how you communicate your invitations, you need to determine how you want your prospects to respond. You may want to send a return card with your invitation letters. Another method is to ask for phone reservations from those who are interested. You may even want to plan follow-up phone calls in the event that your responses fall below your expectations.

Lists

Many advisors who host seminars consistently draw their audiences from mailing lists that are available from list vendors. Review the information in the marketing and prospecting section covered in the direct mail and cold calling topics.

Topics

The content of your seminar should be a blend of technical information and motivational

---

Evaluate Vendor Lists

Use the following series of questions to evaluate your sources of lists:

- What is the source of the list?
- How often is the list updated?
- What selections are possible within the list?
- What is the history of successful usage of the list?
- What is the minimum quantity of names you must purchase?
- What addressing formats are available?
- Is the list in zip code sequence?
- What is the delivery time?
- What will it cost?
- Why is this particular list being recommended?

Essentials of Long-Term Care Insurance

material. How much of each depends on the needs of the prospects you invite. The program should be technically accurate and informative. If you give too much information, however, you may bore your prospects or they may have no need to make an appointment with you. In addition to being educational, the program should motivate attendees to meet with you for more information.

After you decide on a topic, your next step is to figure out whether the material is available or if you must develop it yourself. Many companies have seminar material for their advisors and require them to use it. If your company allows it, you can purchase seminar presentation material. If you decide to develop and write your own seminar material, allow enough time to research your topic thoroughly, and make sure you have adequate resources to produce it. Be sure to allow time for a compliance review by the insurance or financial services company or companies you represent.

Alternatively, you may decide to use the services of a professional presenter or advisor such as a broker, CPA, or attorney. You may even decide to help organize and co-sponsor seminars where other advisors are the seminar leaders. This may be a good choice until you have some experience under your belt. Whether you present the seminar or someone else does it for you, the seminar should establish you as an expert and a professional who can be trusted. Remember to follow your company's compliance procedures for situations in which you bring in an outside speaker

The Time Dimension

The time dimension of seminars has a couple of different meanings. First, effective seminars require a great deal of time to prepare, execute, and follow up. Many advisors who are very successful in seminars contend that a seminar is not a single event but a continuous process. All elements of the process must be carefully planned and implemented, which takes a great deal of time. The good news is that once the elements are satisfactorily developed, the seminar can be repeated time after time, frequently with increasing productivity.

Second, the time aspect of seminars also means selecting the best day and time to hold a seminar. The optimal day and time will depend on the needs of your audience. For example, it may be foolish to hold a seminar for your working prospects during working hours. Similarly, it may not be wise to hold a seminar for seniors late in the evening.

There are factors to consider when choosing a date for your seminar as well. You need to be sensitive to holidays, holy days, and competing events. You may plan a terrific seminar but if it competes with the NBA finals or the county fair, attendance may be adversely affected. You must keep all of this in mind as you look at the available dates and times for the facility where you will hold your seminar and examine your own schedule.

Location! Location! Location!

The site you select should be convenient for the members of your targeted group. Parking may be a critical consideration in urban and suburban areas.

The accommodations you select should match the size of your group. A small group in a large room gives the appearance that a lot of people decided not to come. On the other hand, too small a room may cause some people to leave your seminar because they feel crowded in too small a space.

One successful advisor suggests contacting a reputable LTC facility in the area to co-sponsor the event. The seminar could incorporate a tour of the facility and a presentation by the facility's administrator. This helps prospects appreciate and desire the freedom to choose a reputable facility. It also helps the advisor keep costs affordable.

Facilities

Checking—and rechecking—the facilities you have chosen will help your presentation run smoothly. If possible, try to visit the facility while another meeting is in progress. This action will allow you to determine the level of the lighting, the effectiveness of the sound system, and the visibility of any screens you will use with the overhead projection system. You can assess how well everyone in the room can see the speaker and judge whether the ambiance of the room reflects the feeling you wish to convey to your audience.

Consider what visual aids you will need before you begin calling facilities. If the facility does not provide visual aids, check to be sure that there are ample outlets for computers, projectors, or audio equipment. Double check all equipment prior to the seminar to be sure everything is in working order.

Check with the facility about refreshments, and if you serve refreshments, keep them simple. A basic guide is to serve something wet and something dry. For example, coffee and cookies are usually a hit.

Budget

It is especially helpful to establish a budget and work to stay within this constraint. Food is generally not served, but if you wish to provide refreshments, keep them simple and inexpensive. If you are using a hotel or restaurant, you may need to resist the pressures for lavish meals. Remember, you are selling your services and knowledge, not free food.

Other Details

Consider nametags, pencils, paper, and handouts. These may seem like small details, but it is important to pay attention to the details. They send your prospects a message about you.

For example, handouts of the highest quality that include your name and address send the message that you are professional and that you are willing to put your name on the work you do. Having paper and pencils available sends the message that what you say is important enough to write down.

You also want to plan a feedback mechanism. Some seminar presenters ask attendees to sign in, giving their names, addresses, and phone numbers. Others design an evaluation form that asks the attendees for this information, as well as for feedback on the quality and usefulness of the presentation.

Handouts

Place handouts into a folder. Try not to overdo the number of handouts. Distribute only the essentials, such as:

- *"A Shopper's Guide to Long Term Care Insurance"* (NAIC)
- *"Medicare and You"* (www.medicare.gov)
- Post-seminar Questionnaire
- Your business card
- Blank pages for notes
- Pen/pencil

Presenting a Seminar

If properly presented, a seminar helps to sell you as a competent professional. The following list gives you a few pointers that may help you make an effective seminar presentation:

- Begin and end on time.
- Speak to your audience.
- Get to the point and stay focused. Your audience wants to know what you can do for them. They do not want to hear war stories.
- Keep your goal in mind during your presentation. If you keep your goal in mind, you will stay focused.
- Speak from an outline or note cards, but do not read or memorize your speech.

- Be conversational, friendly, and enthusiastic.
- Use visual aids, if appropriate, but keep them simple.
- Avoid offensive jokes, stories, comments, or language.
- Move around as you speak. Do not remain in one spot the whole time.
- Relax, smile, and enjoy your work. People like to work with professionals who enjoy their work.
- Ask for feedback during your presentation in the form of questions and after your presentation in the form of a critique.

Seminar Follow-up

Most effective seminars are low-key and avoid overt attempts to sell products or specific services. Any one-on-one selling typically occurs after the seminar. It is for this reason that the follow-up phase of the seminar takes on such significance. In fact, many financial advisors who use seminars end their presentation by telling their audience that the advisor will contact each attendee to answer any questions that might have resulted from the seminar.

Telephone

Following your seminar, contact the attendees by telephone or in person to schedule appointments for discussing individual needs. Ideally, this follow-up should occur within one or 2 days of the seminar.

Some advisors try to learn more about the specific interests or needs of the prospective attendees by asking them to complete a confidential fact-finding questionnaire prior to attending the seminar. Among other things, the questionnaire asks attendees about their health and financial situation.

Questionnaire

Other financial advisors rely on post-seminar questionnaires to determine interest. A post-seminar questionnaire can be a very useful tool for determining which of the attendees is most likely to be interested in learning more about your services. (See the accompanying sample post-seminar questionnaire on the next page.)

The mere fact that an attendee takes the time to complete a post-seminar questionnaire is a sign of interest. You can use the attitudinal questions at the end of the survey to gauge each prospect's interest and possible motivations for buying LTCI.

Observation

Still other financial advisors rely on observation and target those people who have asked questions during the seminar presentation for a follow-up call. These advisors mix with the audience during breaks and identify those who seem to be most interested in the presentations. They also ask each of the seminar speakers to give them the names of attendees who asked them questions after the seminar. (Remember that nametags for all attendees will help you and your speakers in this process.)

Contact

Whatever technique you choose for determining which attendees will be your best prospects, try to capitalize on the goodwill and credibility you have cultivated at your seminar by scheduling a personal visit with each of the attendees. Many advisors recommend that you contact nonattendees as well, especially those who previously indicated that they would be in your audience.

Even when these advisors are unable to schedule an appointment with the nonattendees, they keep these prospects on their mailing lists for a specified time. The advisors stay in contact with them regularly, sending them newsletters or bulletins on ideas that might be of interest. These advisors invite these prospects to their next seminar and generally get a positive response. Many advisors find that the prospects become clients after the second seminar.

Contact Information

Since follow-up is critical for seminars, it is important that you have obtained reliable contact information from attendees. If you are doing a seminar for a group of people for whom you do not already have contact information, I have found that you can obtain reliable contact information if you offer a door prize of nominal value (for example, a gift certificate). Most people like to win prizes and will complete the contact information accurately. Tell them you will call the winner to verify his or her name and address. Of course, you need to check with your company's compliance guidelines before you do this.

Post-Seminar Questionnaire

We would very much appreciate your assistance in answering the following questions. Your responses will guide us in improving future seminars and determining if our organization may be of assistance to you in the future.

1. Which speaker did you find the most helpful?

   _____

2. Which subject covered during the seminar was of most interest to you?

   _____
   _____

3. Briefly list any subject areas that were not covered in the seminar that you think should have been covered.

   _____
   _____

4. You may have some questions that you did not have an opportunity to raise during the question-and-answer session. Please briefly list these questions below. We will make every effort to answer these questions for you or to find experts who can provide responses.

   _____
   _____

For the following statements, circle the response that best describes how you feel.	Strongly Disagree		Agree		Strongly Agree
I fear depending on family or friends for my care as I get older.	1	2	3	4	5
If I ever need long-term care, I want the freedom to decide what type of care I will receive and where I will receive it.	1	2	3	4	5
I am afraid I may not qualify for long-term care insurance if I wait too long.	1	2	3	4	5
I want to protect my assets from the potentially high costs of long-term care.	1	2	3	4	5
I am concerned about taking care of my parents or another relative should they need long-term care.	1	2	3	4	5

Name: _____   Address: _____

Phone: _____   _____

Fax: _____   Email: _____

Here are some approaches you might use when you follow up with each seminar attendee on the telephone or in person:

"John, at the seminar you recently attended, we had a question-and-answer period. Since the time allocated for this purpose was fairly brief, I am calling to schedule a time when we could discuss your specific questions or concerns. Would this Tuesday or Thursday work for you or would some time next week be better?"

"Ann, several of the speakers from the seminar you attended this week indicated that you had some excellent comments regarding some of the areas discussed. I'd like to spend some time with you covering those areas. Could we do that?"

Summary

Finally, for seminars to be a cost-effective prospecting tool, you must repeat the program regularly. Only with repeat seminars will you be able to justify the heavy commitment of time that is required to develop a viable seminar process and an effective seminar program. If your seminars acquire the reputation for being informative and valuable, they will be well attended by qualified prospects. The accompanying checklist summarizes the details and logistics you need to consider and plan for to make your seminars successful.

Seminar Checklist

Arranging for a Meeting Room:
- Has the meeting been confirmed?
- Who's your contact?
- Have you met this person?
- Have you seen the facility?
- Have you done a walk-through to see what it will be like for your guests to arrive and go to the meeting room?

Guest List:
- Do you know who will attend?
- Will anyone from your company be there?
- How many guests will your budget cover?

Seminar Promotion:
- Have you arranged a schedule for printing promotional material and material to be distributed during the seminar? Does the schedule include time to proofread printed material to avoid potentially embarrassing errors? Does it allow for delays at the print shop?
- Have letters or formal invitations been sent at least 2 weeks prior to the seminar?
- Have the invitees been called during the week just prior to the seminar to confirm their attendance?
- Have announcements been sent to local newspapers, radio stations, and other media outlets?

Getting There:
- Do your guests know the date and precise time of the seminar?
- Do they have directions to the meeting rooms?
- Will they have to use a special entrance?
- Have you asked the hotel or office complex for directional signs?
- Will you be having a check-in desk?
- How will early arrivals be handled?
- What are the provisions for parking?
- Will your prospects need a means of identification, such as name badges?
- Who will look after late arrivals?
- Will you need a message board?

Meeting Facilities:
- How will the room be arranged?
- Do you want chairs only or chairs and tables?
- Are you supplying paper, pens, and pencils?
- Will you need a microphone? If so, do you have an extra one in case one cannot be located at the meeting facility?
- Will the speakers need help with any equipment during the presentation?
- Is the lighting adequate?
- Will there be an overhead projector?
- Will there be a screen?
- Will you have spare projector bulbs?
- Will you need a flip chart, writing pad, or magic markers?
- Will you need reserved seat signs?
- When the overhead projector is on, do the main room lights need to be turned off? If so, who will do this?
- Have you supplied water and glasses for the speakers?
- Will you need a lectern?
- Who will make the introductions?
- Will there be a coffee break?

Seminar Content/Speakers:
- What topics will be covered?
- Who are the best speakers to address each area?
- How long should each person speak?
- What is the most appropriate format for the presentation (for example, lecture, round table discussion)?
- How much compensation (if any) should the speakers be offered?

Problems:
- Whom do you contact if there is a problem?
- Will the house audio/visual technician be available?
- What do you do if someone becomes ill?
- Where are the fire escapes located?
- Are there any security measures required?
- How will people make outgoing telephone calls?
- Who will handle the incoming calls?
- Do you have a reliable assistant to help you run the meeting?
- Have you thought of everything that could possibly go wrong?
- How will you handle cell phones ringing in the middle of the presentation?

Case History

Prospecting System

Traditionally, case histories tell how a particular sale was made. The following case history is different, however. In it, a multi-line insurance advisor, Ginny Thompson, shares her LTCI prospecting system. Ginny also has a simple selling system as well. She is a strong proponent for systems.

The most important thing for any advisor entering a market is to have a system or a process. That is the key to success.

I target four markets:

- Clients age 45 to 63
- Clients age 64 to 75
- Prospects age 45 to 63
- Prospects age 64 to 75

I use a simple system that consists of a preapproach, an approach, and a way to handle objections.

Clients

I market differently to my current clients because they already have a relationship with me. My preapproach and approach are based on the ongoing insurance reviews I offer to my clients.

Preapproach—I send a preapproach letter that talks about their insurance coverage in general. It says, "Thank you for your business. I hope we're doing what you want us to do. One of those things is to keep you abreast of the gaps in your coverage. I would like to have 30 minutes of your time to go over your insurance coverage with you. I am enclosing a brochure about one kind of coverage I am talking about. I will be calling you in the next couple of days to set up a time to get together."

Approach—I set a reminder for the time it takes for the mail to be delivered. Then my staff person will call and try to set an appointment:

> "Mrs. Client, this is Annette Jones from Ginny Thompson, ABC Insurance Office calling. Ginny recently sent you a letter thanking you for your business. She wanted me to follow up to let you know that she is very sincere about that. She is also very concerned that you have a gap in your insurance coverage. She would like to visit about that LTC brochure she sent you. Would it be convenient for you and Mr. Client to come into the office on Wednesday or would Thursday be better?"

Handling Objections—A part of my system is a strategy for handling objections. For example, if the person responds by saying that they do not have any money for more insurance, my staff person might say:

> "All Ginny wants to do is give you information. You can leave your checkbook at home. She is passionate about this because she has had some personal experiences and she feels that it is very important that everybody knows about the coverage. It will only take 30 minutes."

If the client persists in his or her objection, my staff person will then change tactics. For example, take a person who says that he or she is too young and persists in this objection, my staff person would respond by saying:

> "I understand. You know, a lot of people feel the way you do, but I have to disagree with you. Ginny may send you something to look at and then I may call you back, would that be okay?"

Then I will send an appropriate article from a newspaper or magazine. I clip the article and put a sticky note with my company's logo in the left-hand corner. I write, "I thought you might find this interesting." I set a follow-up reminder for 2 weeks or one month, depending on the level of resistance. Then my staff person will call back and ask, "Did you get the article Ginny sent you on LTCI and the cost of waiting?" Then she starts trying to get the appointment again.

Perpetual Follow-Up—For clients, I follow up for a solid year. At the end of the year, I send another letter that says:

> "During the past year you have heard from me several times but none of the correspondence is more important than what I sent you about LTCI. I am enclosing the booklet again. I really want you to look at it. I am going to be calling you because I think it is so important that you know about this."

I set a reminder to call and start all over again until the person says, "Don't call me again about this. I don't want to hear from you about this anymore."

Prospects

For prospects, my handling is different. I buy leads from a vendor, specifying the age range (either ages 45 to 63 or ages 64 to 75), zip code, home ownership, and a household income of $75,000 or more.

Preapproach—Because I am specifically prospecting for LTCI, I send a preapproved letter along with a booklet on LTCI.

Approach—I then set a reminder to follow up with a phone call. My staff person uses a slightly different word track for prospects:

> "Mrs. Prospect, this is Annette Jones calling. I'm with Ginny Thompson's ABC Insurance office. We recently sent you information regarding LTCI. Ginny would like to visit with you. She wants to inform everyone that this insurance coverage is available. Can she visit with you this week, or would next week be better?"

Handling Objections—Objections are handled the same way as they are handled for clients, except that the article strategy will only be used if the caller seems receptive to the phone call. Typically, external leads are not as friendly as clients. However, often my office staff or I can successfully pivot and sell an auto insurance policy. Then I retry marketing LTCI to these people, this time using the client approach discussed earlier.

Advice to Advisors New to the LTCI Market—My advice is to have a process. You cannot enter the LTCI market unless you have an approach, a time to call, a systematic sales presentation, and a process for follow-up. If you do not have a system or process you will not be successful.

Chapter Two Review

Key Terms and Concepts are explained in the Glossary. Answers to the Review Questions and Self-Test Questions are found in the back of the book in the Answers to Questions section.

Key Terms and Concepts

prospecting
qualified prospect
market segments
   age-based
   couples versus singles
   women
generations
   Generation X
   Baby Boomers
   Silent Generation
target market

prospecting
   referral
   center of influence (COI)
   networking
   seminars
   cold-calling
preapproach
   direct mail
   building prestige
   ten-second commercial
   résumé
approach
   telephone approach
   pivot approach

Review Questions

2-1. What are the four characteristics of a qualified prospect?

2-2. Describe two ways in which prospects in the under age 50 market segment can be approached to buy LTCI.

2-3. Give reasons why the ages 50 to 65 market segment will be the bread and butter market for LTCI for the next several years.

2-4. What is a target market?

2-5. Describe each of the following prospecting methods:
   a. referrals

b. centers of influence
c. networking
d. seminars
e. cold calling

2-6. List four different ways to preapproach a prospect.

2-7. What are the four elements of a good approach script?

2-8. Describe four advantages of seminars.

Self-Test Questions

Instructions: Read chapter 2 first, then answer the following questions to test your knowledge. There are 10 questions; circle the correct answer, then check your answers with the answer key in the back of the book.

2-1. The market segment that probably is the most difficult to sell LTCI to is the

(a) over age 65 market segment
(b) ages 50-65 market segment
(c) under age 50 market segment
(d) business owners market segment

2-2. Which of the following characteristics of a qualified prospect depends on how well the advisor's own characteristics match those of the prospect?

(a) The prospect needs and values the advisor's products and services.
(b) The prospect is insurable.
(c) The prospect can afford to pay for the advisor's products and services.
(d) The prospect can be approached by the advisor on a favorable basis.

2-3. The primary reason given by women for buying LTCI is that they

(a) want to avoid being a burden on loved ones
(b) want to preserve assets
(c) have a higher probability of needing it
(d) know LTC will cost more for them

2-4. Which of the following statements describes the most common mistake that advisors make when working with wealthy prospects?

(a) They emphasize the importance of picking the desired setting for care.
(b) They focus on the emotional nature of LTC.
(c) They assume these prospects want to self-insure.
(d) They assume these prospects want their children to inherit their wealth.

2-5. People born in the Silent Generation are characterized as being which of the following?

I.   Risk-takers
II. Image-conscious

(a) I only
(b) II only
(c) Both I and II
(d) Neither I nor II

2-6. Centers of influence (COIs) typically possess which of the following characteristics?

I.   COIs are viewed as takers.
II. COIs are sought out for advice.

(a) I only
(b) II only
(c) Both I and II
(d) Neither I nor II

2-7. All of the following are pointers to help you make an effective seminar presentation **EXCEPT:**

(a) Get to the point and stay focused.
(b) Be conversational, friendly, and enthusiastic.
(c) Remain in one spot as you speak.
(d) Speak from an outline or note cards.

2-8. Adult children generally will be more receptive to talking about their parents' LTC needs if their own situation is characterized by all of the following **EXCEPT:**

(a) They have young children.
(b) They are from a dual-income family.
(c) They live a long distance from their parents.
(d) They have many surviving siblings.

2-9. All of the following statements comparing LTCI prospects in the over-age-65 market segment with younger prospects are correct **EXCEPT:**

(a) Over-age-65 prospects are much less concerned about protecting and conserving their assets.
(b) Over-age-65 prospects are more sensitive to healthcare issues.
(c) Over-age-65 prospects are more deliberate in their decision-making and very receptive to seminars.
(d) Over-age-65 prospects experience a higher percentage of coverage declinations.

2-10. All of the following are advantages of prospecting using seminars **EXCEPT:**

(a) Seminars are an efficient use of time.
(b) You can meet prospects in a non-threatening way.
(c) Seminars can be used to prequalify prospects.
(d) Seminars require less planning and effort than other prospecting methods.

3

Long-Term Care Caregivers, Settings, and Financing Alternatives

---

Overview and Learning Objectives

Chapter 3 examines the different caregivers associated with LTC. It then looks at the settings in which care is provided, reviews financing alternatives for LTC, and describes the major features of Medicaid and Medicaid Planning. By reading this chapter and answering the questions, you should be able to:

3-1. Describe the four types of caregivers.

3-2. Describe the major delivery settings for LTC.

3-3. Explain the different alternatives for financing LTC.

3-4. Describe the major features of Medicaid and Medicaid planning.

Chapter Outline

Caregivers and Care Settings for LTC

Before we begin a discussion on caregivers and care settings, let's take a minute to review the nature of LTC. LTC deals with chronic conditions and care needed over an extended period of time. LTC can include skilled medical care, however, it primarily addresses custodial and personal care needs that arise when someone cannot perform physical or cognitive activities deemed necessary for "ordinary" living. LTC focuses on maintaining a person's living situation, not on improving his or her health, as is the case for acute care.

LTC is provided by caregivers and delivered in specific care settings. Among the caregivers and the care settings, care progresses from less intensive to more intensive as the care delivered moves from family members to professionals and from the home setting to supportive-living arrangements. This progression is often called a *care continuum*. A care recipient's level of independence, and the care options that satisfy the needs of the care recipient and match a family caregiver's availability and capacity, determine the care recipient's place in the care continuum. The home is usually the best care setting in which to maintain independence. However, it may not be the option selected because of the limits of a family caregiver and

---

Policyowner Perspective on LTCI

Authors' Note: The following is an excerpt from the June 27, 2002 article *Navigating the Maze of Long-term Health Insurance* found at *http://www.cnn.com 2002/HEALTH/06/27/long.term.health.ap/index.html*. Reprinted with permission of *The Associated Press*.

Beth Chapman
Beth Chapman, 58, a self-employed consultant, sees insurance as a tool to maintain her independence. She remembers growing up sharing her family home with her father's father and her mother's mother.

"That set the stage for my father to buy long-term care insurance because he didn't want to be a burden to his kids," she said.

Chapman has saved for her retirement and figures that she's accumulated enough to cover her living expenses after she stops working, but not enough to handle any debilitating illness. She bought long-term care insurance to fill that gap.

"Philosophically, I don't believe the government should pay for my care," she said. "I don't happen to think assisted living is a good model, either. I'd like to stay in my own home as long as possible and get the help there if I need it."

---

the care recipient's need for social interaction and more demanding caregiving that can be satisfied more completely in a supportive-living arrangement. This section describes long-term caregivers and care settings that comprise the care continuum.

Caregivers

Formal and informal caregivers are the two main types of caregivers. In addition, respite caregivers and care coordinators also provide LTC services.

Informal Caregiver

An informal caregiver is an individual who voluntarily cares for a LTC recipient without pay and without formal education and training in LTC. Informal caregivers include immediate family members such as spouses, children, brothers and sisters, and others related to the care recipient by blood or marriage such as aunts, uncles, cousins, and in-laws. Friends, neighbors, and volunteers from churches, charities, and community groups can also be informal caregivers. The informal caregiver, usually a family member, with overall responsibility for a person's LTC is called a *primary caregiver*. All other informal caregivers are *secondary caregivers*.

> **LTC is a family affair.**

Formal Caregiver

A formal caregiver in a LTC setting is an individual who provides care and services as a profession or occupation to LTC recipients. Formal caregivers include physicians, nurse caregivers, other licensed medical personnel, and nonlicensed personnel. Families may retain formal caregivers' services on an individual basis. However, formal caregiver services other than those provided by physicians are often obtained through home care agencies that assist informal caregivers in the home care setting.

Physicians—Physicians are formal long-term caregivers because they usually authorize and direct the medical care and other necessary services provided to LTC recipients. Physicians may treat LTC recipients directly

> ### Talk to Everyone Over Age 50
>
> "Just talk to everyone over age 50 about LTCI. More often than not, these prospects have had a family member or neighbor who has needed nursing home care. If not, they probably at least know someone who has had life turned upside down because of his or her involvement with a relative who has needed some type of LTC."

for acute illness, such as pneumonia, or medically manage a chronic condition such as Parkinson's disease. A geriatric physician specializes in the treatment of the aged.

Nurse Caregivers—A *nurse caregiver* is a registered nurse, licensed practical nurse, or nurse assistant (aide) who is responsible for the medical treatment of actual or potential health problems, with the goal of rehabilitating a care recipient or stabilizing a care recipient's medical condition. A registered nurse supervises the conduct of nursing services that may include custodial services provided in conjunction with medical care. Thus, nurse caregivers also direct the services provided by nonlicensed personnel. Nurse assistants in the home care setting are called *home health aides*. Nurse caregivers are the principal providers of skilled and intermediate care mentioned earlier in chapter 1 and to be mentioned later in this chapter.

Other Licensed Medical Personnel—Other licensed medical personnel are those with special health care skills obtained through training and experience such as therapists, speech-language pathologists, and registered dietitians.

Therapists—A therapist is a trained medical specialist who commonly performs one or more of the following services:

- physical therapy—treatment of physical impairments through the use of special exercise, application of heat or cold, and other physical modalities
- respiratory therapy—treatment that maintains or improves the breathing function through the administration of medications and oxygen and/or the use of ventilator equipment
- infusion therapy—introduction of fluids, electrolytes, or drugs, directly into a vein, tissue or organ
- occupational therapy—functional enhancement of people who have physical, social, and emotional deficits arising from physical injury, illness, emotional disturbance, congenital or developmental disability, or aging

Speech-Language Pathologists—A speech-language pathologist is a professional with advanced training and education in human communications, its development, and its disorders. Individuals with these skills measure and evaluate language abilities, auditory processes,

> The "Magic Question"
>
> "Do you know someone who has needed LTC?"

and speech production and treat those with speech and language disorders.

Social Worker—A social worker is an individual with advanced education in dealing with social, emotional, and environmental problems associated with physical or cognitive impairments.

Dietitians—A dietitian is a professional trained in the application of the principles of nutrition to the planning and preparation of foods to promote health and treat disease.

Nonlicensed Personnel—Nonlicensed personnel are employed to assist LTC recipients with nonmedical tasks that usually relate to activities of daily living (ADLs) such as bathing and feeding and instrumental activities of daily living (IADLs) such as cleaning, laundry, meal preparation, shopping, paying bills, and completing other chores. In the home setting, these nonlicensed personnel are called *homemakers*, *companions*, and *chore workers*. While they are usually unlicensed, some states require that certain categories of these persons be certified. Personnel at this level often obtain training in geriatric care.

Respite Caregiver

A respite caregiver is an alternate caregiver who provides LTC services to relieve a primary caregiver from the physical and emotional stress of providing care over a long period of time and/or to allow some period of personal time. This service is called *respite care*. Respite care may occur in a number of care settings and can be provided by informal and formal caregivers. Respite care can be relatively brief. For example, a neighbor who relieves a caregiver for an hour a day several days a week provides respite care by giving the primary caregiver the opportunity to take a break or pursue personal interests. Respite care can also have an extended duration. Usually the longer the period of respite care, the more likely it is provided by formal caregivers. For example, a care recipient living at home could receive services from a home care agency or be placed in an assisted-living facility for a week or two when the caregiving family takes a vacation.

Care Coordinator

A care coordinator, also known as a *care manager* or *care planner,* assesses an elderly person who shows some degree of physical or cognitive impairment to determine his or her care needs and then develops a care plan to meet those needs. The plan also identifies and assesses the care resources available from the family, including financial resources as well as the resources available in the community. The plan effectively places the care recipient in the care continuum by recommending the proper care setting and appropriate caregivers or combinations of caregivers in a manner that respects the care recipient's independence and needs and the availability and capacity of the informal caregivers. A social worker functioning as the care coordinator typically develops the care plan. The charge for this service is usually on a fee-for-service basis and costs about $100 per hour.

The services of a care coordinator may be requested by a family caregiver, a physician, or may be part of the certification process to determine eligibility for benefits under a LTCI policy. The primary family caregiver or the coordinator can manage the plan by monitoring the quality and effectiveness of care and adjusting the plan as the care recipient's and caregiver's needs change.

Care Settings

Care settings are the environments in which LTC services may be provided to care recipients. Care settings also occur along a care continuum that begins with home care provided by informal caregivers. It advances to supportive-living arrangements outside the home with the use of formal caregivers. As the care recipient's needs become more intensive and complex, more support is needed to maintain the home as the care setting. While supportive-living arrangements outside the home may indicate that the care continuum requirements exceed the capabilities of the home environment, they are often an alternative to the home environment when they involve independent living and assisted-living facilities. As supportive-living settings progress from independent living through assisted living and to nursing home care, they also represent a care continuum. Because the nursing home setting provides the most intensive and complex form of long-term care using formal caregivers, nursing homes often constitute an endpoint on the care continuum. Hospice care, which can be provided in many settings, and hospital care also mark the end of the care continuum for some long-term care recipients.

The key to providing LTC services is to select the level of care and setting that meets the care recipients needs, while maintaining the maximum degree of independence and the most normal living situation possible under the circumstances of the disability or declining health. The assistance provided should meet but not exceed the care recipient's needs and should allow as independent a life as possible.

Home Health Care

Home health care as the name implies takes place where the care recipient resides and encompasses virtually any home environment outside of a nursing home. Home may be the familiar family residence of many years or a new residence acquired for retirement. The proximity of family members and reduced home maintenance and repair burdens are often the reasons seniors relocate, especially as they become less independent or after the death of a spouse. The care recipient's home may also be in a family member's residence, an independent living facility, or an assisted-living facility.

The spectrum of LTC services available in the home setting is quite broad and encompasses medical and custodial services using both informal and formal caregivers. These services are provided to the extent and combination needed to meet the recipient's changing needs and the availability and capacity of family caregivers. Nationwide, an estimated 22.4 million families are providing physical and emotional assistance to loved ones. Caregivers spend about $2 billion each month out of pocket on groceries, medicine, and support services.[1] About 9 million Americans over age 65 live alone and about 2 million have no one to turn to if they need help.[2]

Most care recipients and their families view the home as the ideal care setting, at least when care needs are more easily managed. With familiar surroundings, possessions accumulated over a lifetime, and proximity to established neighbors and friends, the care recipient can flourish and function at a high level of independence despite a disability or chronic condition. To the extent recovery is possible after an illness or injury, recovery is quicker when care is delivered in a preferred setting, such as at home. Assistance may be hands-on or in the form of supervision to make sure these tasks are properly and safely completed. In the home setting, family members to the extent they are available and have the capacity to do so, may provide the needed custodial services by assisting with ADLs, IADLs, and home maintenance.

"Long-Term Care Insurance—You can't stay home without it!"

Many elderly with some disabilities live by themselves and may need only minor assistance at the beginning and end of the day. While the ideal location is the care recipient's own residence, the care recipient may move into a family member's home to make it easier for the family caregiver to provide assistance.

EXAMPLE: Jane's mother, Dorothy, recently widowed at age 78, remains in reasonably good health, but is becoming increasingly frail and suffers from macular degeneration, which restricts her vision. Jane visits her mother two or more times a week to pay bills and handles the financial matters that are now beyond Dorothy's current abilities. When she visits, Jane brings her mother groceries and other necessary supplies. Jane also closely monitors her mother's routine daily activities, such as dressing and bathing, to make sure that she is completing them without major difficulty. Jane's husband cuts the grass, shovels snow, and keeps Dorothy's house in repair.

Jane, as the primary caregiver, and her husband are able to take care of Dorothy's current needs quite well as informal caregivers providing care in Dorothy's home where, despite some limitations, she maintains significant independence. They are providing Dorothy LTC at a relatively low level in the care continuum by assisting with the IADLs and the ADLs, frequently on a stand-by basis, and by providing home maintenance.

As care needs change with increased dependency, a family caregiver may have to seek additional assistance to maintain the care recipient at home. This assistance can include a range of support through home care agencies, adult day care centers, and community services. The services that these groups provide allow a family member to maintain a relative in the home care setting when the relative's increasing needs exceed the availability and/or capacity of the informal caregiver. In the absence of these services, the family caregiver would have little choice other than to turn to supportive-living arrangements.

Home Health Care Agencies—A home health care agency is a private company that specializes in care to the elderly and disabled. These agencies employ a range of formal caregivers that frequently includes those previously listed under the headings of nurse caregivers, other licensed

---

A Buyer's Perspective

"I knew I would buy LTCI someday, but seeing my friend's problems scared me into acting. After all, I'm a single woman on my own. If I needed care, there would be no one to provide it for me. I want the freedom to choose where I will receive care and who will provide it for me. LTCI gives me the ability to choose."

---

medical personnel, and nonlicensed personnel. These agencies can provide medical and custodial services. Specifically, they can provide intermediate nursing services, help with bathing, dressing, and meals and offer socialization and housekeeping. Some agencies, however, specialize in home health aides (nursing assistants) and nonlicensed personnel such as homemakers, companions, and chore workers who may maintain and repair a home.

EXAMPLE: In a continuation of the previous example, Dorothy, fell and broke her hip. After release from the hospital and a less-than-30-day stay in a nursing home, she returned home to complete her recovery. A home health care agency now provides medical services in the form of nursing care services and physical therapy 3 times a week. A home health aide visits every weekday to help with dressing, bathing, and transferring her in and out bed and chairs. Jane has just received a letter from Medicare informing her that Dorothy's recovery is now complete to the extent that she no longer requires nursing care. The services of the home health aide who assisted Dorothy with her ADLs is also no longer covered because Medicare does not pay for custodial care in the absence of a need for intermediate nursing care.

Because Dorothy is left with limited agility after her surgery and is becoming increasingly frail, Jane and Dorothy agree to retain the home health care agency's services for a few hours every weekday to assist with dressing, bathing, and personal hygiene while Jane and her husband are at work. On the weekend and sometimes during weekday evenings, Jane and her husband continue to care for Dorothy as they did before her accident. However, her needs now include hands-on assistance with ADLs that the home health aide provides during the week.

Dorothy has returned to a lower level of care than when she required nursing care during her recovery from surgery. Nevertheless, although Dorothy remains at home, her increased dependency and the continuing services of a formal custodial caregiver has clearly advanced her along the care continuum beyond the point at which Jane and her husband began to care for her.

Home care agencies are usually licensed by the state, although only about half have received federal certification required for payment of services under the Medicare and Medicaid programs. The National Home Care Council, the Joint Commission on Accreditation of Healthcare Organizations, and the Community Health Accreditation Program are three prominent standard setting organizations that accredit home care agencies. State licensure, federal certification, and accreditation are important indicators of the home care agency's staff qualifications and, therefore, the quality of its services.

Adult Day Care Centers—The adult day care center is a relatively new setting that provides social, medical, and rehabilitative services to people with physical and mental impairments. These centers are designed for the elderly, who may be severely impaired but live at home and whose family caregiver is unavailable to stay at home during the day because he or she is working. Without the services these centers provide, many people could not remain in the community.

Adult day care centers are usually open 5 days a week from 6 to 12 hours per day and typically provide a full range of LTC services. Medical services include nursing care, as well as physical, speech, and occupational therapy. Not all centers provide medical services, however. Custodial care is also provided and most of those who receive care at adult day care centers are frail and need help with ADLs. Many have cognitive impairments, including the early stages of Alzheimer's disease. The centers also provide meals under the direction of a dietitian and meet social needs through recreational and educational activities. Many programs offer transportation between home and the center. Daily charges range from around $50 to over $100 if medical services are provided. These centers are frequently sponsored by community service agencies.

Community Services—Community services are described under the headings of community-sponsored programs and services funded by the Administration on Aging.

Community-Sponsored Programs—Almost every community, through volunteers, community groups, charities, churches, and government provides various arrays of services that enhance a care recipient's ability to remain at home and support family caregivers. The development of adult day care centers that has just been reviewed demonstrates the important role community

---

Words of Advice from a Successful Advisor

For advisors who are taking their first steps into the LTCI market, I would recommend the following:

- Immerse yourself in LTCI. Learn about the product and the marketplace.
- Mention LTCI to everybody and talk to anyone between the ages of 37 and 80 about LTCI.
- Educate the younger prospects that LTCI is not for the elderly. Tell these prospects that 40 percent of all LTC services are delivered to people under the age of 65.
- Ask prospects and clients to refer their parents and relatives
- Pivot or open the door with LTCI. It's a great product to use to cement an existing client relationship or to begin a new one.

services can play in LTC. Many communities offer organized classes ranging from art to organized exercise. Other social services include group sightseeing, scheduled transportation to local shopping facilities, and regularly scheduled movies. These services keep seniors not only physically active, but also mentally engaged.

Services Funded by the Administration on Aging—The federal Older Americans Act established the Administration on Aging (AOA), which supports local area agencies on aging (AAAs) through funds provided to each state. Nationwide over 650 area agencies on aging receive funding from their respective states. The AAAs contract with public and private groups to provide services or may provide services directly to support in-home and community services for individuals aged 60 or older. There are several categories of these services[3]:

- in-home services—include the Meals on Wheels program, homemakers, chore services, telephone reassurance, friendly visiting, energy assistance and weatherizing, emergency response systems, home health services, personal care services, and respite care
- information and access services—include information and referral/assistance, health insurance counseling, client assessment, care management (coordination), transportation, caregiver support, and retirement planning and education
- community-based services—include employment services, senior centers, congregate meals, adult day care services, volunteer opportunities
- housing—includes senior housing and alternative community-based living facilities
- elder rights—includes legal assistance, elder abuse prevention programs, and ombudsmen services for complaint resolution

Each community determines its own priorities for the services it offers within these categories and the extent to which they are offered. Consequently, they may differ markedly from community to community. Eligibility requirements may relate both to income levels and care priorities such as the homebound elderly with no family caregiver. Community services, even those with federal funding, do not represent an entitlement program like Medicare or Medicaid. Budgets are limited and often there are waiting lists for those who are otherwise eligible. In an effort to expand the reach of their services, agencies are accepting payments that vary with incomes above their traditional eligibility thresholds.

Families are encouraged to contact local agencies to determine the specific services offered in their communities, as well as eligibility and payment requirements. AAAs are listed in telephone directories, usually under city or county government headings. With funding provided by the AOA, the state and area agencies on aging have established an Eldercare Locator administered in cooperation with the National Association of State Units on Aging. The Eldercare Locator helps elderly adults and their caregivers to find local services for seniors through a toll-free service at 1-800-677-1116 with some locator features available through the Internet at *www.eldercare.gov*. Many churches also have volunteers who are valuable resources for finding local caregiving.

Supportive Living Arrangements

With advancing age, many seniors in generally good health or with only minor limitations become less willing to maintain a home, especially if they live alone. They also may need some degree of assistance from time to time or at least want the security of knowing that it is available. In addition, they may feel isolated living at home and miss the companionship of others, especially after the death of a spouse. At the same time, they wish to remain as independent as possible for as long as possible before entering a nursing home. Supportive-living arrangements for these individuals are available in settings across a care continuum that ranges from independent housing, to an assisted-living facility, and eventually to a nursing home. Which setting individuals or couples may enter is directly related to their level of independence. Because these living arrangements are often available through unrelated facilities on a stand-alone basis, they are described separately. However, in many other cases, a combined facility may offer two or more shared-living arrangements. This discussion excludes adult retirement communities that are typically designed for younger retirees in good health who must provide entirely for their own medical and LTC needs.

Independent Housing—Independent housing is a collective term applicable to a wide range of housing arrangements that include senior apartments, home sharing, and accessory apartments (completely separate living quarters inside a single family home). The living spaces may be a bedroom, an apartment, or perhaps separate units in a complex

> "I have found that when people reach their late 50's and early 60's, they get more realistic about their need for LTC."
>
> —multiline advisor

of buildings. Common areas are usually available for dining, recreation, and meetings. Residents do not require constant supervision. However, these facilities provide nonmedical support services that can be scheduled and not required on demand. Examples of such services are meals, housekeeping, and laundry. Assistance with some routine daily activities such as bathing, dressing, and grooming may be purchased as separate services. Generally, residents are free to come and go as they please. Local transportation to shopping and community events may be available.

Independent housing is usually privately owned, but is frequently developed by not-for-profit groups. While many of these living arrangements are licensed, the regulations governing their operations vary widely as does the quality of the housing and services provided.

Assisted-Living Facilities—An assisted-living facility provides supportive-living arrangements for elderly residents who, despite some degree of impairment, remain independent to a significant degree, but require continuing supervision and the availability of assistance when needed on an unscheduled basis. There may be separate sections of assisted-living facilities devoted to caring for individuals with cognitive impairments such as Alzheimer's disease.

Residents may have single rooms or their own apartments with kitchens or they may live in separate units. Services usually include meals, laundry, housekeeping, personal services (such as a hairdresser or a barber), and transportation outside the facility. Services also include assistance with one or more ADLs and medication monitoring is routine. A nurse may be called for an assisted-living resident who needs limited amounts of nursing care. However, if constant nursing and/or custodial care is required, the resident is no longer a candidate for assisted living.

Assisted-living facilities may serve as many as several hundred residents, although most are smaller. While costs also vary widely, average annual costs are approximately $25,000 or about half the cost of a nursing home. Board and care homes and adult foster care are much smaller in scale than assisted-living facilities, yet provide similar supportive services.

EXAMPLE: In a further continuation of the previous example, Dorothy's accumulating conditions further impair her independence to the point where the home care agency visits that assist with bathing and dressing are insufficient to meet her changing needs. Dorothy can no longer be left home alone.

After performing an assessment, the care coordinator hired by Jane agrees that Dorothy needs a higher level of care that includes continual supervision and hands-on assistance with bathing, dressing, and transferring in and out of bed and chairs. The coordinator recommends either an assisted-living facility or an adult day care center in the community, if Jane is able to take care of Dorothy's needs after work and on weekends. However, if the adult day care center option is taken, Dorothy has to give up her home of many years and move in with Jane to allow her daughter to care for her on a daily basis.

Because Dorothy prefers the independence of a home-like setting, she decides to move to Jane's home. Jane is willing to meet the additional care needs required by having her mother live with her. Dorothy applies and is accepted at the adult day care center. Jane and her husband adjust their work schedules to accommodate the center's hours. They are pleased that Dorothy receives care and supervision throughout the day, makes new friends, and is more active than she was previously.

This arrangement continues successfully for quite some time until Dorothy's needs at home increase to the point that they are more than Jane and her husband can handle. Somewhat reluctantly Dorothy moves to an assisted-living facility where she receives supervision and the availability of support services on a continuing basis.

Dorothy has advanced significantly along the care continuum. Initially, her increased needs were met through a higher level of care at the adult day care center, although the care setting remained the home with informal caregivers also providing more care. With the move to the assisted-living facility, both the setting and the dominant involvement of formal caregivers indicate that she is now at an even higher level on the care continuum.

Nursing Home—A nursing home is a state licensed facility that provides skilled, intermediate, and custodial care services with the care recipient's condition determining the combination and extent of services provided. Nursing homes are classified as *skilled-nursing facilities* when they meet the accreditation criteria required for reimbursement of services provided to Medicare and Medicaid patients. Nursing homes typically have separate sections or units for each level of service.

Hospitals usually discharge patients to nursing homes to complete their recovery from an acute illness or injury. Indeed, approximately two thirds of people discharged from nursing homes stayed for 3 months or fewer.[4] Those who stay longer are often chronic LTC recipients who enter a nursing home when they need more care than a home care setting or assisted-living setting can provide. They need around-the-clock care at least for custodial care and possibly nursing care. Other factors that affect the decision to enter a nursing home include:

- the absence of a willing or available family caregiver
- limitations on the capacity of an available family caregiver to provide home care even with the support of community and professional home care services
- the cost of home care needed to meet the recipients needs makes the nursing home a more economical option

Nursing homes represent the highest level of care and an end point on the LTC continuum. They provide the most intensive LTC services both as a setting and in the array of formal caregivers available on a 24-hour basis.

Combined Facility—A combined facility offers two or more shared-living arrangements that provide the same housing and services described previously under separate supportive-living settings. Some combined facilities provide independent and assisted living, while others provide assisted living and nursing home care. In both of these situations, the combined facility usually gives no assurance or guarantee to the resident regarding access to, or the cost of, the next level of care should it be required. By contrast, a *continuing care retirement community (CCRC),* also known as a life-care facility, provides the full continuum of supportive-living arrangements and is obligated to provide the housing and defined LTC services at each level of care for the life of the resident.

Typically, CCRC residents must be capable of fully independent living upon entry, but are assured of assisted living and nursing home levels of care as their future needs change. The residents may receive periodic home care services when they reside in their independent living accommodations. When a resident needs continuing supervision, he or she is usually required to move to the assisted-living unit of the CCRC. If, however, care needs escalate to the point where skilled care or custodial care is required on a continuing basis, the resident then moves to the CCRC's nursing home facility. Return to assisted-living or independent living remains a possibility if the resident's/patient's condition improves. A resident spouse capable of independent living remains in the independent accommodations where the couple initially resided. Religious and other not-for-profit organizations sponsor CCRCs. Large corporations also develop them.

Hospice Care—*Hospice care* is a system of treatment designed to relieve the discomfort of a terminally ill individual and to maintain quality of life to the extent possible throughout the phases of dying. When hospice care is available, the cost of treating terminally ill patients is usually much less than the cost of institutional hospitalization. It is not designed to produce a cure. Hospice care, only recently considered a long-term care component, has a number of unique patient care features.

First, as the definition suggests, the care emphasizes comfort and palliative treatments to manage the pain, rather than the performance of heroic medical treatment and surgical procedures.

Second, in addition to the formal caregivers and care coordinators described previously, the hospice care team includes psychologists, spiritual advisors, and bereavement counselors. Counseling for the patient and family members by these professionals is a standard component of hospice care.

Third, hospice care can be provided in multiple settings, depending on the needs and circumstances of the care recipient. The home is the typical setting because of familiar surroundings and the likely presence of family members who are often caregivers. Individuals without family caregivers may enter a freestanding hospice facility, which provides a home-like setting, professional staff, and continuous access by family members. Nursing homes and hospitals may also serve as hospice care settings.

Finally, because hospice care is provided at the end of an individual's continuum of care, its duration is usually measured in weeks or months, not years.

NOTES:

1. Philadelphia Corporation for Aging (PCA), PCA Aging Advocacy from Web site at *www.pcphl.org/advocacy.html*, page1, downloaded June 5, 2002.

2. Administration On Aging, The Administration on Aging and the Older American Act from Web site at *www.aoa.gov/aoa/pages/aoafact.html*, page 1, downloaded June 5, 2002.

3. National Association of Area Agencies on Aging, Area Agencies of Aging: A Link to Services of Older Adults and their Caregivers, from Web site at *www.n4a.orgaboutaaas.cfm*, pages 1–4, downloaded June 5, 2002.

4. Centers for Disease Control and Prevention/National Center for Health Statistics, The National Nursing Home Survey, 1997.

Financing Alternatives

The need and cost for LTC was clearly established in chapter 1. In the previous section of this chapter, you were introduced to the different caregivers and care settings, each with its level of financial and emotional costs. Obviously, as you progress through the care continuum, the financial and possible emotional cost to the care recipient and his or her family increases.

Many people will need some level of LTC at some point in their lives. After you understand what the prospect expects in terms of caregiving and care settings, the next question is: How will he or she pay for it?

This section covers the financing alternatives for the cost of LTC. There are three basic sources for payment: self-funding, government programs, or LTCI. A fourth, charity, is not covered.

Understanding the financing alternatives enables you to do two things. First, you will be familiar with them should a prospect want to use any of them in funding LTC. Second, you will be able to give a declined prospect a sense of what can be done as an alternative to the LTCI for which he or she could not qualify.

> Most people are aware of the need, especially those who are aged 50 and above. I feel I need to educate them about the alternatives they have to pay for LTC.
>
> —LTCI advisor

Self-Funding

As you discuss the cost of LTC with your prospects, you will want to know what role they anticipate their personal assets will play in paying for their care. Their feelings, as well as the hard facts of what assets they own, are necessary to determine the solution that will work best for them. You will read about gathering this information in chapter 4, when you discuss the fact-finding interview. For now, we will look at some of the different ways people can self-insure against LTC costs.

Savings and Assets
Savings and assets include monies from savings accounts, CD's, 401(k)s, IRAs, pension plans, mutual funds, stocks, bonds, and so forth. The

concept of using savings and assets is to pay for the costs of LTC from current investment income or the liquidation of investments. For example, one could either make payment from the dividends of a mutual fund or by redeeming shares of the mutual fund.

In this situation, the person is paying for LTC costs as they come due and is paying them dollar for dollar. The advantage of this method is that a person only pays if he or she needs LTC. If LTC is not needed, his or her heirs receive a larger inheritance.

However, the disadvantages lie in the fact that if LTC is needed, it may be possible for the care recipient(s) to spend down all of the family's savings and assets, reducing or eliminating the inheritance considerably and jeopardizing the quality of care available to the care recipient(s).

Annuities

One method of payment is to transfer assets to an annuity. Doing so ensures the annuitant that he or she will have a specified monthly income, presumably to pay LTC costs.

Unfortunately, the initial amount needed to pay for even a modest daily benefit of $100 is substantial and generally will not increase if the cost of LTC increases. In addition, to obtain the maximum annuity payment possible means the annuitant must select a life annuity with no refund. That is not desirable for someone who wants to leave an inheritance.

There are LTC/annuity products available, which are discussed in chapter 5.

Reverse Mortgages

Today's seniors have benefited from the housing market appreciation over the years. For many seniors, their homes are their most valuable asset. Reverse mortgages are a special type of housing loan that allows homeowners age 62 and older to convert equity into cash. This increases cash flow for the homeowner to pay for home health or nursing home care or for whatever else he or she wishes to rise the money. Payments from a reverse mortgage can be in the form of a single lump sum, regular monthly advances, a line of credit, or a combination of these. There are no payments by the homeowner or any obligation to make repayments as long as he or she lives in the home. Note that the homeowner still retains all homeowner responsibilities, such as real estate and property taxes and maintenance.

Using the equity of a home enables someone to continue to live in his or her primary residence while using the value of the asset. Furthermore, the monies received from this arrangement are generally not subject to federal income tax.

On the other hand, using the home in this way reduces the possibility of the person's heirs inheriting the house free and clear. Should they decide to retain it, they would have to repay the loan via a traditional mortgage.

Life Insurance

There are a few different ways to utilize life insurance, including accelerated death benefit riders and viatical settlements.

Accelerated Death Benefits—Many life insurance policies will make cash advances to those who are terminally ill, a benefit that can be added for little cost (some insurance companies will charge the insured nothing to add the benefit but will charge him or her when it is used). A growing number of policies now include chronic illnesses as a legitimate reason to apply for the cash advance, enabling people to use this benefit to pay for LTC.

In this arrangement, the life insurance company pays a specified percentage of the face amount each month, say 2 percent. For example, on a $200,000 policy, the insured would receive $4,000. Because of the Health Insurance Portability and Accountability Act of 1996 (HIPAA), newer policies may specify that the benefit will not exceed the cost of care, mirroring the reimbursement method for paying benefits and allowing the benefits to escape federal income taxation. The arrangement continues until the maximum amount specified by the company is reached. The maximum amount cannot exceed the amount of the death benefit.

Depending on the face amount and the cost of care, the amount payable may not be adequate. Recall that the average cost for nursing home care is over $50,000 per year. Even a $200,000 life insurance policy would not cover the total cost of care. In the example provided, a monthly benefit of $4,000 would use up the policy's death benefit in a little over 4 years. In addition, there is no way to adjust for inflation.

Viatical Settlements—Another way to utilize life insurance policies is through a viatical settlement. Unlike the accelerated death benefit, a viatical settlement involves a third party, typically a viatical settlement company. In general, the terminally ill insured sells his or her policy to the viatical company for a lump-sum payment. The insured receives a percentage of the policy's face amount. The viatical company is assigned the policy and becomes the beneficiary and pays any future premiums. When the insured dies, the viatical company receives the proceeds.

Individual viatical companies may have different eligibility rules. For example, some may require the policy to be at least 2 years old or the insured's life expectancy to be 2 years or less. These and other factors are also used to determine how much the cash advance will be. Other factors include the financial stability of the life insurance company that issued the policy, whether or not the policy includes a waiver of premium, the National Association of Insurance Commissioners (NAIC) minimum guidelines and so forth.

The biggest plus is that the Health Insurance Portability and Accountability Act (HIPAA) provided that, as of 1997, viatical settlements can be received tax free for terminally ill individuals with 2 years or less to live or for chronically ill individuals. In addition, unlike the accelerated death benefit, the transaction is a lump-sum payment and the insured incurs no further premiums. If the viatical company or investor fails to pay the premium, this has no bearing on the insured; he or she already has received the money.

Unfortunately, the viatical settlement can only provide a limited amount of money; a person could conceivably outlive his or her money. The purchase of an annuity can mitigate the odds of outliving the monies, but then you have the problems that face annuity purchasers, namely an inadequate monthly payment and no way to protect against inflation. In addition, the use of a life insurance policy in this manner means it is not able to protect the need for which it was purchased. For example, if the policy was purchased for estate tax purposes, this may create the need to dip into other assets to pay for estate taxes for which the life policy proceeds were meant.

Government Programs

Medicare

Medicare is a federal health insurance program primarily for people aged 65 and older. The Social Security Administration provides information about the Medicare program and handles enrollments. The program is administered by the Center for Medicare & Medicaid Services (CMS), a part of the Department of Health and Human Services that administers

Medicare. It was formerly known as the Health Care Financing Administration (HCFA).

Three Parts of Medicare

There are two parts to the original Medicare program, Part A provides hospital insurance and Part B provides medical insurance. The third part, Part C, is simply an indirect way to access the original Medicare coverage of Parts A and B through insurance companies rather than directly through the federal government.

Part A: Hospital Insurance—Part A helps pay the expense of inpatient hospital care and provides limited benefits for skilled-nursing home care, home health care, hospice care, and psychiatric hospital care. There are no monthly premiums.

Part B: Medical Insurance—Part B helps pay for doctors' services, medically necessary outpatient hospital services, X-rays, and other diagnostic services, durable medical equipment, and some other services and supplies. There are monthly premiums involved and therefore any person may opt out by signing and returning a non-election form that states he or she does not want it.

Part C: Medicare+Choice—In 1999, Part C of Medicare (called Medicare+Choice) went into effect. It allows Medicare beneficiaries to elect benefits through one of several alternatives to the traditional Parts A and B as long as providers of these alternatives (typically HMOs) enter into contracts with the CMS. These plans enroll about 15 percent of all Medicare beneficiaries and must provide all of the benefits available under Parts A and B. However, they may also provide more comprehensive coverage. In the case of the LTC benefits discussed in this section, the coverage provided by Part C is usually the same as the coverage provided under the original Medicare Parts A and B.

Medicare Coverage of LTC

When you see charts for "who pays for LTC" (for example, the one in chapter 1) you will notice that Medicare is listed as a substantial payor. There are provisions in Part A that do pay for the cost of care

> **Choices**
>
> "Ms. Prospect, you have worked hard all of your life in order to have choices. Yet, if you don't plan and take care of the LTC problem, you surrender this right to the government. It will make decisions for you about the type of care your receive and where you receive it."

typically associated with LTC, namely skilled-nursing facility care and home health care. For this reason, we will take a closer look at these two benefits so you can explain them to a prospect who may have questions. In addition, since many LTCI policies cover hospice care we will look at the hospice benefits provided by Medicare as well.

Skilled-Nursing Facility Care—Medicare hospital insurance helps pay for inpatient care in a Medicare-certified skilled-nursing facility following a hospital stay if the person's condition requires nursing or rehabilitation services that can only be provided in a skilled-nursing facility.

It is important to point out, however, that many skilled-nursing facilities in the United States are not Medicare certified. In addition, in order to qualify for Medicare coverage in a certified skilled-nursing facility all of the following must be true:

- the person's attending physician must prescribe a stay in a Medicare-certified skilled-nursing facility for a condition (1) that was treated in a hospital within the past 30 days or (2) that started while Medicare-covered services were being received in a skilled-nursing facility for another reason.
- the person must have been in a hospital at least 3 consecutive days (not including the day of discharge) before being transferred to the skilled-nursing facility.

If a person qualifies, he or she pays nothing for the first 20 days, except for any charges for which Medicare coverage does not apply, such as incidentals. For the next 80 days, the person must make a daily coinsurance payment ($105 in 2003) and Medicare pays all remaining allowable charges. No benefits are available from Medicare after 100 days of care in a benefit period. A benefit period begins the first time a Medicare recipient is hospitalized and ends only after the recipient has been out of a hospital or skilled-nursing facility for 60 consecutive days. A subsequent hospitalization begins a new benefit period.

Covered items and services include the following:

- room and board in semiprivate accommodations. (Private rooms are covered only if required for medical reasons.)
- nursing services (except private-duty nurses)

- use of facility supplies and equipment, such as oxygen or wheelchairs
- medications ordinarily furnished by the facility
- diagnostic or therapeutic items or services
- rehabilitative services, such as physical, occupational, or speech therapy
- medical social services
- dietary counseling
- ambulance transportation, when necessary, to the nearest supplier of needed services that are not available in the skilled-nursing facility

Medicare Skilled-Nursing Facility Coverage (for 2003)	
Days	Insured Pays
1-20	$0.00
21-100	$105 per day (total of $8,400)
101 +	Full cost

Medicare does not cover custodial nursing home care services. Unless the person is in need of daily care that can only be administered by a medical professional, Medicare will not cover the care. Assistance with ADLs, such as getting from bed to chair, feeding oneself, going to the bathroom, and bathing, are not covered.

Home Health Care—If the person needs skilled health care at home for the treatment of an illness or injury, Medicare pays for covered home health services furnished by a Medicare-certified home health agency. A home health agency is a public or private agency that specializes in giving skilled-nursing services and other therapeutic services, such as physical therapy, in the home. In addition, Medicare will pay 80 percent of the cost of durable medical equipment such as walkers and wheelchairs.

Medicare pays for home health visits only if

- the care needed includes intermittent skilled-nursing care (not 24-hour care)
- the person is confined to home
- the person is under the care of a physician who determines the patient needs home health care and sets up a health plan to provide the care

- the person's condition is improving
- the home health agency providing the services is Medicare-certified

If all of these conditions are met, either hospital insurance or medical insurance will pay for medically necessary home health services.

Hospice Benefits—Hospice benefits are available under Part A of Medicare for beneficiaries who are certified as being terminally ill persons with a life expectancy of 6 months or less. While a hospice is thought of as a facility for treating the terminally ill, Medicare benefits are available primarily for services provided by a Medicare-certified hospice to patients in their own homes. However, inpatient care can be provided if needed by the beneficiary. In addition to including the types of benefits described for home health care, hospice benefits also include drugs, bereavement counseling, and inpatient respite care when family members need a break from caring for the ill person.

To qualify for hospice benefits, a Medicare recipient must elect such coverage in lieu of other Medicare benefits, except for the services of the attending physician or services and benefits that do not pertain to the terminal condition. There are modest copayments for some services.

The benefit period consists of two 90-day periods followed by an unlimited number of 60-day periods. These periods can be used consecutively or at intervals. However, the beneficiary must be recertified as terminally ill at the beginning of each new benefit period. A beneficiary may cancel the hospice coverage at any time (for example, to pursue chemotherapy treatments) and return to regular Medicare coverage. Any remaining days of the current hospice benefit period are lost forever, but the beneficiary can elect hospice benefits again, if he or she is recertified as terminally ill.

Medicare Supplement Policies (Medigap)

Medigap policies are usually designed specifically to cover deductibles and any coinsurance required by Medicare coverage. For all states but a few (for example, Wisconsin and Massachusetts), Medicare supplement policies are standardized and each plan is denoted by a letter A through J. All such plans offer a basic coverage for:

- co-payment or cost sharing of Part A benefits for the 61st through the 90th day of hospitalization and the 60-day lifetime reserve days. In addition, coverage is extended 365 additional days after Medicare benefits end.

- Part B percentage participation for Medicare-approved charges for physicians' and medical services.
- payment for the first three pints of blood each year.

All of the Medigap plans except A and B will pay for the Part A copayment for days 21-100 of a skilled-nursing facility stay.

In addition, plans D, G, I, and J provide an at-home recovery benefit that pays for an at-home provider to assist with ADLs while a beneficiary qualifies for home health care benefits (a physician orders it). There are some limitations: First, the plans provide only $40 per visit. Second, the cumulative limit for this benefit is $1,600.

Medicaid and Medicaid Planning

The Medicaid Program

Medicaid is a joint federal and state program to provide medical assistance to the poor. If an individual meets certain income and resource tests, the state of residence may consider an individual a qualified Medicaid beneficiary. Medicaid is approximately 57 percent (estimates vary) federally funded, with the states picking up the balance.

Nursing home and home health services are provided through Medicaid, which has paid for about 45 percent of the total cost of care for persons using nursing home or home health care in recent years. Unlike Medicare, Medicaid does pay for custodial care. States have the option of offering other non-facility LTC services, such as personal care services, adult day care, and case management.

State Medicaid programs generally pay the Medicare premiums, co-payments, and deductibles for all Medicare beneficiaries below the poverty line. Eligible individuals generally receive free Medicare benefits.

Some individuals with limited resources and no insurance need extended-care assistance. In order to qualify for Medicaid, these people must either already be poor or impoverish themselves by spending virtually all of their assets. That happens to approximately half of the people who enter nursing homes as private-pay patients. These individuals, though not initially poor, depleted their resources to the poverty level as a result of the high cost of LTC. As reported in HIAA's

Consumer's Guide to Long-Term Care Insurance, those who pay for nursing home care out of their own pockets are often impoverished within 6 months to one year. Then they must turn to Medicaid to pay part or all of their expenses. In some cases the spending down of assets was planned, but in most cases it is due to a lack of planning.

Eligibility

Each state sets its own qualifications for this assistance. It also determines the type, amount, duration and scope of covered services, within federal guidelines. The state sets the rate of payment for services and administers its own program. To qualify, a recipient generally cannot have access to any financial resources, such as bank accounts, stock and bond accounts, or mutual funds. Individuals applying for Medicaid must prove that they do not have the financial means to pay for their care.

Income Rules—As a general rule, all income, earned and unearned, received from any source is counted and must be applied to the cost of care. This includes income from work, Social Security, trusts, retirement plans, and investments. A small amount called the personal needs allowance (usually no more than $30 to $50 per month) is left for the Medicaid recipient to cover personal expenses. Medicaid pays the balance of the costs, up to its limits, that the recipient cannot pay.

The income eligibility rules vary widely from state to state. Approximately 40 states have established a *medical needy* category in their Medicaid program, which will qualify a person for benefits if his or her monthly income is lower than monthly medical and LTC expenses. If this is the case and the applicant becomes eligible, Medicaid simply makes up the difference between the individual's income that must be devoted to LTC and what Medicaid would pay in the absence of this income. There is no specific income limit in medically needy states.

The remaining states, known as *income cap* states, use a special income-level option to extend Medicaid to the "near poor" in LTC settings. In an income cap state, a Medicaid applicant meets the income qualification test only if individual income is less than three times the Supplemental Security Income (SSI) benefit level ($1,656 per month in 2003). If income is above that level, Medicaid eligibility is denied, even if the individual has no assets and cannot afford to pay for LTC. Qualifying for Medicaid is much easier in states with a medically needy program than in those states with an income cap test.

Asset Rules—To determine Medicaid eligibility, some assets are counted and others are not. Assets are basically anything that could be used to pay for nursing home care. Medicaid divides assets into two classes:

- countable assets
- noncountable assets (also called exempt)

Countable assets—Before a person can qualify for Medicaid benefits, he or she must exhaust *countable assets* such as

- cash, checking and savings accounts
- stocks, bonds and CDs
- all general investments
- all qualified plans, like pensions, 401(k) plans, and IRAs, if the person has access to and can liquidate the account
- deferred annuities
- life insurance cash surrender values, if face amount exceeds $1,500
- vacation property and second vehicles
- investment property
- every other item not specifically listed as exempt by Medicaid.

Countable assets are used to determine Medicaid eligibility and must be reduced to $2,000. Asset exceptions vary by state.

Noncountable assets (Exempt)— Medicaid has determined that certain assets are not counted toward Medicaid eligibility. A person may keep these assets, no matter how much they are worth, and still be eligible for benefits.

- a small sum of money (usually $2,000-$3,000)
- a primary residence and household furnishings
- a prepaid funeral and burial plot worth up to $1,500
- term life insurance
- business assets and real property, if the person earns a livelihood from them
- all personal property (such as clothing and jewelry) up to reasonable limits
- one engagement and one wedding ring, regardless of value

- one automobile, limited to $4,500 in value, unless medically equipped (then there is no limit)

Although a person's home is considered noncountable, if he or she leaves it to go into a facility, it would be considered countable and would need to be sold to pay for care, unless:

- the person is expected to return there to live
- the person's spouse continues to live in the home
- a blind, disabled or minor child lives in the home
- a child lived in the home and cared for the person for at least 2 years
- a sibling lived in the home and maintained an ownership interest for at least one year

Depleting Assets—Some people who are not poor become poor by spending nearly all their income and assets on care. This is not a good solution to the problem of paying for LTC for most people. It is an unattractive means of last resort for those who have no other options.

Generally, a person can have no more than $2,000 of assets to qualify for Medicaid. If both spouses are in a nursing facility, they may keep no more than $3,000.

Community Spouse-Spousal Impoverishment—The community spouse (the spouse who remains in the community) is allowed to maintain a reasonable amount of resources to live. The community spouse may retain any income of his or her own. In addition, most states allow the spouse to keep half of the couple's assets that generate income such as dividends or rent.

To protect the community spouse from impoverishment, the community spouse is allowed to have an amount of assets that would not cause the sick spouse to be ineligible for Medicaid. This amount is known as the Community Spouse Resource Allowance (CSRA). When the obligation of the sick spouse to "spend down" is calculated, a monthly payment to the community spouse is allowed, reducing the amount that must be spent down. This monthly payment is referred to as the Community Spouse Income Allowance (CSIA). Although these amounts vary by state, for 2002 the CSIA must be at least $1,452 a month, and not higher than $2,232 a month. This means that if the community spouse's own monthly income is less than the floor amount, he or she can receive enough of the income of the sick spouse receiving care to make up the difference. Or he or she can retain enough of the couple's assets to generate income to make up the difference. The assets that can be retained (CSRA) can be anywhere from $17,856 to $89,280 for 2002. States vary in how this amount is calculated. These concepts (CSRA and CSIA) are similar, although technically different, from the concept of minimum monthly maintenance needs allowance (MMMNA) for the community spouse. The MMMNA has two components: basic needs and housing needs.

EXAMPLE: Shortly after Chuck and Ann's 50th wedding anniversary, Chuck's growing dementia and physical frailties caused him to enter a nursing home. Their household income is based on Social Security payments of $1,500 per month to Chuck and $1,200 per month to Ann. In addition, Chuck has a monthly income of $1,000 from a trust fund. Chuck applies for Medicaid and meets his state's medically needy income test: his total income of $2,500 per month is far less than the average private-pay rate for nursing home care of $5,000 per month.

The community spouse income allowance in Chuck's state is $2,232 per month. However, Ann will receive only $1,032 of this amount from his income because she has $1,200 of her own income. This leaves $1,468 that must be applied to the cost of Chuck's care, less personal and medical expenses.

Asset Transfer—Some people reduce their assets to Medicaid eligibility limits by giving the assets to their family members or others. The purpose is that family members or others can enjoy the assets and perhaps even share them. Medicaid rules require liquidating them or spending the money on care. Medicaid's rules require the state to withhold benefits from those who transfer assets by gifting or transferring them at less than fair market value.

"Look-Back" Rules—The U.S. government has tried to close the loophole of transferring assets to qualify for benefits by creating a period of ineligibility for Medicaid. If assets are transferred for less than their market value during a specified period before receiving benefits for nursing home or home or community-based services, ineligibility results. The "look-back" period is 3 years (36 months) for outright transfers and 5 years (60 months) for transfers into trusts. This period of time is measured from the date of the application for benefits. The period of ineligibility is measured by dividing the value of the transferred assets by the average monthly cost of nursing home care in the person's community (determined by the local Medicaid office). The result equals the number of months of ineligibility, beginning from the date of transfer. Some states are using a 5-year look-back for all transfers. This period of ineligibility for benefits is also known as the disqualification or penalty period.

EXAMPLE: Fred transfers assets worth $100,000 to his children 24 months before entering a nursing home and applying for Medicaid. Since this transfer falls within the "look-back" period of 36 months, benefits will be disqualified. The $100,000 transfer is divided by the average private-pay rate for nursing home care of $5,000 per month, resulting in a 20-month disqualification of Medicaid benefits.

Medicaid Planning

Medicaid planning involves methods used by elder law attorneys to qualify their clients for Medicaid benefits. Such planning can assist those with modest assets, pre-existing medical conditions, or who cannot afford LTCI. Simply put, it is turning countable assets into inaccessible assets, by giving them away or transferring them into a trust.

Additionally, for Medicaid planning there are issues relating to estate recovery, transfers of assets, joint property, guardianship, powers of attorney, and medical directives.

Medicaid Trusts—Attorneys specializing in elder law have often used plans transferring assets to achieve Medicaid eligibility. Legally, the client no longer has those assets. Because of the look-back rules, estate recovery rules, and other legislation enacted over the last decade, it has become more difficult to effectively do this. For those who desire to transfer assets, the transfer must be done 36 or 60 months prior to applying for Medicaid. Additionally, one would have to follow the income and asset eligibility rules stated above.

Trusts are an important elder planning vehicle. Trusts can save income and estate taxes, relieve people of financial planning responsibilities, create an income stream, and carry out an estate plan after the trust grantor's death. There are several Medicaid issues to be considered in preparing trusts with Medicaid in mind; how the trust's income will be treated, whether part or all of the trust corpus is an available asset for Medicaid purposes, whether creating the trust is a transfer and if so, how long the penalty period will be, and whether the trust corpus, at the Medicaid recipient's death, will be subject to estate recovery. We will review some trust basics in chapter 7.

Estate Recovery Rules—When Medicaid planning efforts were successful in the past, a person could have his or her LTC costs paid by the taxpayers, and at death still leave a sizable estate to his or her beneficiaries. In an effort to overcome this unfairness, the estate recovery rules were instituted.

Estate recovery rules allow the government to recover from the estate of the Medicaid recipient an amount equal to the cost of care. After a Medicaid recipient dies, the state will likely freeze all bank accounts, put a lien on the home, and void a change in ownership of a transferred asset. States have a right to collect insurance and annuity proceeds from beneficiaries. Even money that was transferred to a person before the look-back period took effect can be recovered under some circumstances—there is no statute of limitations or grandfather clause in these instances.

For Medicaid estate recovery, the definition of estate is broader than probate estate, so that jointly held property that passes directly to the surviving spouse or joint property held in trust may be recovered. Medicaid cannot recover a decedent Medicaid recipient's home before the death of a surviving spouse, or if a child under 21 and blind or disabled is living in the home. There are protections for other surviving children and siblings in the recovery of the home.

To recover monies from an estate, the state uses the mechanism of a lien. A lien is placed on the property while the Medicaid recipient is still alive to prevent its sale. When the Medicaid recipient dies, the lien is foreclosed, the property sold, and the state recovers an amount up to what was paid in Medicaid benefits to the deceased spouse. Heirs receive their inheritance only after Medicaid's claim is paid.

Criminalizing of Medicaid Planning—It was once a common practice for people to divest themselves of all assets to qualify for Medicaid payments of their LTC expenses. No current law prohibits this practice. Under the Health Insurance Portability and Accountability Act of 1996, anyone who knowingly and willfully disposed of or advised another person to dispose of assets to meet Medicaid eligibility was subject to a fine and imprisonment. This provision, known as the "Granny goes to Jail Bill," was very unpopular and was repealed. This concept was changed by a provision to impose criminal liability on any person who, for a fee, counseled or advised a Medicaid applicant in making transfers in certain circumstances. This became known as the "Send Granny's Lawyer to Jail Bill." The provision is considered by some to be unconstitutional and it is not being enforced. There is no current risk of prosecution for giving your prospects and/or clients advice about Medicaid planning.

Disadvantages of Depending on Medicaid

Medicaid offers an opportunity to these unfortunate persons to receive good quality health care. Those who are considering qualifying for Medicaid by spending down should consider a number of disadvantages:

Loss of Financial Independence—A person who has worked hard all of his or her life and has been independent and self-supporting is forced to become indigent and depend on the government and relatives for financial support. Although transferring assets does not guarantee immediate Medicaid eligibility, it does guarantee that the individual is now without legal control of those assets. Many people who have transferred assets have found themselves in a position of having to ask their children or relatives for money.

Demoralizing Loss of Dignity—Now that the person is impoverished, he or she is without financial worth and must depend on others and the government to provide basic needs. This is also generally known as "welfare."

Loss of Choice Regarding Facilities and Care—Medicaid offers only facility nursing home care. There is limited home care, assisted living, or adult day care services in many states.

Financial limitations are placed on providers because Medicaid pays less than private patients. There are so many people in nursing homes on Medicaid because institutional care is the *only* care setting for which most state Medicaid programs will pay.

Most people hold a high regard for having a choice in important decisions such as this. Choosing Medicaid as a LTC financial alternative can have a number of consequences impacting choice and access to quality care. For example:

- Some nursing homes do not accept Medicaid patients. Superior facilities are in high demand and may be unavailable to lower-paying Medicaid patients.
- Nursing homes that accept Medicaid may only have a limited number of beds for Medicaid patients. For better facilities there may be a long waiting list for Medicaid patients. One may be forced to enter a less-desirable facility, especially if the need for facility care is urgent. This place may be far from home, away from family and friends. Although it is illegal to evict a Medicaid beneficiary from a nursing home that accepts Medicaid, this does not mean that a nursing home is obligated to take them.

Ethical Questions Concerning Medicaid Planning

The use of Medicaid planning to become eligible for the payment of LTC costs creates moral, ethical, and malpractice risks for attorneys and other financial advisors. The Medicaid eligibility requirements and transfer and income rules are fairly complex, vary from state-to-state, and are constantly changing. Even experienced attorneys can become confused by state and federal policies regarding Medicaid.

Furthermore, an advisor needs to ask the question: ethically, is it proper for middle-class people to use health care benefits intended for poor people? The problems from doing this may result in poorer care for nursing home residents, a reduction in benefits available to those who truly need them, a financial strain on nursing homes who receive a reduced Medicaid reimbursement payment, and taxpayers having to pay for nursing home costs for the middle class rather than the needy.

Veterans' Programs

The Department of Veterans Affairs (VA) provides care in its own facilities to veterans in need of skilled and intermediate nursing care. The VA also provides both skilled and intermediate care to veterans through contracts with community nursing homes. Although the VA does provide nursing home care to some veterans, there is no entitlement for this service. Eligibility is based on a prioritized group status and is provided first to veterans with service-connected injuries. Care is provided to veterans on a space-available basis.

For specific information on these programs, see Volume I of the VA guide to LTC and services resource guide or contact your local VA office for more information.

Long-Term Care Insurance

With the exception of Medicaid, none of the other alternatives mentioned is designed to cover the cost of LTC and using one of them to do so is the equivalent of using a screwdriver to hammer a nail into a wall. It can be done. Sometimes it will even work. But if you have a hammer and a screwdriver at your disposal, which would you use? If LTC is a concern for your prospects and/or clients, the product of choice should be LTCI. In the following chapters, we will discuss how to uncover the need for LTC and how to explain the LTCI solution.

Chapter Three Review

Key Terms and Concepts are explained in the Glossary. Answers to the Review Questions and Self-Test Questions are found in the back of the book in the Answers to Questions section.

Key Terms and Concepts

informal caregiver

formal caregiver

respite care

care coordinator

home health care

adult day care

reverse mortgage

viatical settlement

accelerated death benefit

skilled-nursing facility

assisted-living facility

nursing home (care)

continuing care retirement community
    (CCRC)

hospice care

Medicare
  Part A: Hospital Insurance
  Part B: Medical Insurance

medigap policy

Medicaid
  eligibility
  income rules
  asset rules
     countable/noncountable (exempt) assets
     depleting assets
  community spouse

look back rules

estate recovery rules

Review Questions

3-1. Describe each of the following caregivers:

    a. informal caregiver
    b. formal caregiver
    c. respite caregiver
    d. care coordinator

3-2. Describe each of the following care settings:

   a. home health care
   b. adult day care centers
   c. independent housing
   d. assisted-living facility
   e. nursing home
   f. combined facility
   g. hospice care

3-3. Name the four major sources used to pay for LTC expenses.

3-4. Explain how life insurance might be used to pay for LTC expenses.

3-5. Jane, aged 67, has Medicare Parts A and B. She recently fell and broke her hip, causing her to be hospitalized for a week. She now needs physical therapy and skilled-nursing care in a nursing home to recover from her injury. Will Medicare pay for Jane's nursing home care, and if yes, for how long?

3-6. Jack, Jill, and June have Medicare Parts A and B, and they all need LTC services. Jack needs custodial care because he is unable to perform several ADLs due to a chronic physical condition. Jill needs skilled care to rehabilitate her broken leg. June needs supervisory care because of a cognitive impairment. Explain whether Jack, Jill, and June are eligible to receive Medicare benefits to cover their LTC needs.

3-7. Joe, aged 67, is single and receives Social Security of $1,100 per month, a pension of $1,888 per month, and interest payments of $300 per month. If Joe, who is placed in a nursing facility costing more than his monthly income, wishes to qualify for Medicaid benefits, what portion of his income will he be required to spend on care if he lives in

   a. a medically needy state?
   b. an income cap state?

3-8. Joe's assets include his residence in which he has $100,000 worth of equity, household furnishing and personal effects valued at $5,000, a car valued at $3,000, stocks and bonds worth $80,000, and $500 in cash. In order for Joe to qualify for Medicaid, which assets will he

   a. first have to liquidate and spend on care?
   b. be allowed to keep without affecting his eligibility?

Self-Test Questions

Instructions: Read chapter 3 first, then answer the following questions to test your knowledge. There are 10 questions; circle the correct answer, then check your answers with the answer key in the back of the book.

3-1.   Which of the following is a formal caregiver?

    (a)   a home health aide
    (b)   a community volunteer
    (c)   parent
    (d)   friend

3-2.   Continuing care retirement communities (CCRC) are required to

    (a)   allow new residents to enter the CCRC at any stage of the care continuum
    (b)   accept new residents whose primary source of payment is Medicaid
    (c)   provide housing and defined LTC services at each level of care for the life of the resident
    (d)   have Medicare-approved home health aides on staff

3-3.   Medicaid is a government-funded program designed to provide medical assistance for

    (a)   retired government employees
    (b)   low-income people who meet certain asset and income limitation tests
    (c)   elderly people who are not covered by Medicare
    (d)   disabled people who do not have Medigap coverage

3-4.   Informal care is most often provided by

    (a)   medical professionals
    (b)   unlicensed home health care workers
    (c)   social workers
    (d)   family or friends

3-5.   Which of the following best describes custodial care?

    (a)   rehabilitative care provided after surgery
    (b)   assistance with the activities of daily living
    (c)   therapy provided at least four days a week
    (d)   environmental care provided in the home

3-6. An assisted living facility is designed to provide living arrangements for those who

   (a) are severely ADL dependent
   (b) may have some impairment but are independent to a significant degree
   (c) are free from any ADL dependency
   (d) require some acute care

3-7. Which of the following statements regarding hospice care is (are) correct?

   I. The home is the typical setting for this care.
   II. It is provided at the end of the care continuum.

   (a) I only
   (b) II only
   (c) Both I and II
   (d) Neither I nor II

3-8. Which of the following statements regarding the Medicaid look-back period is (are) correct?

   I. It is measured from the date of the application for benefits.
   II. It is 36 months for transfers into trusts and 60 months for outright transfers.

   (a) I only
   (b) II only
   (c) Both I and II
   (d) Neither I nor II

3-9. All of the following eligibility rules must be met in order for home health-care benefits to be covered by Medicare **EXCEPT**:

   (a) A physician prescribes and periodically reviews the need for home health care.
   (b) The patient is homebound and the care provided is intermittent or part-time.
   (c) The care is provided by a skilled nurse who works for a Medicare-certified home health-care agency.
   (d) The patient requires constant custodial care.

3-10. All of the following are considered to be exempt assets when determining an applicant's eligibility for Medicaid **EXCEPT**

    (a)   a wedding ring
    (b)   a prepaid burial plot
    (c)   an individual retirement account
    (d)   reasonable household furnishings

4

Meeting with the Prospect

Overview and Learning Objectives

Chapter 4 discusses the techniques and strategies necessary to conduct an effective initial LTCI interview with prospects. Pre-qualifying and qualification of prospects according to insurers' underwriting criteria as well as the NAIC model legislation will be explored. A great deal of emphasis is focused on effectively communicating with prospects and conducting meaningful fact and feeling finding that support their need and motivation for purchasing LTCI. Finally, there will be a list of useful responses that can be used to answer some of the most commonly encountered objections used by prospects to avoid their buying LTCI. By reading this chapter and answering the questions, you should be able to:

4-1.   Describe the purpose and goals of the initial interview with the prospect.

4-2.   Identify the sections and techniques of an effective fact-finding interview.

4-3.   In general terms identify a strategy to explain the need for LTCI.

4-4.   Qualify the prospect based on general underwriting guidelines.

4-5.   Identify the questions in a LTC fact-finder form.

4-6.   Identify objections to the purchase of LTCI.

Chapter Outline

Preparing for the Interview

What to Expect in the LTCI Sales Process

The demystification of the long-term care insurance (LTCI) sales process requires that those myths perceived as obstacles to making sales be compared with the realities of the current environment. An understanding of the potential pitfalls of marketing and selling LTCI will better prepare you for handling the prospect's misconceptions about the sales process. Such an undertaking will no doubt make a favorable impression on the prospect and improve your chances of making a sale.

Myths Versus Realities

Perhaps the biggest misconception about selling LTCI is that the sales process takes far too much time to complete. The reality of the marketplace today is that the sale of LTCI can be accomplished in a much shorter time frame if the prospect has been identified as a result of a pre-qualification process. A well-designed pre-qualification process considerably shortens the amount of time spent trying to make a sale. Concentrating on selling to those prospects who have been pre-qualified (that is, meet certain income and health standards) makes for a much more efficient sales process because it decreases the number of interviews you complete with prospects who ultimately will not be able to pass the underwriter's scrutiny. In addition, the prospects for LTCI are typically older, have higher incomes, and are better educated. These characteristics translate into better informed insurance buyers who have a more realistic idea of what they need, want, and can afford. Our challenge as advisors is to identify and qualify those prospects who are ready to buy.

Another myth about LTCI prospects is that they are going to do extensive comparisons of many companies' products. While it is true that the typical shopper's guide advises prospects to obtain several different premium quotes, most people do not have the time or desire to do such a comparison. LTCI products are constantly evolving and therefore are difficult to compare, let alone evaluate. Many prospects find that the more they attempt to evaluate various product features, the more complex and overwhelming it becomes. This is where you come into the picture. You can help prospects wade through the confusing terminology and technical language associated with LTCI. By doing proper fact-finding and feeling-finding with prospects, you can formulate several affordable policy options for them to choose from in order to best address their needs.

Today's Policies—The overall quality of LTCI policies is better today than it has ever been. The evolution of LTCI products has been dramatic with respect to the magnitude of the changes and the speed with which these changes have occurred. Newer policies being marketed today cover more types of care in various settings and offer the insured greater flexibility in using the policy to pay for that care. These changes have greatly improved the quality of LTCI being sold today, as well as the credibility of the companies that market the coverage.

Considerable change has also taken place at the federal level with the passage of the Health Insurance Portability and Accountability Act in 1996. This law, referred to as HIPAA, provides favorable tax treatment to "tax-qualified" LTC policies that meet certain standardized requirements.

The changes in LTCI policies sold in the last few years have led to a new generation of policies that not only contain more comprehensive benefits than previously, they also provide these benefits at a much lower premium than ever thought possible. In fact, many potential prospects dispel the notion of buying LTCI because they perceive that it costs too much. Some prospects even confuse the dollar figures associated with the cost of LTC with that of LTCI. Furthermore, many do not understand what LTC costs are covered by Medicare, how Medicaid functions with regard to LTC, and what some popularly touted trusts can achieve. Because of these misconceptions, you as an advisor have not only a tremendous opportunity to market products that are increasingly superior, you also have a responsibility to inform and educate the buying public about today's LTCI.

The LTCI Selling Process

Part of your job as a financial advisor is to guide prospects through the selling process by executing the same due diligence that you would expect if you were the buyer. This process involves (but is not limited to):

- Meeting with the prospect personally
- Explaining the need for LTCI
- Dispelling alternative funding sources
- Addressing comparative shopping issues (to be discussed in chapter 6)
- Qualifying the prospect
- Gathering information:
  - Fact-finding
  - Financial information
  - Feeling-finding
- Begin formulating the potential LTCI plan design
- Securing a discovery agreement
- Addressing the prospects concerns and objections

The remainder of this chapter will address each of these topics in the order listed above.

The Initial Interview

The purpose of the initial interview is to build the foundation for a collaborative relationship with the prospect, not to make a sale. In fact, many successful advisors have said that if you collect the information from the prospect during the initial interview, including his or her needs, values, feelings, goals, and objectives, as well as facts and figures, this will result in much less resistance to making a sale and implementing the solution. The systematic process of building a lasting client-advisor relationship begins with this initial meeting and is comprised of the following four steps:

- Establishing rapport and credibility
- Utilizing effective communication techniques
- Identifying the prospect's needs, wants, qualifications, and concerns*
- Reaching an agreement to work together to address the prospect's needs, wants, and concerns*

[*These topics will be addressed later in this chapter.]

Establishing Rapport

Client building begins with establishing rapport. People want to work with professionals who build meaningful relationships with them and listen to what they want to accomplish. If rapport and credibility are developed in the process of exchanging information, then the product options and amounts you recommend will more likely be reflective of their real insurance needs and values. In order for prospects to buy LTCI from you, they must first trust you. Trust is the intangible aspect of selling that must be gradually cultivated and earned. You must prove that you are there to help them, not simply to sell them something. Thus, your objective in the initial interview is to establish rapport by creating an environment that promotes prospect openness by

- Alleviating the prospects' concerns
- Responding to the social style of prospects
- Communicating effectively with prospects
- Mutually agreeing to an agenda for the interview

Alleviating the Prospects' Concerns—Various barriers that can create tension between you and your prospects during an initial meeting must be removed if rapport is to be established. These barriers can be divided into four major categories:

Distrust of Salespeople—Many people have a negative image of salespeople and avoid meeting with them for fear of being talked into buying something they do not want or need.

Fear of Making a Decision—Decisions involve risk, and many people avoid risk especially when money is involved. Also, fear of making the wrong decision or potential buyer's remorse can cause avoidance of stressful decision-making situations.

Need for Status Quo—Many people are complacent and resistant to change because they prefer familiarity.

Time Constraints—At today's increasingly hectic pace of life, busy prospects are reluctant to commit their time.

Being aware of prospect stress can help you identify opportunities to alleviate it and to establish rapport. Here are some tips.

- *Do not impose.* Schedule your initial meeting at times that are convenient for the prospects.
- *Watch your verbal pace.* Talk in an unhurried, businesslike manner. Never interrupt when prospects speak. Listen carefully to what they say. As we will discuss shortly, listening is your best tool.
- *Remember nonverbal behavior.* You might be surprised to learn that as little as 7 percent of a first impression is based on what is actually said. The remaining 93 percent is based on nonverbal and vocal behaviors, such as physical appearance, body language, voice quality, and tone.
- *Encourage prospects to talk.* Having prospects talk is not only a great tool for getting feedback, but it is also a common way for them to relieve stress. Encourage prospects to do most of the talking.
- *Control your anxiety.* Several studies have shown that a person who is already anxious becomes even more so when talking with someone who displays nervousness or anxiety.

Responding to the Social Style of Prospects—Establishing rapport is your responsibility. This means you should be able to detect what each prospect wants in a sales relationship, and to use your versatility to shape the discussion and your responses to his or her respective needs.

Psychologist Dr. David Merrill described the characteristics of four different social styles:

- Driver
- Expressive
- Amiable
- Analytical

When you adapt to a prospect's social style, you make him or her feel at home and less threatened. Listening closely and observing carefully during the first few minutes of the initial interview gives you an idea of how to treat the prospect. The chart on page 4-9 "Responding to Prospects' Social Styles" summarizes the characteristics of each social style and indicates how you can best establish rapport with a person who has that style. Listen carefully and observe your prospect to determine which set of characteristics most closely describes him or her and then establish rapport by responding in an appropriate manner throughout the interview.

EXAMPLE 1: If your prospect, Jane Weston, enthusiastically talks at length about the plans she has for the new business she is starting, she would be classified as an Expressive. To establish rapport, respond to her by taking time to listen and ask about her plans.

EXAMPLE 2: If your prospect, Ben Hammer, tells you where to sit when you enter his office and looks at his watch when you ask about the photograph of the sailboat on his wall, he would be classified as a Driver. To establish rapport, respond to him by immediately getting down to business and explaining the purpose, process, and benefits of the appointment.

What would happen if you responded to Jane Weston by going directly into an outline of the agenda for your meeting? What would happen if you tried to share your sailing exploits with Ben Hammer?

Here are two more examples to review.

EXAMPLE 3: If your prospect, Bob Hinds, greets you with a worried smile, apologizes for being 15 minutes late, and says that he could not get away from his last meeting where they were planning a retirement party for his administrative assistant—a wonderful woman who has been with him since he started the company—he would be classified as an Amiable. To establish rapport, respond to him by taking time to ask about his retiring administrative assistant.

EXAMPLE 4: If your prospect, Dr. Patricia Gibbons, stands to greet you from behind her desk when you are ushered into her office, waits for you to take a seat, and immediately asks you what the maximum gift is that she can give tax free to each of her grandchildren she would be classified as an Analytical. To establish rapport, respond to her by taking the time to answer her question with a detailed and documented reply.

What would happen if you responded to Bob Hinds by launching into a discussion of gift taxes? How would Bob Hinds respond if you took a few moments to tell him about seeing old friends at your high school reunion last weekend? What would happen if you tried to tell Dr. Gibbons about your high school reunion?

If you are able to identify and respond appropriately to a person's social style in a sales situation, you will be able to establish rapport more quickly and will facilitate the relationship-building process.

Responding to Prospects' Social Styles		
Social Style	**The Prospect's Style Characteristics**	**Your Best Response**
Driver	Forceful, direct	Focus on objectives
	Will not waste time on small talk	Move right along
	Wants to be in control	To get decisions, provide options
Expressive	Outgoing, enthusiastic	Focus on dreams
	Enjoys telling about personal projects and dreams	Take time to listen
	Wants to be recognized	To get decisions, provide incentives
Amiable	Easy-going, dependent	Focus on relationships
	Enjoys telling about personal relationships	Be personal
	Wants to be accepted	To get decisions, provide personal assurances
Analytical	Logical, quiet	Focus on principles and thinking
	Is uncomfortable with small talk	To get decisions, provide evidence
	Wants to be accurate	Be accurate

Communicating Effectively with Prospects

To help solve prospects' problems, financial advisors must be effective communicators. Some advisors think effective communication only means they have to be able to explain insurance products to prospects. In fact, being able to explain insurance products to prospects is important to advisors, but one of the most important aspects of being an effective communicator is learning to also be an effective listener. Failing to hear what your prospect is really saying can cost you dearly. Developing good listening skills will result in increased sales and the sense of a job well done.

Moreover, your ability to be a good listener is vitally important in personal communications. Your prospects are more likely to accept your recommendations if you demonstrate an interest in them as individuals, listen to their hopes and dreams, and help them prioritize their goals. In other words, the most important part of communication is listening.

Active Listening—Your goal as an advisor should be to become an active, understanding listener—one who attempts to understand the prospect from the prospect's perspective. If you can state in your own words what the prospect has said and meant to communicate, and the prospect accepts your statement as an accurate reflection of what he or she said and felt, active listening has occurred. If you develop this skill, you will be in the best position to solve the prospect's problems with a plan or sale.

Active listening is hard work and requires intense focus and concentration. Years of not listening have made most of us poor listeners. We as salespeople often spend too much time talking and not enough time listening. We cannot listen to what the prospect is saying if we are too busy talking. It is easy to become distracted or to prejudge the prospect's meaning before the prospect is finished speaking. It is also too easy to form a response before hearing the prospect's question or comment. Thus, the prospect's message can be easily missed.

Effective listening is a genuine skill worth developing. To become an active listener, you must believe in the importance of each prospect's needs. Then you must commit to hearing and understanding what each prospect is saying. If you put aside your prejudices, opinions, and preconceived notions about a subject and the prospect, you can be objective and open-minded.

It should be obvious to you that a successful fact-finding session requires you to be an effective listener to learn essential information

> The most important part of communication is listening.

about your prospect in order to make the best recommendations. Yet, how often do you find yourself asking questions but not listening to the prospect's responses? You may have decided what is best for the prospect based on your own thinking. By critically listening to the prospect's answers to your questions, you will not be as likely to mistake your preconceived ideas for the prospect's wants or needs.

Learning the difference between sympathy and empathy is also important for an advisor. Despite the general use of the word "empathy," most people still do not fully recognize the difference between sympathy and empathy and the application of the words in the world of selling. Sympathy means you feel like another person feels; you share the same feelings. By contrast, empathy means you understand how the other person feels, though you do not feel the same way. While you cannot sympathize with all of your prospects, you can learn to be empathetic.

> **Empathy means you understand how another person feels, though you do not feel the same way.**

Body language is another aspect of active listening. Gestures that are made in silence can often give you, the listener, more of an indication of what the prospect is communicating than words can. A person's facial expressions, posture, and body stance can be very informative to the observer. By watching people's eyes and hands, you can often determine what signals they are conveying.

Questioning—In any fact-finding session, you will ask questions and your prospects will answer them. If you can help your prospects feel comfortable talking about themselves, you will learn what is important to them. The more you know about your prospects' feelings, the better job you can do. Asking questions and being an active listener allows you to control the direction of the fact-finding conversation without being too obvious about it. Prospects then feel they are a part of the process.

> **Prospects will not be interested in buying LTCI from you until they trust that you really care about helping them achieve financial independence over the long term.**

In fact-finding interviews, you will want your prospects to communicate facts and figures. However, in order to be effective, you must know your prospects' feelings as well. Feelings are often difficult to uncover in a question-and-answer format where you are cast into the role of an interviewer. While your goal should be to listen more than talk, there are times when only a well-phrased question will elicit the information you are seeking.

Finally, it is important to keep in mind that the primary reason for gathering data from prospects is to make suitable recommendations. Each time you meet with your prospects, it is important that your communication be directed at uncovering as many facts and feelings as possible so that you can assure your prospects of the suitability of the products you recommend.

Summary

The intangible by-product of establishing rapport, tuning into the prospect's social style, and actively listening during the interview process is the emergence of your credibility. Your credibility combined with your compassion and understanding eventually lead to trust. Once a prospect trusts you, he or she will be willing to do business with you. Winning a prospect's trust does not come easily. You have to work hard to achieve it, so be patient.

Interviewing Your Prospect

Your job is an ongoing and continuous process. You will spend considerable time with your prospects to determine their financial goals and objectives—their needs. Once this is done you will use the information gathered—the facts and feelings that you have discussed—to make recommendations. Each meeting with prospects should be productive and accomplish specific objectives.

At the beginning of the initial interview with the prospect, you set the tone for the entire meeting by establishing expectations for both you and the prospect. This requires that three specific topics be addressed in the introductory phase of the interview: establishing an agenda, identifying the decision-makers, and setting the stage for obtaining referred leads.

> **Setting proper expectations for the meeting helps build rapport and gets the initial interview off to a positive start.**

Establishing an Agenda

It is a good idea to follow a set agenda for each fact-gathering session. This lets the prospects know what is expected of them and reduces anxiety and discomfort concerning what will happen during the meeting. It is wise to involve your prospects in setting the agenda.

Setting proper expectations for the meeting helps establish rapport and gets the initial interview off to a positive start. You can reduce any initial tension that exists in an interview with a prospect whom you have never met before by outlining the steps involved in your approach to LTC planning. The highlights to be covered involve explaining the steps of the planning process, which are to

1. Assist the prospect in forming goals and objectives.
2. Help the prospect identify existing resources for meeting goals and objectives.

3. Analyze the gap between goals and objectives and existing resources.
4. Devise a plan for bridging the resource gap.
5. Implement the plan.
6. Monitor the plan.

You should have an agenda for every sales meeting. In presenting the agenda you should

- Communicate what you intend to accomplish during the meeting.
- Explain how you will work with the prospect.
- State the benefit for the prospect.
- Check for acceptance.

In the initial LTC planning session, you might propose the agenda by saying something like this to the prospect:

Purpose	*What You Say*
Communicate what you intend to accomplish during the meeting.	During this meeting, we will discuss some life planning issues that may be of concern to you.
Explain how you will work with the prospect.	First, I'll tell you a little about who I am and the company I represent.
	Then we'll talk about your concerns, goals, and desires regarding long-term care planning.
	Next, we will look at how your financial status currently stands in regard to your net worth, cash flow, and budget.
	Finally, I'll identify any problems or gaps in your current long-term care plan.

State the benefit   That way you can determine whether it will be
for the prospect.   of value for us to move ahead and develop an
                       LTC planning strategy tailored for you.

Check for   How does that sound?
acceptance.

By proposing the agenda in this way, stating the benefit to the prospect, and checking for acceptance, you are sharing control of the interview with your prospect, which helps you to establish rapport.

Also, as an afterthought, it may be advisable to reassure the prospect of your continuing commitment to the process by adding the following:

"If in the course of our work together we should discover that you have a need for LTCI, I'll assist you in devising a customized plan that addresses your individual concerns. I'll then help you to implement that plan and promise to monitor and service that plan in the future."

After you present your agenda, ask for any other concerns that your prospect wishes to discuss. Write them down and be sure to cover these concerns in your discussion. Do so even if the concerns fall under categories you had on your agenda. Your prospect's input is an important first step in the open exchange of data and feelings.

Identifying Decision-makers in the Process (Children, Attorneys, and Other Advisors)

The next step you will want to take in the interview is to attempt to identify the decision-makers in addition to the prospect who may be involved in the potential purchase of LTCI. This could include professional advisors such as the prospect's attorney, or other immediate family members such as siblings or adult children. Ask the prospect if there are any advisors that he or she will consult before making the buying decision. If so, it is best to try to elicit their personal involvement as soon as possible. From a sales standpoint, you cannot deal effectively with potential objections or concerns that may arise unless you are able to speak directly with that person. There is far too much technical language and professional jargon used in the LTCI sales process that the prospect might be unable to explain or interpret for these other decision-makers. There is also too much at stake for you to not ask the prospect to at least arrange for open lines of communication with his or her other professional or personal advisors. Ideally, however, have the prospect invite them to participate in the interview.

Paving the Way for Referrals

As mentioned in chapter two, many financial advisors use the early part of their initial interview with new prospects as an opportunity for mentally preparing them for the fact that they will be asking for referred leads. If the prospects are pleased with the service you have performed for them, whether or not they actually do business with you, you will have earned the right to ask them for referrals at some point during the selling process since you performed a valuable service by educating them about LTC needs. You could say the following:

> "One of the ways that I am compensated for the work I do is by receiving personal introductions from people like yourself to others you know. Now, I wouldn't expect you to have any idea whether these people are in the market for LTCI, or for that matter any insurance or investment-related products. However, if you find yourself pleased with my professionalism, I would appreciate it if you could refer me to several people you know so that I may have the opportunity to help them also. Does this seem reasonable to you?"

Explaining the Need for LTCI

The transition from the initial exchange of amenities and acknowledgment of the agenda to the qualification portion of the interview is facilitated by a relatively short section during which you describe your company, yourself, your services, and the general problems facing individuals today in financing the increasing costs of LTC.

This part of the initial interview deals with explaining, in general terms, the need for LTCI. Various methods are used to accomplish this objective. This is when you discuss the global financial problem of potentially needing LTC, and then briefly describe how LTCI is the most desirable remedy for solving this looming financial problem. You should then categorically disqualify the adequacy of various financing alternatives and government programs as workable solutions. You should also give each prospect *A Shopper's Guide to Long-Term Care Insurance* if you have not already done so.

Clarifying Motives and Goals

Your first meeting with a prospect presents both an opportunity and a challenge. The opportunity is to address the prospect's interest in LTC planning. The challenge is to develop a climate of cooperation so you can learn enough about the prospect's financial planning goals and buying motives in order to individualize a plan of action that best addresses his or her circumstances.

In setting the stage for explaining the need for LTC planning, you must take time to establish what prospects know and what they think they know about LTC. For example, one advisor simply asks: "What does LTC mean to you?" (By the way, the answer to this question almost invariably contains something along the lines of this response: "It's care for when you go into a nursing home.") Asking this or a similar question is a great way to begin a discussion of LTC for the purpose of establishing certain definitions used in describing such items as types of care, the cost of care, and what various government programs do and do not cover. It also requires uncovering the prospects' presumptions about the myths and misunderstandings of what LTCI is and how it works. You have to ask questions to establish a baseline of commonality in the language of LTC. You have to elicit feedback from prospects regarding their level of knowledge about LTCI and seek acknowledgment of their understanding of insurance terminology. Only when you are speaking the same language with prospects can you begin to understand their objectives in purchasing LTCI.

Methods

In order for you to enhance your credibility with your prospects, it is important that you explain the need for them to buy LTCI. This often begins with a strictly verbal discussion that can lead to the use of other tools and techniques (which of course must be approved by your company's compliance department) that you as an advisor can draw upon to help you. These various tools and techniques should be contained in a LTCI sales presentation binder that you develop.

Using Visuals—Getting your prospects to look at a visual is a useful technique. People tend to actively listen to what is being said when they are involved in the communication, and it is your responsibility to make sure that your prospects are kept involved and are actively listening throughout the data-gathering process. Asking questions and asking for their opinions while they look at visuals keeps them involved in the process. The physical act of putting visuals in front of them indicates where you are going with the discussion and helps to focus their attention.

Keep in mind that any materials presented to prospects must have the prior approval of your company. Because of this requirement, it is a good idea to have one or two prepared presentations that you use consistently with all your prospects. This consistency helps to facilitate your compliance with the applicable regulations.

Third-party Substantiation—In addition to simple pictures, your company probably has pre-approved LTCI marketing brochures, product fact sheets, and even third-party testimonials available for your use. You should become familiar with these and selectively decide which ones to include in the LTCI sales presentation binder that you develop.

Statistical Evidence—Many financial advisors will want to use charts, graphs, and statistics about the cost and trends of LTC. Other resources are reprinted magazine articles and slides or powerpoint presentations. You need to develop and update your own inventory of useful visual materials that are designed to appeal to the prospect's emotions regarding his or her need for LTCI.

Real-life Stories—Many advisors also find it useful to develop a repertoire of real-life stories and case histories that they can draw upon to verbally illustrate the need for LTCI. While this technique may not be appropriate for every advisor since some are better storytellers than others, it is but one more resource in the advisor's inventory of tools and techniques for making a

---

An excerpt from the real-life story of one advisor:

"I am on a mission because I can't believe what this has done to the lives of my wife and me. I feel like I have a part-time job because of how much time I spend dealing with the frustrating financial and administrative problems of having my father-in-law in a nursing home…and money is the solution like it is in life insurance. If you have money pouring in, it makes life much simpler. Five or six thousand dollars per month coming in to help provide for LTC is going to relieve a lot of stress in the lives of all parties concerned."

sale. The anecdotal allusion to an actual claim situation where the need for LTC arose suddenly can help to shift a prospect's complacency about the need for LTCI into one of heightened personal awareness.

A Shoppers Guide to Long-Term Care Insurance—To assist consumers in determining whether LTCI is appropriate for them, the National Association of Insurance Commissioners (NAIC) has developed *A Shopper's Guide to Long-Term Care Insurance.* This publication is intended to help consumers understand LTC and the various insurance options that are available to help pay for LTC services. By state law, insurance companies through their advisors must give this guide to prospects to help them understand LTCI and to decide which, if any, LTCI policy to buy.

The decision to buy LTCI is very important, but one that is not right for everyone. However, according to the NAIC shopper's guide, a prospect should consider buying LTCI if he or she

- has significant assets and/or income to protect
- wants to control his or her LTC choices
- wants to preserve his or her sense of dignity
- wants to stay independent of the support of others

Clearly, the need for LTCI goes beyond strictly financial considerations. Those seeking to maintain control of their LTC choices, to preserve their sense of dignity, and to remain independent of family caregivers or government bureaucracies are potential candidates for LTCI.

The Problems: Cost and Probability of Needing Care

The greatest single predictor of the need for LTC is advancing age and the gradual deterioration in physical and mental abilities that accompany it. The increased longevity that Americans enjoy has concurrently increased the probability of needing assistance with the activities of daily living (ADLs). People in this country who live to age 65 can expect to live an average of 18 more years. With increased longevity comes the increased probability of needing assistance in the ADLs. LTC costs can be very expensive. A level of sustained cost would be a real financial hardship for many families. The financial strain borne by the more than 20 million families who provide some type of informal, unpaid care for an older relative or friend who either lives with or is visited by the caregiver is increasing. How will the cost of LTC services be paid?

Individuals and their families pay one-third of all nursing home costs from their own funds. Many people use their life's savings and investments. Some people sell assets such as their homes to pay for their LTC needs. The financial devastation of paying for LTC with personal assets, the physical and emotional stress of providing informal care to relatives, and the personal indignity of depending on Medicaid can be circumvented by owning LTCI.

Financing Alternatives to LTC

How to Pay for LTC—A helpful technique for selling LTCI coverage is to ask the question: Should the need arise, how will you pay for LTC? Many prospects will exhibit a total lack of knowledge concerning this topic. There are many misunderstandings and myths regarding LTC services and the resources available for financing them. As financial advisors, you will need to be prepared to educate your prospects on the shortcomings of the various personal financing alternatives to LTCI and the applicable government programs. As if to underscore the need for LTCI, this education process will often require you to completely dispel the erroneous beliefs about the usefulness of these alternatives as LTC funding vehicles.

Personal Financing Alternatives—A detailed discussion about the various financing alternatives to LTCI was presented in chapter three. Using personal savings and assets and relying on family members, reverse mortgages, and/or viatical settlements are all unlikely or unacceptable solutions to the LTC problem. Should questions about these financing alternatives arise in the initial interview with a prospect, you should be prepared to address them by explaining just how undesirable they are as solutions to the problem of LTC.

The Medicare Program and/or Medicare Supplement—One of the biggest misconceptions that many LTCI prospects have is assuming that government programs such as Medicare and/or Medicare Supplement insurance will cover their LTC costs should the need arise. Believing this assumption can be a costly and disappointing mistake. You should be knowledgeable about the shortcomings of these government programs and be prepared to disqualify them as viable methods of paying for most LTC costs. A brief overview of these programs and their relationship to LTC will demonstrate their inadequacies when it comes to providing LTC benefits. This is more fully explained later in this chapter in the section titled, "The Circle of Health Protection."

The Medicaid Program—Medicaid, which is another government program, does provide extended-care assistance to seniors who have extremely limited resources and no insurance. However, these benefits come at a terrible price. In order to qualify for Medicaid, an individual must be impoverished. Assets accumulated over a lifetime must be "spent down." When only minimal assets remain, the Medicaid program will step in to cover the costs of care. Most people find the prospect of becoming destitute—spending down all of their assets to qualify for Medicaid—distasteful at the very least. But, unfortunately for some, it may be the only solution.

The price paid for Medicaid coverage is more than financial. Clearly, there is also a psychological price to pay for impoverishment. Moreover, many commentators point out that a quality of care issue is often involved. Health care providers participating in Medicaid must accept Medicaid payments made to them as payment in full. Medicaid reimbursement rates are usually lower than the rates paid by LTC insurers or by private patients, and therefore this often translates into a lower quality of care.

The Solution: LTCI

This leaves LTCI as the most viable option for most prospects. Premiums can be budgeted and assets can be legitimately protected from the ravages of LTC costs. Living standards can be maintained for healthy family members while those needing it can receive the quality care they desire.

The only sensible answer to financing the costs of LTC is to transfer the risk to an insurance company. This solution provides many advantages:

- LTCI enables your clients to preserve their independence.
- LTCI provides for financial security and independence of the healthy spouse.

- Benefits are available when needed. Care is not delayed because it might cause financial hardship.
- Freedom in choosing LTC options is provided.
- Wealth and assets that have accumulated are preserved for a spouse, children, charity, or other purposes.

Qualifying the Prospect

After you have generally discussed the need for LTCI and the probability of needing some type of care, you should make sure that your prospect, and his or her spouse if applicable, potentially qualify for coverage before you proceed to personal information gathering. The only truly acceptable reason for a person failing to insure himself or herself against the risk of LTC is that he or she does not qualify medically or financially for the coverage. If this is determined to be the situation, the LTCI selling process is finished.

In the ideal scenario, qualified prospects are identified before private face-to-face meetings are established. As was mentioned in chapter 2, many successful advisors prequalify prospects on the telephone once they have agreed to an appointment. However, in many instances, a face-to-face meeting occurs before you know whether or not you are dealing with a qualified prospect. These meetings take time. The more time you spend with qualified prospects the greater the number of sales you will close. Therefore, consider the following four-step approach to increase the amount of time you spend with current qualified prospects:

- Begin qualifying your prospect with LTCINS links.
- Demonstrate the "Circle of Health Protection."
- Conduct a "Financial and Personal Resources Review" fact finder (if necessary).
- Attempt a trial close before conducting a full analysis.

LTCINS Links
LTCINS (which stands for LTC insurance) is an acronym for key information that you obtain from asking a series of questions. When the information is linked together, you can make a relatively quick judgment about whether it is possible to underwrite a prospect. Using LTCINS, you have a sense of whether the prospect is insurable. You will also have a barometer of the prospect's finances and if there are sufficient funds to pay for LTCI.

Qualified prospects for LTCI possess four basic characteristics. They are people who

- need and value your products and services
- can afford to pay for LTCI
- are insurable for LTCI
- can be approached by you on a favorable basis

If these four conditions are satisfied, then the next step is to secure a preliminary agreement to proceed to the full fact-finder. If these four conditions are not satisfied, you must have a contingency strategy to either pivot to another product, outline a plan for future contact with the prospect when he or she is better qualified, or gracefully exit the interview and move on. Some pivoting ideas are discussed later in this chapter.

L=Life Span—The first questions you ask the prospect are: "When were you born?" and "Can you provide me with an exact date?"

This information will let you know immediately whether or not your prospect is young enough to be underwritten by your company. If the prospect is too old, you will have to pivot to a discussion of other products and referrals. Knowing the exact date of birth also enables you to provide the prospect with a quote of the approximate premium costs. This information also provides you with the data necessary to motivate a prospect to save money by purchasing now rather than waiting past a birthday/premium increase date.

T=Time in Hospital—The next line of questions begins with: "Have you ever spent time in the hospital?" If the answer is yes, then: "Was it during the past 5 years (or other appropriate threshold date set by your carrier)? What was the reason? How long did it take you to recover?"

You should be prepared to pre-qualify prospects for the product to see if they would be medically eligible for coverage. A few simple medical questions can quickly determine whether there may be a medical underwriting problem.

Most applications contain a series of between 4 and 10 questions that are designed to pre-qualify prospects for coverage. The length of the list of questions will be much longer for insurers that have stringent underwriting standards. If a prospect answers "yes" to any of these questions, then he or she will be disqualified, and you are advised not to submit the application.

You should become aware of conditions that are "red flags" to an insurer. This will save time and avoid disappointment and hurt feelings if potential declination is spotted early in the process. If you determine that the prospect is insurable, continue with your LTCI presentation. If the prospect fails to qualify for LTCI for either medical or financial reasons, you should have a plan for pivoting to other products that will also enhance the prospect's financial plan. In addition, whether the prospect qualifies or not, you should ask him or her for the names of other people they know who might also be prospects for LTCI.

C=Children—The next line of questioning for the prospect deals with the family: "Do you have children?" If the answer is yes, then: "What are their ages? Do they live nearby? Do you speak to them often?"

Many seniors refuse to make decisions without input from their adult children. Getting a sense for the ages of these children provides you with information about other potential prospects. LTCI is often bought by two generations of family members, particularly if a relative has suffered a lengthy illness or has had to pay for expensive nursing home care.

If adult children are part of the decision–making process and you believe the prospect will pre-qualify, offer to postpone the remainder of the interview until they can be present. Otherwise, you risk having the senior prospect make a presentation on your behalf to his or her children. This can result in the children ignoring what is being proposed or seeking the advice of another advisor. Either way, the result may be a lost sale.

Viewing the potential purchase of LTCI from the perspective of adult children enables you to better understand why they may have several valid reasons for assisting their parents in purchasing LTCI. First of all, you can assume that children want their parents to have the highest possible quality of care. The parents may require their children's assistance in evaluating the various and sometimes confusing policy options. The children may want to assist their parents in paying for the coverage, so it makes sense for them to understand what they may be partially financing. Moreover, adult children have a vested interest in seeing that their parents have LTC coverage because it can protect against the

---

According to one LTCI advisor:

"I won't discuss a LTCI policy with senior prospects unless their adult children are in the room every time I talk to them... When I give a presentation to the whole family, I usually find that the children advocate the purchase of this product for their parents."

---

depletion of assets they may eventually inherit, or it can protect them from having to use their own assets to pay for LTC services their parents may ultimately need. Also as a part of the policy, the children may be the third party who is to be contacted if the LTCI coverage is about to lapse or terminate because someone forgot to pay the premium.

I=Insurance Proposals—This next line of questioning for the prospect deals with potential competition: "Are you weighing other LTCI proposals?" If the answer is yes, then: "Are you already working with another advisor?" If the answer is yes, then: "Who is the advisor and what company does the advisor represent?"

The prospect's answers to these questions will tell you whether you are in competition for making the sale. You should expect that the subject of competition will come up during the interview process, and you should not shy away from dealing with it. On the contrary, you should be prepared to address the subject of competition from a multidimensional perspective. Some of the comparative concerns that a prospect may have are categorically discussed later in chapter 6.

Some move on to other prospects. Some insist on being the last to present a full-scale proposal. Those with access to several insurance carriers typically offer to compare products across company lines. Captive advisors sometimes promote other product lines and point to the advantages of dealing with one insurance carrier. Here there is no one right or wrong answer. Use the approach that works best for you.

N=Nursing Home Experience—This line of questioning for the prospect deals with his or her exposure to nursing homes: "Has anyone in your family or any close friends ever been confined to a nursing home?" If the prospect answers yes, then: "How do you regard these experiences?"

The purpose of these questions is twofold. It helps you gather facts about the prospect's experiences with and fears about nursing homes. Furthermore, you may learn more about health issues that can potentially impede the underwriting process. For example, you may learn whether there is a family history of Alzheimer's, heart disease, and/or cancer. Also, this line of questioning just might motivate the prospect to take

---

Competition:

When asked if competition presents a problem to marketing LTCI, one advisor said: "My first reaction is that there is no competition. As a result of the conversations and the relationship I build with the prospect's family and my involvement in explaining the coordination of LTC services with their finances, I preempt the competition.

I sell my ability to be the family's LTC coach for the rest of their lives! I also stress the financial strength and integrity of my company."

---

action. Prospects are reminded of what are frequently unpleasant memories. The desire to avoid institutionalization and possibly even impoverishment is reinforced.

S=Savings Level—The final line of questioning for the prospect deals with his or her ability to pay for the coverage: "Do you have savings? Do the savings amount to over a million dollars? Are they in the range of $500,000? Do they amount to $100,000, $50,000, or less? Are you able to add to savings? Have you recently been forced to dip into savings? If you have, why was it necessary?"

The answers to these questions will help to tell you whether LTCI is appropriate for the prospect and whether he or she is able to afford premium payments. In other words, the answers provide enough information to make an initial judgment about whether the prospect should proceed with the purchase of LTCI, or should rely on planning alternatives other than insurance to meet LTC costs. To help determine whether the prospect is financially qualified to purchase LTCI, the NAIC has established the minimal financial suitability guidelines, which state that 1) premiums should not exceed 7 percent of income, and 2) if an applicant wishes to purchase the coverage for asset protection, he or she should have a least $30,000 in assets. In fact, your company may have its own higher specific income and saving level guidelines for determining whether LTCI is an appropriate and suitable product for your prospect.

The purchase of LTCI may not be financially suitable for wealthy prospects. Some would argue that wealthy people can afford to pay for LTC without a great deal of asset erosion or financial hardship. Alternatively, others would argue that wealthy people have automobile and homeowners insurance, so why should they not recognize LTC as an equally legitimate risk that needs to be managed?

Insurers will not issue a policy to someone who violates their financial suitability guidelines or the guidelines established by the NAIC without obtaining from the prospect acknowledging documentation to the contrary. These guidelines are designed to protect the public at large.

However, in addition to the objective suitability guidelines for buying LTCI, there are also subjective reasons for buying it that cannot be overlooked. Some of the main reasons that prospects cite for buying LTCI are to preserve their independence, to maintain control over their assets, and to keep their sense of dignity regarding their care. It is important to bear in mind that the sale of LTCI is not just about dollars and cents. Many people believe they will never be disabled and reject the idea that they will ever need care. Therefore, the decision to purchase LTCI is often a very emotional one. Consequently, this is something that you need to be sensitive to as you ask feeling-finding questions in the interview. These types of questions will be discussed later in this chapter.

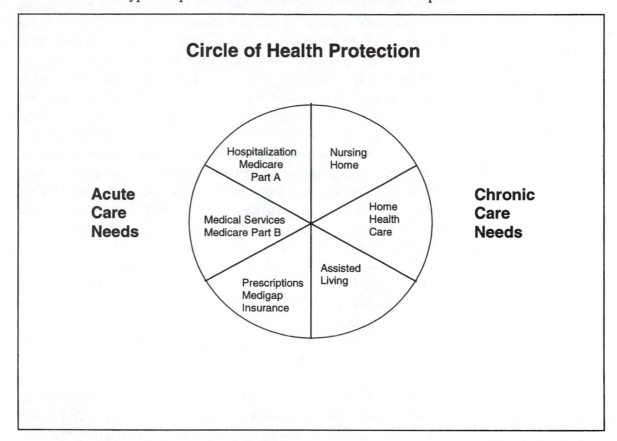

The Circle of Health Protection

After you have gathered information using LTCINS links, you can provide your prospects with information about their health care coverage with the help of a graphic called the "Circle of Health Protection." The circle is made up of two halves, each with three sections. The first half of the circle represents protection for acute health care needs. In this case, a patient receives medical care for a relatively brief period of time for a severe episode of illness (such as pneumonia), an accident or other trauma, or recovery from surgery. Acute care is given in a hospital. The other half of the circle represents protection for chronic health care needs. Chronic health care needs are the needs covered by LTCI, and they represent the broad range of medical, custodial, social, and other care services to assist people who have an impaired ability to live independently for an extended period of time.

Acute Care Needs—Use the acute care half of the circle to discuss Medicare Parts A and B as well as medigap insurance. Many prospects are already covered by Medicare or will certainly qualify for it at retirement. The purpose of this explanation is to dispel misconceptions about government programs. (This same discussion is also applicable to group and individual medical expense policies such as Blue Cross and managed care contracts that only pay for acute care services. Their discussion may be more meaningful for your younger prospects.) You can provide your prospects with a brief overview, not a detailed analysis, of Medicare hospitalization, outpatient benefits, and medical services. This may also give you an opportunity to cite the shortcomings of the various financing alternatives that your prospects may bring up for discussion. (Many advisors find that giving prospects the Health Care Financing Administration's current *Guide To Health Insurance for People with Medicare* very useful for making reference to Medicare and medigap plans.) To help keep prospects focused during the discussion, you may wish to use a highlighter to color the Medicare Parts A and B portions of the circle.

You may also wish to use some of the following points in your discussion with the prospect:

Medicare does not cover strictly custodial nursing home care services.

Medicare—Medicare does not cover strictly custodial nursing home care services. Unless you are in need of daily care that can be administered only by a medical professional, Medicare will not cover the care. Assistance in the specific activities of daily living (ADLs), such as getting from bed to chair, feeding oneself, going to the bathroom, and bathing, are not covered.

Skilled-Nursing Facility Care—Medicare hospital insurance helps pay for inpatient care in a Medicare-participating skilled-nursing facility following a hospital stay if the person's condition requires nursing or rehabilitation services that can only be provided in a skilled-nursing facility. It is important to point out, however, that many skilled-nursing facilities are not Medicare approved.

Medicare and LTCI—One of the most important things to know about Medicare is what it does not provide. It does not provide for nursing home care unless it is required as the result of a medical condition requiring hospitalization. It does not provide benefits solely for custodial care. This last restriction by itself will give you the opportunity to discuss LTCI coverage with your prospect.

Medicare Supplement Policies (Medigap)— Medigap policies are usually designed to cover deductibles and any coinsurance costs the insured who has Medicare coverage is required to make. If Medicare excludes the required LTC needed by a covered insured, it will also be excluded by medigap insurance policies. While these policies provide beneficial protection, they are not the answer for LTC needs.

> **Reliance on government:**
>
> - Don't let clients become complacent believing that Medicare will take care of their needs.
> - Don't let clients become lulled into believing that Medicaid planning can adequately solve the LTC problem for less than the cost of LTCI.
> - Educate your clients about the pitfalls of relying on government programs for LTC needs.

Use the medigap portion of the circle to alert your prospect to the deductibles, copayments, and prescription drug costs that are not covered by Medicare. Once again, the objective is to provide a brief overview. Sometimes, a prospect may already have a medigap policy or similar coverage. If so, you may wish to color this portion of the circle to demonstrate the extent of the prospect's current coverage. If you are using a highlighter, half of the circle should now be fully colored. It is now time to turn the discussion to chronic care needs.

Chronic Care Needs—Use the chronic care half of the circle to discuss nursing homes, home health care, and assisted living facilities. Begin the discussion by repeating that Medicare does not cover the bulk of these costs. (Ordinary group or individual managed care health insurance policies also do not pay for chronic care services.)

Nursing Homes—Point out that at best Medicare will cover 100 days of nursing home care. Then refer to the cost of nursing homes in your community. For example, you may indicate to the prospect that nursing home costs in your community average $175 a day, which is over $63,000 per year. Then ask the questions: "Have you considered how you or your family would pay for these costs? Would you be able to pay $63,000 a year for nursing home care from savings? If you could pay it, how long would your savings last?" The prospect's answers to these questions can provide you with insight into his or her thinking.

Home Health Care—Move next to home health care. Ask the prospect if he or she would prefer to stay at home in the event of a major illness. Expect a yes answer. Most prospects want to remain in their homes until they die, so point out that there are costs associated with this option. "Someone may have to clean and cook for you and may have to help bathe and dress you. You might even need help just getting out of bed. In our vicinity, these costs can amount to roughly $120 for an 8-hour day, which is less than the cost of a nursing home, but it is still a lot of money for many of us to pay. Would you be able to pay for home health care? One hundred twenty dollars a day does not sound like very much money until you consider that for a 5-day week that amounts to $600. Would your family be able or willing to provide weekend care, or would they prefer to spend the additional $240 for that as well? If so, that brings the cost of care to $840 a week, or over $3,000 a month."

Assisted Living—Next, move the discussion to the final section of the circle—assisted living. Provide a brief explanation of what is meant by assisted living, indicating that it provides personal care and support services, such as help with bathing, dressing, meals, and housekeeping, to people with physical or cognitive impairments. Point out that for many individuals assisted living represents a preferable alternative to nursing home care since it provides far greater independence. Once again, shift the discussion to costs by indicating that assisted living costs in your area range anywhere from $1,500 to $4,500 per month. Then ask: "Do you or your family have this extra money? Would you want money spent this way, or would you prefer to consider a more practical alternative that can cover all these costs for a reasonable monthly premium?"

Allow prospects time to think about these questions and their answers. Let them visualize their alternatives. Sometimes you will be able to begin filling in the application right at this point in the interview. If the prospect conveys the proper buying signals and the willingness to apply for LTCI, then by all means proceed with quantifying the needed parameters of coverage discussed later in this chapter in the sample "Long-Term Care Fact-Finder" and complete the application.

However, on most occasions you will find that the Circle of Health Protection serves as an introductory educational tool and that you will still want to further probe a prospect's needs and preferences using a mini fact-finder such as the "Financial and Personal Resources Review."

Financial and Personal Resources Review

The *Financial and Personal Resources Review* is a short and simple fact-finder designed to uncover information and potential objections to purchasing LTCI. At the same time, it can also serve as an additional motivator for the purchase of LTCI coverage. The use of this mini fact-finder is optional, but you may find it very helpful.

A copy of this mini fact-finder is found on page 4-33 for your use, but please be sure to first obtain your company's approval.

Preliminary Discovery Agreement

By the time you have successfully discussed the need for LTCI, asked the LTCINS pre-qualification questions, demonstrated the "Circle of Health Protection," and completed the financial and personal resources review, you should expect that a qualified prospect is ready to take the next steps toward purchasing LTCI. These steps begin with the completion of a more thorough fact-finder and feeling finder so that an appropriate LTCI plan can be designed. At this juncture, you may consider using a trial close or preliminary discovery agreement such as the following:

> "Mr. and Mrs. Prospect, based on your answers to my questions up to this point, it is apparent that you would want quality care if you needed ongoing assistance with the basic activities of daily living. You also do not want to be a financial, physical, or emotional burden to your heirs and would rather preserve your legacy for them. If I can design or formulate a plan that would enable you to accomplish the goals you've expressed at an affordable cost to you, would you be interested in working together to construct such a plan?"

(If the answer is no or unsatisfactorily negative, see the section on the next page, titled "Handling Prospects Who Fail to Qualify," for optional pivoting strategies you may consider using depending on the type of situation you encounter.)

If the answer is yes, you have a qualified prospect with whom you can proceed. As mentioned previously, depending on the prospect's receptivity and willingness to purchase LTCI, you can begin to take the application for coverage at this point in the interview. You will still need to ask the prospect questions regarding the five areas of LTCI benefits (found later in this chapter in the section titled "Begin Formulating the

Potential LTCI Plan Design") in order to complete the application. If the prospect strongly views LTCI as a single-product need and displays positive buying signs, then sell the product now, rather than jeopardize the opportunity to make the prospect your client. However, if based on your sales experience and judgment you perceive that the prospect is interested in a comprehensive financial plan that includes LTCI, then you should proceed with completing the LTC fact-finder that is displayed later in this chapter.

Transitional Phrase—The transition into the actual fact-finding form is usually facilitated by asking for the prospect's permission to proceed by saying something like this:

"In order for me to do a proper job analyzing your financial well-being, I'll need to ask you some personal questions. I can assure you that the information I gather will be held in the strictest confidence. With this in mind, is it alright to proceed?"

It should be noted that it might be necessary to schedule a second interview to complete the actual fact-finder. This decision is a judgment call that is based on the following factors: how well you know the prospect; how well educated he or she is about LTC issues; the length of time that the previous segments of the interview have taken; and how fatigued the prospect is.

Handling Prospects Who Fail to Qualify

You will encounter some situations where you are prepared to make the transition into completing the comprehensive fact-finder only to discover that the prospect does not qualify for LTCI. There are many reasons why a prospect may fail to qualify. However, whatever the reasons are, you should first attempt to pivot to another product sale using the fact-finder to gather the necessary information.

Pivoting Options (if the Prospect Does Not Qualify)—When a prospect does not qualify for LTCI, you must tell him or her but you do not necessarily have to lose the prospect. Pivoting involves delicately suggesting to the prospect that he or she consider an alternative approach to financing LTC needs. Likewise, if the prospect is able and wants to fund LTC costs but is uninsurable, you can propose an alternative by saying:

Financial and Personal Resources Review

Prepared for: _____

1. Health Coverage
   Do you believe your current health coverage adequately covers

A. hospitalization costs?	Yes	No
B. nursing home costs?	Yes	No
C. home health care costs?	Yes	No
D. assisted living costs?	Yes	No

2. Health Care Preferences
   If you suffered a long-term disability, where would you prefer to receive care?

A. Nursing home?	Yes	No
B. Your own home?	Yes	No

3. Financial Resources for Health Care
   If you faced a nursing home bill of $50,000 right now, how would you pay for it?

A. From savings?	Yes	No
B. Bank loan?	Yes	No
C. Other sources?	Yes	No

   How long could you personally afford to pay this $50,000 bill from these resources?

A. One year?	Yes	No
B. 2.5 years? (Most nursing home stays average this length.)	Yes	No
C. 5 years or longer?	Yes	No
Would your children be able to help you pay for this care?	Yes	No

   How would you prefer to pay for this care if you had a choice?

A. Private resources?	Yes	No
B. Insurance benefits?	Yes	No

   If your answer is insurance, is there a reason why you have not purchased it?

4. Personal Resources for Health Care
   If you became ill tomorrow, would your family

A. be trained to provide you with at-home medical care?	Yes	No
B. have the time to provide you with at-home care		
For one week?	Yes	No
For one month?	Yes	No
For 9 months?	Yes	No
For one year or more?	Yes	No
C. be physically able to provide long-term care?	Yes	No
D. be able to quit working to provide care?	Yes	No

5. Goals for Financial Resources

Would you like to leave an estate to your children?	Yes	No
Would you like to help pay for your grandchildren's educations?	Yes	No
Would you want your estate to be depleted by LTC debt?	Yes	No

Pivoting:

One advisor builds pivoting into his interviewing process:

"During the first interview, I give all the relevant players assignments to do. I assign the prospects' adult children to look up bank accounts and talk about their parents' finances among themselves. Then, to discuss what the children uncover about their parents' finances, I schedule a second interview.

The children sometimes find money that the parents didn't know they had. For example, the children once found enough money for their parents to buy a $100,000 immediate joint and survivor annuity. This provided enough money to pay for LTCI and then some!

However, if one or both parents are uninsurable, the found money goes into a Section 529 education-funding plan for the grandchildren."

"I'm sorry to tell you that you will not be able to obtain LTCI at this time due to your medical condition. However, you may be able to cushion some of the potential costs of paying for LTC by developing a strategy that employs alternative financial resources. If we can construct a plan of action within your budget to cover some of the potential costs of LTC, would you be interested?"

The following are several categories of prospects who fail to qualify for LTCI along with strategies for dealing with them:

- hostile or uncooperative prospects
- uninsurable prospects
- prospects with insufficient funds
- prospects shopping for a better deal

Uncooperative Prospects—If a prospect is hostile or is generally uncooperative during the pre-qualification process, you should move on and concentrate your efforts with those people who will appreciate your expertise and assistance. There are too many qualified prospects in the LTC marketplace who do not own this product and would be more than willing to purchase it if they were properly guided through the selling process. Your precious time needs to be spent with them.

Uninsurable Prospects—If a prospect is uninsurable for LTCI, you may want to serve as a resource person and refer them to an elder care attorney for additional LTC planning. However, you may also want to pivot to another product that he or she should consider. Many prospects for LTCI, especially those who are in or near retirement, are likely to have considerable assets in savings that they are seeking to protect with LTCI. Mutual funds and annuities are two products that you can sell without worrying about underwriting rejections. Explain your company's concerns about the prospect being uninsurable and then open the discussion on how these other product lines can be used to defray some of the costs of LTC services.

In fact, when the discussion centers on financing alternatives to LTCI, your creativity can build your credibility in the prospect's eyes, and this can lead to the sale of other products as well as referrals to other family members.

Prospects with Insufficient Funds—Some prospects simply cannot afford LTCI. Not everyone who needs LTCI is qualified to purchase it. The "no money" objection is one of the basic disqualifying criteria in financial services selling. The sooner you discover that the prospect cannot afford LTCI, the sooner you may be able to pivot to another product that he or she can afford. For example, someone with modest savings might be a prospect for a small life insurance policy or a deferred annuity. Furthermore, he or she may also become a source of leads to other prospects who may be more qualified for LTCI.

Prospects Shopping for a Better Deal—Many prospects have hidden objections. They are not interested in completing a comprehensive fact-finder or establishing a long-lasting client/advisor relationship. Sometimes they even spend years waiting for the illusive better deal while they remain uninsured. Nevertheless, these prospects can be cultivated slowly over time, if you have the patience.

Education can sometimes be the solution to overcoming this procrastination. These are excellent prospects to invite to an LTC seminar that you may be conducting. The education you provide may help them confront and overcome their reasons for procrastination. A seminar is a low-key way for you to maintain contact with these prospects. When they are ready to buy LTCI, your name should come to mind. In the meantime, these prospects may purchase other products from you or become a source of referrals.

Keeping in Contact with Qualified Prospects

Do not forget to maintain contact with qualified prospects who do not buy LTCI from you initially. Also, remember to stay in contact with your clients once a sale is made. Seminars, newsletters, birthday and holiday cards, and periodic reviews are all methods of maintaining contact. Your LTC clients are prospects for other products. If you are conducting a seminar on a topic other than LTC, invite them. A seminar is an excellent way to maintain face-to-face contact and to invite cross-selling opportunities in a time-efficient manner. Newsletters are less personal but still remind clients of your expertise. Sending birthday and holiday greeting cards also keeps your name in front of clients and prospects and can lead to repeat business and referrals, may help to build relationships, and is usually appreciated by them. Periodic reviews offer a way of uncovering sequential sales opportunities while staying in touch with your clients' changing needs.

The Fact-Finding Process

After you have qualified the prospect and obtained a preliminary discovery agreement, the actual fact-finding and feeling-finding portion of the selling process can take place as a continuation of the initial interview, or it can be done as a separate interview. This is your option. However, it's important to be mindful that the prospect might be fatigued. The discussion of finances can be very exhausting to some people. You will want to make certain that your prospect is still alert and attentive to your questions if you decide to continue the initial interview into the fact-finding process.

There are two basic approaches to the personal information gathering process. One approach is deductive while the other is inductive.

Total Financial Needs Analysis to the Dominant or Single (LTC) Need—(the Deductive Approach)

This approach is characterized by using a thorough and lengthy fact-finding form that broadly covers all the prospect's financial needs. This method would cover life insurance, disability, retirement, investment, estate and education planning needs, as well as LTC needs. The process requires quantifying these various financial planning needs and asking the prospect to prioritize them. The category of needs with the highest priority should be determined first. You should then try to cover this most important category of needs by selling the prospect the appropriate product or products.

The Dominant or Single (LTC) Need to Total Financial Needs Analysis—(the Inductive Approach)

This approach is the converse of the approach to information gathering described above. This method starts with a dominant or single need, such as the need to cover LTC. It then broadens into a full-blown comprehensive financial needs analysis where several financial planning needs are identified and prioritized. This broadening into a comprehensive needs analysis may very well be done only after the dominant or single need has been covered by a particular product sale, and it could take several interviews to complete. However, sometimes, as was discussed earlier in this chapter under the "Preliminary Discovery Agreement" heading, the dominant or single need product, such as LTCI, may be the only product you ever sell to the prospect, so that a total financial needs analysis may never transpire.

We do not necessarily endorse one approach over the other. Your company can provide you with guidance in this area that is consistent with its own marketing strategy. Some companies using the inductive or dominant needs approach will focus on using LTCI as a door opener in the seniors market in the hope of becoming involved in the prospect's retirement and estate planning. Other companies using the deductive or comprehensive financial planning approach attempt to position the sale of LTCI somewhere in the prioritized sequence of financial planning needs. For purposes of the discussion here, we have extracted those fact-finding and feeling-finding questions that can be used with either approach to enhance your LTCI sales opportunities.

Fact Finders

There are numerous fact finders available for collecting data. Your company has probably already provided you with one that you are using. Nevertheless, we have included a sample LTC fact finder that you are welcome to use with the permission of your company's compliance department. The important point to remember about using the fact finder is to not limit yourself to asking just the questions on the fact finder. You should also ascertain your prospect's feelings and values. Asking only the questions on the fact finder will not collaboratively involve your prospect and will not reveal his or her important feelings and values. Your company's fact finder may provide a space for listing the prospect's feelings and values. If it does not, be sure to jot down the feelings and values revealed during the fact-finding process.

Your prospects must be collaboratively involved in the sales process. Since the prospect is buying your LTCI product and services, he or she should make the decision to buy based on knowledge obtained from you during the interview. This involves more than just being told what LTCI policy design to buy because it is the best one for him or her. By making a knowledgeable decision to buy, the prospect develops a sense of ownership in the process and will truly become your client for other products.

A formal LTC fact-finder can be divided into three distinct discovery components. These components are

- factual
- quantitative
- attitudinal

Factual—Questions in this section of the LTC fact finder are closed-ended and are designed to find out simple data that the prospect can easily identify or remember. Many questions in this section begin with "who is," "when did you," "when do you," and "what are" or "what is." These questions can be asked and answered rapidly in an almost staccato fashion.

Spaces are provided for filling in the prospect's and his or her spouse's name, date of birth, Social Security number, phone numbers, and children's names, ages, and locations. There is also a question that asks for the names, addresses, and phone numbers for the prospect's professional advisors (that is, attorney, accountant, insurance advisor, bank or trust officer, and securities broker). Additional questions ask about the documents prepared and the services performed by these advisors for the prospect. There are also several questions that ask about the prospect's hobbies, when he or she plans to retire or actually did retire, or whether he or she has any parents, children, or grandchildren who require special care. All these questions combined will only take a few minutes to answer and are a good warm-up for the more difficult questions that follow.

Transitional Phrase—Then you should transition into the next section of the fact finder by letting the prospect know that his or her cooperation in providing answers to questions about personal details is appreciated and necessary in order to get a clear understanding of the present financial situation. Begin by saying: "I appreciate your cooperation in providing the answers to personal details about you and your family. Now with your permission, I'd like to ask you some questions about your finances that are necessary in order for me to get a clear picture of where you stand so that any recommendation I may make will be suitable for your circumstances. Therefore, if you have no objection, may I continue?"

Quantitative—The objective of this section of the LTC fact finder is to have the prospect provide information about his or her most recent income statement and personal net worth (balance sheet) statement. If the prospect has not already prepared an income statement or personal net worth statement, then he or she will have to obtain the information by looking at income tax records, checkbook receipts, and other documents.

The questions in this section of the fact finder are comprised of closed-ended factual questions that may have to at times be combined with open-ended questions that help to clarify reasons behind the existence of the quantitative data. Many questions in this section begin with phrases like "how much" or "what's the amount of." For example, you may ask how much they have in mutual funds followed by a question that explores their feelings about risk and diversification. Another example could involve asking what their mortgage balance(s) is/are and following it with questions about how they feel about paying down their debts.

In filling out this section of the fact finder, you are asking for personal financial information. Even though you have already told the prospect that you need it and why, completing this section will take a considerable amount of time especially if there are no existing financial statements. All the while you are also gradually building trust with the prospect as he or she answers each question.

Obtaining a Dollar Commitment for the Premium that the Prospect Can Afford—It is while completing the quantitative section of the LTC fact finder that you should obtain a dollar commitment from the prospect concerning the amount that he or she can afford to spend on LTCI premiums. It does not have to be a specific dollar figure per se. You could attempt to elicit a "range of affordability" in terms of monthly or annual cost. In any event, you will want to make sure that the prospect does not exceed the NAIC 7 percent of income suitability rule. Therefore, while all the financial information is still fresh in everyone's mind, you may want to say something like this to the prospect:

"Mr. or Ms. Prospect, assuming you have a need and a desire for LTCI, I would like you to consider how much you could comfortably afford on a monthly basis to address that need. I don't expect you to have a specific dollar figure in mind, but if you have some idea of what you can afford, I assure you I will do everything possible to customize a LTCI plan that fits within your budget. Does this make sense to you?"

Begin Formulating the Potential LTCI Plan Design—Sometime during the data gathering process, you will need to obtain information from the prospect that outlines the types and levels of care that he or she is interested in receiving should the need arise. (It is recommended that this be done at the conclusion of the quantitative section of the fact finder, but you could do it just as well at the very end of the attitudinal section.) Specifically, you need to acquire information about five different policy benefits before attempting to design a plan of coverage. You will have touched upon some of these benefits earlier when you completed the "Financial and Personal Resources Review," but now is the time to let the prospect articulate the specific benefits he or she wants in a LTCI policy. This requires you to ask the following questions about the five benefits.

- Elimination Period—How long is the prospect willing to wait before collecting benefits from the policy: zero days, 30 days, 60 days, or 90 days?
- Care Settings—In which of the following care settings would the prospect like to have benefits paid to him or her if they are needed: nursing home only coverage, home health care only coverage, or both?
- Daily Benefit Amount—How much coverage does the prospect feel is adequate for his or her needs? The average daily cost is $150. What is the cost in your area, and what percentage of that cost does the prospect want to insure?
- Benefit Period—How long does the prospect want benefits to last: 1 year, 2 years, 3 years, 5 years, or unlimited?
- Inflation Rider—Does the prospect want the daily benefit to increase with the rate of inflation: simple interest inflation rider, compound interest inflation rider, or none at all?

> **Your objective is to make it easier for your prospect to buy the LTCI policy that you recommend and that achieves his or her financial goals and aspirations.**

The chosen amount of each of these five benefits will of course affect the cost of the policy. Therefore, it is necessary to zero in on the precise amount of these benefits that the prospect wants, and that is relevant to his or her individual needs. To determine a starting point from which you can develop an individual LTCI policy, ask the prospect to prioritize the available benefits. Later, as you fine-tune the plan to fit his or her budget, you can adjust the benefits accordingly.

By the time you have completed the quantitative section of the fact finder, you should have set the stage for the all-important attitudinal section.

Transitional Phrase—Again, the progression into the next section of the interview should be prefaced with a transitional phrase. You should confirm the prospect's annual and monthly cash flow amounts as well as his or her net worth amount so that you are both in agreement on the figures. This confirmation of figures is a good way of punctuating the completion of this section of the fact finder. Then, at this point in the interview you may want to compliment the prospect on his or her cooperation by saying: "You've been very cooperative and forthcoming with information about your personal finances, and I truly appreciate your help. Now I'd like to ask you some questions about your feelings concerning the potential need for LTC. There are no right or wrong answers to these questions, but the more open and honest you are with me, the better I'll be able to serve you. Does this sound reasonable?"

This preface should probably be accompanied by a change in your posture to nonverbally indicate to the prospect that you are about to begin a more intimate and conversational portion of the interview. You could, for example, sit back and cross your legs in a more leisurely fashion while directly facing the prospect. This type of body language speaks volumes toward making the prospect feel more relaxed and comfortable.

Attitudinal—Values are a person's beliefs and attitudes about a given subject. Feelings reflect a person's values. When you learn about your prospect's dreams and aspirations, you begin to understand him or her. Values are the basis of a person's behavior, and they influence a person's priorities in life. Discovering your prospect's priorities is the key to understanding what he or she will spend time and money on achieving.

Involving the prospect in the fact-finding segment of the sales process gives him or her an ownership interest in your LTCI policy recommendations. The very process of discussing and examining his or her feelings leads the prospect to self-discovery. In fact, the prospect is far more likely to expend the necessary time and money on buying an LTCI policy that he or she played a role in designing.

Your objective is to make it easier for your prospect to buy the LTCI policy that you recommend and that achieves his or her financial goals and aspirations. The prospect brings all his or her life experiences, education, product knowledge, and personal values to the interview, and your function is to integrate these with new knowledge, data, examples, and illustrations. If properly done, the prospect will be ready to purchase the LTCI policy that you are recommending and he or she helped to design.

The questions used in this section of the fact finder are almost strictly open-ended. You are attempting to elicit feelings and emotions that are reflective of the prospect's attitudes and values about LTC. You will need to proceed slowly here because many of the prospect's emotions will be brought to the surface at this time. The questions asked here often begin with words such as, "why," "how do you feel about," "what would you want to," or "have you ever." The prospect's subjective responses to them provide insight into his or her underlying motivations for buying LTCI. Your use of open-ended questions invites the prospect to give his or her answers in a multiple sentence discussion format. This sensitive discussion provides you with valuable information that can help you design an LTCI plan that will allay the fears and concerns of the prospect while giving him or her peace of mind.

Conclusion and Summary—When you have completed all three parts of the LTC fact finder, you should then be equipped to analyze and digest the information so that an appropriate and acceptable LTCI plan can be designed.

The order in which you proceed through the fact finder depends on your level of comfort with questions that need to be asked. You can do each section separately or integrate all three of them together. This is a matter of advisor preference and personal interviewing style. For example, the questions in the attitudinal section are meant to conclude the fact finder, but many advisors insist on asking these questions at the beginning of the LTC fact-finding interview in order to encourage the prospect to think as early as possible about his or her potential need for LTC. However, it is probably easier to stay more organized and focused if you do each section sequentially. Other advisors will find it more conversational to mix the questions from all three sections together. The point to remember is that comprehensive information gathering requires the completion of all three of the fact finder components.

> The order in which you proceed through the fact finder depends on your level of comfort with questions that need to be asked.

Since an enormous amount of data may be collected during the fact-finding process, it may be a good idea to review and confirm each section as it is completed. Or you may choose the close of the interview as the best time to review all the information you have recorded.

You should review and summarize your interpretation of the prospect's feelings about LTC issues and give him or her a chance to agree with your assessment or to clarify any aspects you may not have accurately understood.

By reviewing the facts and feelings that you have recorded, you not only check your understanding of what the prospect told you, you also show the prospect that you were paying attention to what he or she said. Be sure that the prospect concurs with your interpretation of his or her feelings. An LTCI plan will not be effective if it is based on inaccurate information or on assumptions that you, rather than the prospect, made.

Mutual Agreement to Work Together

The fact-finding process is often a very complex one. More than one meeting may be necessary before the entire process is complete. At the beginning of any subsequent meetings, be sure to review and confirm the information gathered at the previous meetings. Always be sure that you and the prospect are thinking along the same lines.

Discovery Agreement—Finally, many financial advisors conclude the initial fact-finding interview by summarizing in writing the expressed goals of the prospect. This practice, known as the discovery agreement, can also be done verbally. When the discovery agreement is done verbally, you should ask the prospect to prioritize or rank his or her financial goals so that he or she can confirm which ones are most important.

However, it is more effective to send a letter subsequent to the meeting that acknowledges not only the gist of what was discussed, but also provides a blueprint for proceeding through the next step(s) in the sales process. This implied contract is an essential ingredient for establishing the foundation of a true client/advisor relationship. This agreement to work together toward mutually acceptable solutions to the prospect's LTC financial concerns establishes a climate of trust and partnership.

Summary

The client-focused selling philosophy is the basis for creating and building a personally rewarding clientele. The third and fourth steps in the selling process outlined in chapter 1, which are to meet the prospect and to gather information, are described in this chapter as a way of making this philosophy practical. Contacting the right people means that you will have more appointments with prospects who are qualified. By focusing on your prospect's needs and values during interviews, you will build the trust needed to generate a higher volume of sales and an ongoing supply of referrals. These are some of the essential ingredients of a selling process that will help you develop a thriving business.

Long-Term Care Fact-Finder

Factual Section

Your Name _____   Your Spouse's Name _____

Social Security # _____   Social Security # _____

Date of Birth _____   Date of Birth _____

Home Address

Street _____

City _____ State _____ Zip _____

Home Phone _____ Your Business Phone _____

Your Cell Phone _____ Spouse's Cell Phone_____

Your Fax _____ Spouse's Fax _____

Your E-mail _____ Spouse's E-mail _____

Children

Name	Address	Age
_____	_____	_____
_____	_____	_____
_____	_____	_____
_____	_____	_____

Will any of your children be involved in your decision to purchase long-term care insurance?

_____

_____

Do any of your children or grandchildren require special care? What about your parents?

_____

_____

What career accomplishments are you most proud of?

_____

_____

When do you plan to retire or when did you retire?

_____

Do you plan to remain in your current home during retirement?

_____

Are there any recreational activities or hobbies that you enjoy?

_____

_____

What are the names, addresses, and phone numbers of your professional and personal advisors?

Adviser	Name	Address	Phone
Attorney	_____	_____	_____
Insurance Advisor	_____	_____	_____
Securities Broker	_____	_____	_____
Accountant	_____	_____	_____
Banker	_____	_____	_____
Trust Officer	_____	_____	_____
Others	_____	_____	_____

Have you taken the time to have any of the following documents prepared? If so, by whom and when?

Document		Prepared By	Date
Will	Yes / No	_____	_____
Living Will	Yes / No	_____	_____
Durable Power of Attorney	Yes / No	_____	_____
Health Care Directive	Yes / No	_____	_____
Revocable Living Trust	Yes / No	_____	_____
Irrevocable Trust	Yes / No	_____	_____
Financial Plan	Yes / No	_____	_____
Estate Plan	Yes / No	_____	_____

What other services have any of your professional advisors performed for you?

_____

_____

Quantitative Section

Do you know how much the average daily costs are in your area for the following?

Nursing Homes $ _____   Assisted Living $ _____

Home Health Care $ _____   Adult Day Care $ _____

Have you purchased insurance coverage to protect against all other types of risks except for long-term care?   Yes / No

What kinds of insurance products do you own?

_____

_____

Have you ever been approached about the purchase of long-term care insurance before?

_____

_____

If so, why didn't you buy it?

_____

_____

Net Worth Statement

ASSETS   MARKET VALUE

Savings accounts   _____

Checking   _____

CDs and money market   _____

Stocks & bonds   _____

Life insurance (cash values)   _____

Annuities (surrender values)   _____

Pension(s) & profit-sharing plans   _____

IRAs (Traditional & Roth)   _____

Mutual funds   _____

Principal residence & vacation home   _____

Investment real estate   _____

Business interests   _____

Personal property (autos, furniture, jewelry, etc.) _____

Collectibles (antiques, art, etc.)   _____

Other assets   _____

Total Assets $ _____

LIABILITIES

Mortgages (1st, 2nd, home equity lines of credit) (balances) _____

Automobile loans   _____

Credit card balances   _____

Installment loans   _____

Business debts   _____

Other debt   _____

Total Liabilities $ _____

Total Assets   _____

Minus Total Liabilities   _____

Equals **TOTAL NET WORTH** $ _____

Do you have assets that you would be willing to spend in order to provide for long-term care?

_____

_____

How do you feel about taking investment risks?

_____

_____

Would you consider yourself a successful investor? Why or why not?

_____

_____

Do you worry about outliving or depleting the assets you've accumulated in your life's savings?

_____

_____

Income Statement

INCOME

Wages, salary, commissions, bonuses, etc.:

    Your Own _____

    Your spouse's _____

Interest _____

Dividends _____

Rental & investment property _____

Social Security _____

Pension benefits _____

Profit sharing & IRA _____

Annuities _____

Life insurance benefits _____

Trusts _____

Other _____

Total Income $_____

EXPENSES (fixed and variable)

Housing (rent, mortgage payments) _____

Household maintenance (fuel, utilities, repairs, etc.) _____

Food _____

Transportation (gas, parking, maintenance, public transit, etc.) _____

Medical care (doctors, dental, prescriptions) _____

Debts (budgeted debt liquidation, revolving credit payments) _____

Insurance premiums:

    Life, health, disability income, medigap _____

    Homeowners & automobile _____

Savings and investment _____

Education funding & childcare expenses _____

Taxes:

    Income _____

    Property _____

EXPENSES (discretionary)

Entertainment & restaurants _____

Travel, recreation, & vacations _____

Charities & gifts (church, donations, holidays, birthdays, etc.) _____

Home improvements and furnishings _____

Personal / miscellaneous _____

Total Expenses $_____

DIFFERENCE   (Total Income minus Total Expenses) $_____

Dollar Commitment:
How much would you be willing to set aside on a monthly basis to provide for your long–term care needs?

_____

_____

If we could design the ideal long-term care insurance package for you, which of the following benefit selections would you want included?

- **Elimination Period**—How long are you willing to wait before collecting benefits from the policy?

Zero days_____ 30 days_____ 60 days_____ 90 days_____Other_____

- **Care Settings**—In which of the following care settings would you like to have benefits paid to you if they are needed?

Nursing home only coverage _____
Home health care only _____
Both _____

- **Daily Benefit Amount**—How much daily benefit coverage do you feel is adequate for your needs? The national average daily cost is $150. The average daily cost in your area is $_____.

What percentage of this cost do you want to insure?

100% _____80% _____60% _____Other_____

- **Benefit Period**—How long do you want benefits to last?

1 year _____ 2 years _____ 3 years _____ 5 years _____Unlimited _____

- **Inflation Rider**—Do you want the daily benefit to increase with the rate of inflation?

Simple interest _____Compound interest _____None at all _____

Attitudinal Section

Why are you considering the purchase of long-term care insurance today?

_____

_____

Have you ever personally known someone who needed long-term care?

_____

_____

What happened to that person to cause him or her to need long-term care?

_____

_____

How did you feel about the circumstances surrounding the care needed and received by that person?

_____

_____

Have you ever needed to provide care or assistance to someone close to you?

_____

_____

Do you plan for family members to care for you as you age?

_____

_____

Ideally, as you age, in what type of setting would you like to live if you needed care?

(i.e., current residence, continuing care retirement community, assisted living facility, nursing home)

_____

_____

What would have to happen to cause you to enter a nursing home?

_____

_____

If you needed professional chronic care, how much financial hardship would you endure to pay for it?

_____

_____

Objections—Managing Resistance

Objections to the sale of LTCI are abundant. However, experience shows that most of the objections that prospects express tend to disguise the real reasons they fail to buy LTCI. The real reasons that most people do not buy LTCI (assuming they can afford it) are that they do not believe they need it today, and they do not believe they will need it in the future. In fact, most of the objections discussed below are variations of these two common themes. Just as the impetus to buy LTCI is sparked by emotion, so is the resistance to buying it. Prospects do not imagine themselves needing assistance with normal everyday activities. Their pride and vanity can get in the way of their logic and reason.

Objections are liable to surface at any time during the selling process, not just at the close of the sale. Therefore, you need to have a general strategy in place to deal with prospects' concerns as well as specific responses to handle their objections categorically whenever they surface.

Handling Concerns and Objections

The first step in handling an objection is to listen to the prospect. No one likes to be interrupted or feel that he or she is not being taken seriously. Listening to what the prospect has to say will help you understand the objection. Therefore, encourage the prospect to explain how he or she feels about the issue.

Give yourself an opportunity to confirm your understanding of the prospect's objection by restating or rephrasing it. This gives you an opportunity to learn more about the exact nature of the objection, and it also puts you in a better position to counter it.

The sales process should build momentum until the inescapable conclusion is reached that the prospect needs the protection and he or she should buy it immediately. Each step in the process supports the one that follows. By the time the prospect begins to raise concerns and objections,

> **A well prepared sales presentation can reduce the number of objections encountered by anticipating and dealing with them before they are raised.**

you should know enough about his or her personal and financial situation, and his or her attitudes and feelings that you can address them directly, honestly, and convincingly.

A well-prepared sales presentation can reduce the number of objections encountered by anticipating and preparing for them. For example, if you satisfactorily obtain a dollar commitment from the prospect early in the interview, this will prevent the "no money" objection from surfacing later. You can also reduce the number of objections by

- Developing rapport and trust (combats the "no confidence" objection).
- Getting an agreement at each step in the presentation (reduces the "no need" objection).
- Focusing on the benefits of your recommendations (forestalls the "no hurry" objection).

Naturally, prospects may raise objections to purchasing LTCI. This is a natural reaction to the thought of spending money. Many objections stem from the thought of spending money and/or not getting sufficient value for it. People hate to spend money needlessly or wastefully on something they think they do not need or want that has little value.

As you talk with prospects, use "trial closes" such as, "Other than affordability, do you feel this is the best product to suit your needs?" Overcoming objections takes practice and experience, so it is important not to get discouraged if at first you are not successful.

Techniques for Dealing with Prospect Resistance

Acknowledge, Clarify, and Resolve

There are a few commonly used methods for dealing with objections. One is a three-step technique for responding to prospect resistance. It simply acknowledges a concern and then clarifies and resolves it.

1. Acknowledge a Concern—You validate the prospect's thoughts and feelings by acknowledging his or her concern. If you do not acknowledge the concern but instead take it head on and try to wrestle it down, all you will succeed in doing is putting more distance between the prospect and you.

Responses such as "I understand how you feel," or "I can appreciate that" show your prospects that you are listening to them and care about what they say.

2. Clarify—Clarifying a vague or negative response from a prospect is often necessary before it can be effectively resolved. Any statement that is too global, vague, or overreaching needs to be clarified and explored. Clarification can take many forms, such as "Could you please explain that?" or "I don't understand what you mean. Can you give me an example?"

3. Resolve—Once a prospect's concern is acknowledged and clarified, you can resolve the concern by making appropriate recommendations. This may involve educating the prospect on some point by clarifying and repeating what has already been covered.

Feel, Felt, Found

Another popular three-step technique used to deal with objections is to use the words feel, felt, and found in three successive sentences as demonstrated below:

- "I understand how you **feel**."
- "Many of my prospects have **felt** the same way."
- "Until they **found** that . . . . (Briefly state a benefit. For example, explain how the plan was a good solution for their specific situation.)

Notice that this technique uses the acknowledgment step of handling objections that is mentioned above. Empathetic acknowledgment puts the prospect at ease since his or her feeling was common to others until the others found that the solution provided them with a desirable benefit. This neutralizes the situation and gives you an opportunity to remain poised as you address the prospect's specific concern or objection by explaining the benefit that is being provided.

Common Objections

Objections to Purchasing LTCI

Objections to purchasing LTCI fall into one of four general categories. They are

- No need
- No money
- No hurry
- No confidence

We will discuss 13 common objections according to their appropriate category. Then we will explain the tactics for dealing with each of these objections.

No Need

Not Me—The thought of living in a nursing home or being old and at least partially incapacitated frightens people in our society. In fact, very few people want to even think about the possibility of needing assistance with the normal activities of daily living (ADLs). Denial rules here and it is often difficult to get prospects to seriously consider that the risk of needing LTC is real and that they could be affected. The reality is that over 40 percent of those people over age 65 will need LTC sometime during their lives.

I'm in Great Health—Citing good health as the reason for not purchasing LTCI is another hollow objection. The outright rejection or at least postponement of the decision to purchase LTCI presents several possible problems. As with life insurance, the cost of LTCI increases with age, and the prospect's insurability is likely to be an even more important factor later in his or her life if a health problem develops. Eligibility and standard issue rates can be threatened by many health conditions. So the fact that the prospect is in great health is an excellent

> **One advisor states:**
>
> "It's not that there are objections per se. I view the prospects' questions as opportunities to educate them and their families on the inherent obstacles and problems in obtaining quality LTC. I also work hard to build my relationship with them. By the time my prospects buy LTCI, they know exactly what the policy will do for them and why they are buying it."

reason to purchase LTCI *now* while it is relatively inexpensive, rather than a reason to delay it.

The Odds Are in My Favor—Although a prospect may believe that the odds are in his or her favor, the fact is they are not. While it is true that health care advances are translating into increased longevity, this does not mean that all these added years are spent in good health. The number of seniors reaching age 85 and beyond is increasing dramatically. Unfortunately, with increased age comes the increased likelihood of chronic illness and the need for LTC. Forty-three percent of Americans aged 65 and older can expect to spend some time in a nursing home. Roughly three-fourths of nursing home residents are aged 75 or older. The odds are that the longer a person lives, the more likely the person will need LTC services of some kind.

The Cost of Care Is Not that Expensive—Another favorite objection prospects use is to question why they should buy LTCI when the cost of LTC is not that expensive. Use statistical evidence (such as the figures cited in chapter one) to counteract this argument. While many prospects may simply be ignorant of the real costs involved in LTC and have had no reason to think about or explore them, the potential financial drain on the middle class family who needs LTC can be emotionally devastating. For example, the average annual cost of nursing home care today is around $50,000 (although it can be much higher). By 2030, it is estimated that the annual cost of nursing home care will rise to about $200,000. Paying LTCI premiums will always be less costly than paying for LTC services.

You may want to ask the prospect, "Does it make sense to work hard all your life setting aside money for retirement only to see it all disappear to pay for LTC?"

My Kids/Family Will Take Care of Me—Historically, families in many countries have taken care of their own members rather than institutionalize them. When this country was younger and very rural, care by other family members was the rule. However, as the nation has grown older and become more industrialized, families have become more geographically dispersed. This has resulted in adult children being unable to take care of dependent parents or other aging relatives. However, with the benefits in today's LTCI policies, such as home health care, you can explain to the prospect how he or she could avoid leaving home for care and still receive benefits. LTCI can ensure that parents receive quality care in any setting including their daughter's or son's home. In those situations where the adult children feel a responsibility to care for their parents, they are often willing to help pay the premiums.

In any event, caregiving on an extended basis can be an enormous emotional, physical, and financial burden. If the parent without LTCI needs to move in with the child, resentment of the situation can affect all concerned. In these situations, this objection is not thought out properly. For instance, suppose the prospect's children have moved across the country or the prospect has retired to another state. You will also want to pose some of the following questions to those prospects who raise this objection:

- Do your children have the time?
- Can your children afford to stop working?
- Do your children have the necessary medical skills?
- Are you psychologically prepared to be dependent on your children for your most basic needs?
- Do you want to burden your children with this kind of responsibility?
- Have you and your children talked about this issue and made specific plans?

The Government Will Pay—The "government will pay" objection presents an opportunity for you to both educate the prospect about the relationship between government programs and LTC benefits and build credibility in the process of doing so. Do not let the prospect be lulled into the complacency associated with thinking that government programs will adequately take care of his or her needs. Ask your prospect just what costs he or she believes the government will pay in the area of LTC. Then you can respond by addressing each misconception as it arises. (The shortcomings of Medicare and Medicaid have been discussed previously in other sections of this book.)

You should also remind your prospect that unlike government programs, LTCI provides nursing home and home health care benefits regardless of the amount of assets he or she owns. The prospect's accumulated assets can be spent enjoying life or can be preserved for his or her heirs. Therefore, legal maneuvers aimed at preserving assets can be avoided.

Finally, make the point that care options are greatly expanded when a person owns LTCI. In many communities, nursing home entry becomes easier when private money (instead of government funds) is being used to pay the cost. Home health care options are also broader and more varied with LTCI than when having to comply with government rules aimed squarely at restricting such options.

I'll Stay at Home—I'm Not Going into a Nursing Home Under any Circumstances—Nursing homes are not the only form of LTC, although they are certainly the most expensive. If some form of home health care is desired, you can point out to the prospect that this option can cost as much as $25,000 per year or more.

Also point out that many features in an LTCI policy assure that the insured as well as family members are given options and alternatives to nursing home care that may not otherwise be available. The expenses for these alternative treatments would also be covered by LTCI. Another fact worth mentioning is that, although very few people enter a nursing home willingly, it may be the only alternative available to those concerned.

I'll be Wasting my Money if I do not Use It—Many prospects understandably have a fear of wasting their hard earned and limited funds. A healthy 65-year-old female prospect may think, "What if I pay LTCI premiums for 20 years and then drop dead from a heart attack? I would rather leave that money to my children, instead of wasting it on insurance premiums."

This is where a return of premium rider (discussed in chapter 5) may come in handy. Also, more companies are offering life/LTCI combination plans. A life/LTCI combination is a hybrid plan that provides permanent life insurance death benefits and accumulates cash values that can be used for LTC costs.

No Money

The Insurance Is too Expensive—This is the second most common objection after "I want to think about it." The key to overcoming this objection is to bring it up during your presentation, which should include information on the high cost of waiting to purchase LTCI. For example,

- If you wait 3 years it will cost you 24 percent more a year for the rest of your life.

> The motto of one LTC insurer is: "Long-term care insurance—it's not an expense, it's an investment."

- If you wait 5 years it will cost you 68 percent more for the rest of your life.
- If you wait 8 years it will cost you 128 percent more for the rest of your life.

Also, comparing the amount of money spent on LTCI premiums to LTC costs is eye opening. For example, if the premium for $150 a day of LTCI coverage is $1,800 per year, you can point out that nearly $55,000 of nursing home costs would be provided per year under such a policy. That is equivalent to 30 years of premiums. These types of contrasts are dramatic.

Additionally, if expense is an objection for an older prospect, you may counter this objection by attempting to orchestrate an arrangement where the prospect's adult child or children help to finance the cost. This simple yet creative approach is most helpful for older prospects who have fixed incomes. Sharing the cost with relatives can ease their financial discomfort of paying for LTCI.

No Hurry

Let Me Think about It—This is the classic unspecific objection that probably is a smokescreen hiding the real reason or reasons for not continuing the buying process. This objection usually hides something that the prospect does not want to tell you or simply cannot articulate. The earlier in the sales process that you uncover this objection the less frustrating it will be for you because you cannot combat buyer ambiguity.

You can ask the prospect why he or she wants to think about it or what specifically he or she wants to think about, but this can be adversarial and not reveal the real reason for hesitation. The revelations surrounding the reality of thinking in the first person about the unpleasantness of needing LTC can emotionally overwhelm some prospects. You need to be sensitive to their emotions and to their prerogative to not take action now. So unless you can elicit the real objection, the best way to deal with this situation is offering to stay in touch with the prospect, putting the paperwork in your tickler file, and moving on to other prospects.

It's Too Early to Plan—There are several risks involved in waiting to purchase LTCI. These risks include the possibilities that the prospect may not be insurable and the premium will be higher. You could offer several responses such as:

Response 1: "Will you be able to qualify for LTCI coverage when you need it? Even if you could, if your health has declined, it's likely to cost you far more than it would today, all else being equal."

Response 2: "I suggest we compare the costs between buying today and waiting until tomorrow. Typically, you can buy more LTCI coverage for less at your current age than if you wait just a few more years."

I Would like to Shop around a Little More—When the prospect raises this objection, it is important to

1. Acknowledge it and not pressure him or her into making a decision.
2. Emphasize what factors he or she should consider in shopping, such as price versus value, personalized service, company strength, and policy benefits.
3. If it is feasible, ask if he or she would allow you to help make policy comparisons.

This is a competitive market where several quotes from different companies offering LTCI should be presented. Find out if there are any companies that the prospect is particularly interested in. There may be competition, which is often the case in this market. Not offering alternative plans and companies leaves you vulnerable to this objection.

However, bear in mind that this is a relationship-based sale. Therefore, shopping may simply involve the comparison of several different policy options available from the single insurer you represent. Ask the prospect if providing this type of policy comparison would satisfy his or her desire to shop.

> **According to one advisor:**
>
> "Adult children are often willing to help pay for the cost of LTCI in order to protect their legacy as well as to mitigate their potential expenses if they are called upon to help pay for their parents' LTC."

No Confidence

I'd like to Talk with (My Kids, Attorney, Physician, CPAs)—Early in the sales process you should try to find out who will be involved in making decision and seek their participation. You may be surprised to find that advisory professionals or even family members are supportive of the concept of responsibly planning ahead for the probability of needing LTC. Not only will LTCI protect the insured's assets it will also allow him or her to maintain control of how he or she is cared for and enhances the sense of independence in choosing care options when they may be needed. Family members may even be interested in helping to finance the cost of LTCI. LTCI can reduce their anxiety regarding how they might find the time to care for a parent, acquire the skills necessary to provide for a parent, take time off from work, or psychologically deal with the role reversal of caring for a dependent parent.

Case History

Real-Life Story:
"A Very Lucky Guy"

When it comes to thoughts about LTC, the first images that come to mind for most of us are extremely aged and frail people scattered through the halls and patient rooms of nursing homes. This causes us to automatically associate the need for care with being old and helpless.

It is only in the recent past when the disability of some high profile celebrities has come to light that this has begun to change. Muhammad Ali was diagnosed with Parkinson's disease in his early 40s. Christopher Reeve was tragically injured in a fall from a horse at age 42. Michael J. Fox first realized the symptoms of Parkinson's disease at age 31. All three of these men require varying degrees of care and assistance with the activities of daily living. They are highly visible examples of the fact that you do not have to be old to need LTC.

So if the need for care can strike at any age as these examples show, why is it that so few people own LTCI? Some people say they don't believe they will ever need it. Others say they can't afford it. However, there is another reason why more people don't buy it. The need for LTC hasn't yet touched them personally. Which is why I'd like to share my own personal experience with you regarding a friend and colleague named Charlie.

I got to know Charlie back in the mid 1980s when I was a trainer for a large insurance company. Charlie was a student at that time in the initial week of "boot camp" for advisors' training, and I was one of the teachers. Over the years we stayed in touch, and in 1995 Charlie also became a trainer in a nearby office. Consequently, as colleagues we attended several meetings together each year and became good friends.

In the latter part of 1999 Charlie returned to the field to do what he loved best—be a financial advisor. Within 2 years he was doing fabulously well and was among the top 10 percent of all advisors in our company.

In June 2001, the building that housed Charlie's office was flooded, and he had to temporarily relocate to my office to transact business. To thank me, Charlie insisted on taking me to lunch. During lunch I asked how he was doing and he told me of his success in the business and of how well his children were doing. He spoke about plans to again take his family on a 2-week vacation to the Outer Banks of North Carolina as he had done every year previously. When I asked him to what he attributed his outstanding success, he said, "I guess I'm just a very lucky guy."

Charlie took his family to North Carolina and on August 3, 2001, the third day of his vacation, he became very ill with respiratory discomfort and was rushed to a nearby hospital in an ambulance.

What ensued was a nightmare. Charlie was in and out of a coma for 7 weeks with an ailment that the doctors couldn't exactly pinpoint or diagnose. There was serious doubt as to whether he would survive the ordeal. Friends in his hometown organized a fund-raising benefit to help ease the financial burden on his family and to demonstrate their support for Charlie.

Charlie's family stood vigil for weeks at the hospital's intensive care unit. The financial and emotional costs to the family were devastating. They were in a state of upheaval with the trips back and forth between North Carolina and Pennsylvania.

Finally in late September, Charlie emerged permanently from the coma and was returned to his home in Pennsylvania. It was determined that he would undergo a slow and painstaking recovery from this mysterious pulmonary disease with respiratory complications.

After weeks of treatment and various regimens of medication, Charlie's doctors finally identified Charlie's illness as Legionnaire's Disease. What followed was another 7 months of respiratory and physical therapy. Then, in April 2002, Charlie was allowed to return to work on a limited, part-time basis.

Charlie is fully recovered now and he is slowly putting the pieces of his life and his career back together. Since Charlie is only 45 years old, he will have no problem rebuilding his life.

This case demonstrates that we never know if or when we are going to need LTC. Many of us see people from afar who are disabled and it has no effect on us. However, once you attach the name and face of someone you know to LTC problems, it becomes all too real and very personal. Charlie needed convalescent and rehabilitative care at an unthinkably young age. For those of you who think you have to be old to need LTCI, just remember this story about Charlie. He could have died from his medical ordeal—but Charlie is a very lucky guy.

Chapter Four Review

Key Terms and Concepts are explained in the Glossary. Answers to the Review Questions and Self-Test Questions are found in the back of the book in the Answers to Questions section.

Key Terms and Concepts

active listening

acute care

alternative funding sources

chronic care

circle of health protection

client-focused selling

deductive approach

discovery agreement

effective communication

financial and personal resources review

inductive approach

LTC fact-finder

LTCINS links

objections: four categories

pivoting

social style

Review Questions

4-1. In a two-interview sales approach, what is the main purpose of the initial interview?

4-2. List the four social styles and describe the characteristic that best explains what a prospect with a particular style wants.

4-3. Identify the steps involved in the LTC planning process.

4-4. What are some of the sales presentation tools and techniques that can be used by an advisor to help explain the need for LTCI?

4-5. Explain what the initials LTCINS stand for and how the acronym can help an advisor obtain key information from a prospect.

4-6. What are the four characteristics of a qualified prospect for LTCI?

4-7. Explain why some prospects fail to qualify for LTCI during the fact-finding interview.

4-8. What are the three district discovery components of a formal LTC fact-finding form?

4-9. What is the name of the implied contract that you should secure at the conclusion of the fact-finding interview that represents mutual consent between the prospect and you to continue working together?

4-10. Describe two three-step techniques for responding to prospect resistance.

4-11. Identify the four general categories of objections to purchasing LTCI.

Self-Test Questions

Instructions: Read chapter 4 first, then answer the following questions to test your knowledge. There are 10 questions; circle the correct answer, then check your answers with the answer key in the back of the book.

4-1. The most important part of effective communication is

(a) talking
(b) listening
(c) understanding
(d) responding

4-2. The approach to information gathering that is characterized by using a fact-finding form that broadly covers all the prospect's financial needs and narrows the discussion to prioritized, dominant needs is the

(a) deductive approach
(b) inductive approach
(c) single-need approach
(d) dominant-need approach

4-3. At the end of which section of the LTC Fact-Finder form is it recommended that the advisor ask plan design questions about five different types of benefits?

(a) the factual section
(b) the quantitative section
(c) the attitudinal section
(d) the feeling section

4-4. The *Financial and Personal Resources Review* is a short, simple fact finder designed to

(a) quantify the need for LTCI
(b) take the place of the LTC Fact-Finder
(c) uncover information and potential objections to purchasing LTCI
(d) persuade the prospect to make a buying decision when using it

4-5. Which of the following objections to purchasing LTCI is (are) from the "no hurry" general category?

   I.   Let me think about it.
  II.   The odds are in my favor.

(a) I only
(b) II only
(c) Both I and II
(d) Neither I nor II

4-6. Which of the following statements regarding effective communication with prospects is (are) correct?

   I.   The most important part of communicating with prospects is asking a lot of questions.
  II.   Silent gestures may be a better indication of what prospects are communicating than words.

(a) I only
(b) II only
(c) Both I and II
(d) Neither I nor II

4-7. All of the following are components of the initial fact-finding interview with a LTCI prospect **EXCEPT**

(a) explaining the need for LTCI
(b) qualifying the prospect
(c) securing a discovery agreement
(d) making a sale

4-8. The Circle of Health Protection includes a discussion of all of the following topics **EXCEPT**

(a) Medicare
(b) Medicaid
(c) nursing homes
(d) assisted living facilities

4-9. In presenting the agenda for the initial interview, you should do all of the following **EXCEPT**

(a) communicate what you intend to accomplish during the meeting
(b) state a benefit for the prospect
(c) check for acceptance
(d) pave the way for getting referrals

4-10. In order to establish rapport in the initial interview, you must create an environment that promotes prospect openness by doing all of the following **EXCEPT**

(a) alleviating the prospect's concerns
(b) responding to the social style of the prospect
(c) talking most of the time with the prospect
(d) mutually agreeing to an agenda for the interview

5

The Long-Term Care Insurance Product

Overview and Learning Objectives

Chapter 5 provides an overview of the LTCI product. It also discusses the impact of the Health Insurance Portability and Accountability Act (HIPAA) on LTCI products. By reading this chapter and answering the questions, you should be able to:

5-1. Explain the principal features, benefits, and provisions of your LTCI product to a prospect.

5-2. Describe LTCI combination products.

5-3. Describe the main provisions and policy definitions of HIPAA.

5-4. Explain the tax treatment of LTCI premiums and benefits for tax-qualified and non-qualified policies.

Chapter Outline

The LTCI Product

Policy Characteristics

Differences Among Products

LTCI is a relatively new and rapidly developing product. It is a complex product, with many variations among companies. As LTC needs have changed, so have LTCI contracts. Policy innovations introduced by one company spread to and are adopted by other companies, with the process continually evolving.

Pricing for these diverse policy features varies greatly. Because LTCI is new, many insurers have little claims experience on which to base premium cost projections. Therefore, their related experience with life and disability insurance provides the basis for determining how to offer, price, and structure LTCI policies. This helps to account for many of the differences found in pricing this coverage, as each company uses different actuarial assumptions and claims experience in underwriting this product.

Adequate and competitive pricing has been a serious issue for insurers as well as state regulators. A balance between adequate and competitive pricing must allow insurers to provide affordable benefits to policyowners, cover expenses, and generate a profit for the company while remaining competitive. Otherwise, company insolvencies and/or premium increases would be inevitable. Conversely, there must be protection for the public against unfair pricing and excessive profits by insurers. Lacking a solid record of claims experience and with insurer liabilities stretched far into the future, the ability of companies and regulators to set prices has been difficult at best.

Price increases are very undesirable because they threaten a policyowner's ability to continue premium payments, and they erode the public's confidence in the products being offered by the industry. Underpricing may be even more undesirable since it may make future rate increases inevitable, or it may threaten a company's ability to pay its contractual obligations, or even to remain in operation.

For many types of insurance, policy provisions are relatively standardized. For LTCI the opposite is true. Significant variations in policy provisions and definitions, and therefore cost, exist from one insurance company to another. A prospect can choose from several different policy provisions. Consequently, properly comparing any two LTCI policies is usually a challenge. Complicating this process even further, many companies offer more than one comprehensive policy, or they offer riders that effectively convert a basic comprehensive policy into an enhanced one. It is difficult for a prospect, as well as an inexperienced advisor, to grasp the many variations in policies and be able to compare them completely and fairly. This, coupled with the wide number of options available to a prospect, makes the evaluation and comparison of LTCI policies more difficult than the evaluation and comparison of most other types of insurance.

When comparing policies, be sure to look carefully at the definitions of policy features. There can be a wide variation in definitions and coverage, and these can usually be tied to price. The general rule that you get what you pay for applies here, at least with respect to policies purchased relatively close in time. There may be some policies that are "on sale" (that is, being sold below market value) for reasons other than price, but typically if a policy is inexpensive, it probably is so for a good reason. For example, its benefits may not be as generous as those in higher-priced policies. In lower-priced policies, the benefits are usually not as favorable for the insured as those in higher-priced ones. If a policy is priced well below market, be cautious and investigate the reasons for its low price. Never assume those reasons—always read the policy to discover them.

Types of Care Covered

There are many types of care for which benefits may be provided under a LTCI policy. By broad categories, these can be identified as facility care, assisted-living, and home and community based care. A LTCI policy may provide benefits for one, several, or all of these types of care.

Facility Care (Nursing Home)—Nursing home care is a term that encompasses skilled-nursing care, intermediate care, and custodial care. All types of care can be thought of as on a care continuum from acute to chronic. An emerging, more sophisticated integration of care techniques and facilities can accommodate people along the continuum and offer a wide variety of services for different levels of care. As more need for these services evolves, we can expect the levels and types of care to improve and advance.

For many, the term *nursing home* has a negative connotation, thus the reference to *facility care*. It is for many the place that they would like to avoid, but for some it may be the only option for their families. It may be the best option if there is no one to care for the person at home. The nursing home is a place where the person will receive attention, be close to medical services, and be able to socialize with others. You should visit nursing homes in your area to become familiar with them, what they offer, and what they cost.

Although some people enter a nursing home for rehabilitation or convalescence after a hospitalization, most people who enter a nursing home for longer stays are experiencing a chronic condition. They may need services for conditions such as dementia, Alzheimer's disease, multiple sclerosis, or severe health conditions resulting from heart disease, stroke, diabetes, or arthritis. They may have lost their ability to perform ADLs, or become too sick or difficult for family members or others to care for them.

To ensure that appropriate care as well as quality care is being provided, insurers require that the nursing homes, as well as most other care providers, be properly licensed. Assessment is part of the licensing and license-maintenance procedure for nursing homes, and they must meet high standards on an ongoing basis.

Assisted-Living Facility Care—Assisted-living facility care is provided in facilities that care for those who are no longer able to care for themselves but do not need the level of care provided in a nursing home. The number and types of these facilities are growing rapidly. Assisted living facilities are intended to foster independence, dignity, privacy, and the ability to function at the maximum level while maintaining connections with the community.

Assisted living facilities offer a more home-like atmosphere than a nursing home. Their relatively recent appearance as a LTC provider has witnessed explosive growth because they offer an effective form of care in the LTC delivery system. Both insurance companies and government are behind them because there is a need for affordable alternative settings to the traditional nursing home. We simply cannot afford to put everyone who needs more care than can be provided at home in a nursing home—we need alternatives. Assisted living serves as an intermediate stage of care, between home and community care and a nursing home. It provides cost-effective services for people who need some assistance, yet it does not provide the more intensive care of a nursing home.

Home and Community-Based Care—Home health care provides for part-time, skilled-nursing care by registered and licensed practical nurses. It also provides for occupational, physical, and speech therapy as well as part-time services from licensed home health aides under the direction of a physician. Services typically include administering prescription medication, monitoring blood levels, wound care, diabetic care, incontinence management, and injections. Most people desire care at home because it provides an important foundation of emotional well-being, control of one's lifestyle, security, familiarity, privacy, and the other comforts we all associate with home.

Home and community-based care may also include benefits for one or more of the following:

- *medical equipment, emergency alert systems,* and *modifications to the home*, such as a ramp for a wheelchair or bathtub grab rails can be purchased, rented or installed. Insurers find that the cost of equipment or making minor modifications to the home is less than the cost of receiving care in a nursing home. This type of care allows the person to stay in his or her home, rather than going to a facility. These plans usually provide a benefit for equipment or modifications that is between 20 to 50 times the *maximum daily benefit (MDB)*. This may cover such things as wheelchairs, special beds, and monitoring devices. For a $150 per day policy, a benefit of 30 times the MDB would provide $4,500 for medical equipment.

- *respite care* provides for temporary institutional or home care for a person while the informal caregiver takes vacation or break time. This benefit allows occasional full-time care for a person who is receiving home health care. Respite care can be provided in a person's home or by moving the person to a nursing facility for a short stay. Insurers limit the number of days this benefit is payable. There is a separate policy maximum expressed as a maximum number of days or a dollar amount. The benefit is calculated on an annual basis and renews each year. Originally only 7 to 14 days were offered, but realizing the need and appreciation of this benefit, policies have increased this benefit to an average of 30 days.

- *adult day care* facilities offer weekday custodial care to people with light to moderate impairment. They function much like child day care, providing a supervised, safe environment for people who lack informal caregivers during the day and, therefore, cannot stay at home and function on their own. Medicine administration, meals, and some skilled nursing services are provided. Generally, people who attend adult day care need to be able to move about and toilet independently, but need some assistance with other ADLs. This, however, will vary greatly from facility to facility depending on their staff's qualifications and skills. For example, some facilities could accept wheelchair bound people and those who are catheterized for bowel and bladder movements. People with Alzheimer's disease or senile dementia may also be appropriate candidates.

- *caregiver training* provides training for a family member or friend in how to give safe and effective care, so that an insured in need of care can remain at home. Insurers recognize that it is more cost effective to train an informal caregiver than have the insured go to a nursing home. The amount payable typically is limited to a maximum of three to five times the MDB. For example, if a policy had a $100 MDB amount, the informal caregiver training would pay upwards of $300 to $500. This is normally a one-time maximum benefit.

- a *homemaker companion,* or *home health aide*, is normally an employee of a home health care agency who assists with homemaker services such as cooking, laundry, shopping, cleaning, bill paying, or other household chores. This benefit also provides personal care services in daily living, such as grooming, personal hygiene, and taking medications.

- *hospice care* does not attempt to cure medical conditions but rather treats terminally ill persons by easing their physical and psychological pain associated with death. In addition to providing services for dying people, hospices may also offer counseling to family members to help them with the physical, psychological, social, and spiritual needs of coping with the terminal illness and subsequent death of a loved one. While a hospice may be a separate facility, this type of care can also be provided on an outpatient basis in the dying person's home. Most comprehensive LTCI policies that provide benefits for hospice care make no distinction in the setting. However, some policies provide benefits only for care in a facility because Medicare provides home care benefits for those persons eligible for Medicare. In fact, Medicare pays for hospice care only when the dying person has a life expectancy of less than 6 months. If the person lives beyond the 6-month period, Medicare will continue to pay until death, provided the person's life expectancy remains at 6 months or less. The 6-month standard is now being more stringently enforced than it was in the past.

Where Care Is Provided

There are almost as many variations among LTC policies as there are insurance companies writing the product. Much of this variation is related to the types of care for which benefits are provided. These benefit variations fall into three broad categories: facility-only policies, home care only policies, and comprehensive policies.

Facility-Only Policies—Many early LTC policies were designed to provide benefits only if the insured was in a nursing home. This type of policy was frequently referred to as a *nursing home policy*. Today, however, these policies are practically unavailable in their original form. Their more modern counterparts provide benefits for care in not only nursing homes, but other settings as well, such as assisted-living facilities and hospices. While the term *facility-only policy* is often used to describe this broader type of coverage, in its most generic sense it also includes nursing home policies.

Home Health Care Only Policies—Home health care policies were originally developed to be used either as an alternative to nursing home policies or to complement such policies if more comprehensive coverage was desired. A home health care policy is designed to provide benefits for care outside an institutional setting. Some home health care policies also provide benefits for care in assisted-living facilities, and this is one area in which they often overlap with facility-only policies. While a few insurers still write stand-alone home health care policies, most other insurers have exited this market or write the coverage as part of a broader comprehensive policy.

Comprehensive Policies—Most LTCI policies written today can be described as comprehensive policies. A comprehensive policy, sometimes referred to as an integrated policy, combines benefits for facility care and home health care into a single contract. However, variations exist within this type of policy with respect to what is covered as part of the standard policy and what is an optional benefit that the prospect may select. For example, some policies cover almost all care settings as part of their standard benefits; other policies provide facility-only coverage as a standard benefit, with home health care covered as an option for an additional premium.

Originally, facility polices covering nursing homes paid benefits by offering a maximum number of days that benefits would be payable. With these indemnity (per diem) policies it was easy to understand and determine just how long the policy would pay benefits when the insured entered a nursing home. Since these policies paid a fixed-dollar amount per day regardless of actual charges, a 3-year policy meant that the insured had access to a maximum of 1,095 (3 x 365) days of benefits.

As policies began to offer comprehensive and integrated benefits covering nursing home, home care, assisted-living facilities, and more, the *pool of money* method was introduced to determine total plan benefits, regardless of where the services were provided. Today, the pool of money method is the predominant approach to determining maximum policy benefits.

Comprehensive plans base their total benefits on the total sum of money in the pool that can be paid under the policy. Although days are used, it is not in the strict sense of actually counting days of benefits, but as a way of determining the maximum dollar amount payable under the policy. The maximum dollar amount can be calculated by multiplying the number of days (years) of coverage times the MDB amount. For example, if an insured has a 2-year benefit period (730 days) and a $150 MDB amount, the pool of money is $109,500 (730 x $150 = $109,500).

As benefits are paid for the actual charges incurred up to the MDB, the pool of money is reduced by the actual dollar amount of benefits paid. There is in reality no need to count the number of days that care is received. The benefit maximum will be measured on actual dollar benefits paid, rather than the number of days of coverage used by the insured. For example, if an insured had a $150 MDB amount but only used $75 for home care expenses, the pool would be reduced by the $75 paid, not the $150 that could have been used that day. In this way, the insured has an incentive to find the least expensive care and manage the pool, since the lower the cost of care, the longer the pool will last. If the insured had a 2-year, $150 MDB amount, but only used $75 a day, the policy would in fact last 4 years. If the insured did not receive care every day, the coverage would last even longer.

Benefit Amounts

The prospect purchases the level of benefits he or she desires up to the maximum amount the company will provide. Typically, benefits are sold in increments of $10 per day up to $200 or $250 or, in a few cases, up to as much as $400 or $500 per day. Most insurance companies will not offer a MDB amount below $40 or $50.

Rather than restricting benefits to a maximum daily amount, some policies base benefits on a weekly or monthly benefit amount, such as $1,000, $2,000, or $3,000 or more. This can dramatically affect the amount of benefits paid. A MDB is the most that would be paid by the policy for any given day of benefits, even if the insured receives multiple services or incurs multiple costs on a given day. A person may receive both care from a home care agency and adult day care on a single day. On another day that same person may receive no services and/or incur no expenses. When services are actually received depends on the scheduling of services and the availability of caregivers. Insurers with a weekly maximum allowance may multiply the daily limit times seven to create a weekly amount, or simply have a weekly amount with no reference to a MDB. If a policy is paid on a weekly basis with a MDB, for example $100 per day, the insured could incur up to $700 of covered expenses on the same day and they would all be paid by the LTCI policy, provided the total amount of expenses for the week did not exceed $700. If the monthly benefit is $3,000, based on a $100 MDB amount, the insured could have up to $3,000 of paid services (30 times $100) for the month regardless of the $100 MDB amount. Alternatively, the monthly maximum benefit could be $3,000 without any reference to a MDB. In this case any covered expenses up to the $3,000 monthly maximum would be paid.

Here again, as with almost all features of LTCI policies, there is a great deal of variation in how companies measure benefits. To complicate matters further, some companies sell different policies that measure benefits differently. The way benefits are measured may be part of the basic policy, or it may be found in an optional rider. For example, a company may have a MDB, but still offer benefits on a weekly or monthly basis as a rider for an additional premium. With longer measuring periods for benefits, it is more likely that an insured will receive reimbursement for most, if not all, of his or her LTC expenses. As the measuring period increases, so will the premium.

The same level of benefits is usually provided for all levels of institutional care. Most comprehensive policies now allow prospects to select home health care equal to 100 percent of the MDB for institutional care. If a policy provides home health care benefits only, then the MDB for that coverage is what the prospect selects. Insurers today generally permit prospects to select different amounts of MDB for different types

---

"This Is Not For Us"

I met with a couple in their early 50's that were referred to me. They were in excellent health and had no history of health problems. I went through my usual sales process and could tell their reaction was " This is not for us." Needless to say they did not buy the coverage.

The prospect's father was in excellent health--a kind of physical fitness guru--very fit, very active, a "picture of health." The prospect and his father were traveling to Australia to hike and enjoy outdoor activities. Six or 7 months later I got a call from the prospect asking me to see him and his wife again. It seems that a few weeks after returning from Australia, the prospect's father had a major stroke without any warning. In addition to cognitive impairment, he was totally paralyzed on his right side and the family saw no alternative but to place him in a nursing facility that cost about $5,000 to $5,500 a month. Needless to say, when we met this time, the couple bought a LTCI policy. It's sad, but sometimes it takes a tragedy to get people to realize the need, accept the need, and do something about the need.

of providers. For example, a prospect can select a $200 MDB for nursing home care, a $150 MDB for assisted living, and a $100 MDB for home care. These MDB amounts could also be selected on a percentage basis, so that assisted living is 75 percent of the nursing home MDB, and home care is 50 percent of the nursing home MDB. Other insurers simply have a single maximum amount that is paid for all services under their LTCI policies.

Policies pay benefits in one of two ways. Some policies provide benefits on an *indemnity (per diem) basis*. This means that the full daily benefit amount is paid regardless of the actual cost of care. Benefits typically range from $50 to $500 per day. The earliest LTCI policies were of this type. For example, if the cost of a nursing home under an indemnity (per diem) policy is $150 and the insured has a MDB amount of $200, then the full $200 will be paid. Indemnity (per diem) policies are seldom coordinated with benefits that are payable under Medicare. If home health care benefits are provided by an indemnity (per diem) policy, benefits are paid after the need for home health care is certified. A few insurers will even pay if a family member provides the care at no charge, although this will increase the premium. Because indemnity (per diem) policies pay the MDB amount, regardless of the actual charges, they tend to be more expensive than comparable reimbursement policies with the same MDB amount.

The majority of newer policies pay benefits on a *reimbursement* basis. Such contracts reimburse the insured for actual expenses up to the specified policy limit. For instance, in the previous example, if the insured has a reimbursement policy instead of an indemnity (per diem) policy, only $150 per day would be paid, instead of the $200 that the indemnity (per diem) policy would pay. A tax-qualified policy that provides benefits on a reimbursement basis must be coordinated with Medicare, except when Medicare is the secondary payer of benefits. The lifetime maximum pool of money for benefit dollars can last longer under a reimbursement policy, since the insured is only using money from the pool when actually needed to cover costs. There is a trend, however, by some insurers to offer an indemnity (per diem) rider with a reimbursement policy to cover the home and community care expenses. This type of policy gives a prospect more choice in designing LTCI coverage.

Period of Benefits

To determine the period of benefits under a LTCI policy, it is necessary to look at the elimination period and the maximum duration of benefits.

Elimination Period—The prospect needs to select a period of time that must pass after LTC commences but before benefit payments begin. The majority of LTC insurers refer to this period as an *elimination period*, but some insurers call it a *waiting period* or a *deductible period*. Most insurers allow the prospect to select this period from several choices. For example, one insurer allows the choice of 20, 60, 100, or 180 days. Choices may be as low as 0 days or as high as 365 days.

In a comprehensive policy, there normally is a single elimination or waiting period that can be met by any combination of days during which the insured is in a LTC facility or receiving home health care services. However, some insurers have separate elimination periods for facility care benefits and home and community care benefits. The two elimination periods may be for the same length of time, and days used for one elimination period may or may not be used to offset each other. Generally for a day to count towards an elimination period, the insured must be responsible for paying someone or someplace for LTC services.

Some policies require the insured to meet the elimination period for each separate stay in a LTC facility or for each separate period of home health care. These policies may or may not allow the carryover

---

Two retired Connecticut residents participating in a joint LIMRA/HIAA study said:

Retiree 1: "Most insurance is pretty easy to understand. You have auto insurance, you have a car crash and get a check for the amount. If you buy a $100,000 life insurance policy, you know what you are going to get if you die. Most insurance policies are pretty easy to understand except for LTCI policies. They all have different amounts they'll pay, different waiting periods, and different benefits. The industry has made LTCI too complicated. It's expensive, yes, but I suspect more people would buy it, even with the expense if they could understand it. And because the policies are hard to understand you can't really compare them as far as I'm concerned. Maybe if you took a week and laid them all out and had a pad and pencil, maybe you could understand them. But nobody wants to do that. People take more time planning their vacation than planning their insurance needs. So I think the problem is that LTCI is too damn complicated."

Retiree 2: "Yeah, yeah, I may be dumb but I'm not stupid. I can't make heads or tails out of them. Sure I know basically what they say, but if you were to put three or four down in front of me and say `which is a better policy?' I'd have to throw a dart to determine it. So one of the problems is you don't want to buy a bad policy just like you don't want to buy a bad car or a bad house. But you can't tell. I can't tell, and I don't think anyone at this table could tell if the policy was good or bad. It's not that it's too complicated. It's that it's a new concept. Do I really need this? Is this something I can afford? You have to convince people it is a necessity and that's where the problem lies."

of days that were applied to a prior elimination period, which was not satisfied, to satisfy a new elimination period. Newer policies, however, typically do not require that more than one elimination period be satisfied during the insured's lifetime.

Some policies have an accumulation period. This gives the insured a period of time in which to satisfy the elimination period. If the insured is unable to satisfy the elimination period before the accumulation period expires, he or she has to start over and satisfy a new elimination period. For example, the policy may state that the insured has two or three times the elimination period to accumulate the days needed to trigger benefits. This can vary widely and account for premium differences. However, most new policies have no defined time limit over which days of care must accumulate. They can accumulate indefinitely until the elimination period is satisfied. As can be seen, the more restrictions placed on satisfying the elimination period, the less favorable the provision is to the insured, and it will be more difficult to qualify for benefits.

There are two ways that home health care services can be counted toward the elimination period: days of service and calendar days. Policies that follow the days of service method count only those days when actual services are received for which charges are made. For example, if an insured receives services three days during the week, this counts as three days. So if the insured's policy has a 60-day elimination period, benefit payments would not begin until the insured has been receiving services for 20 weeks (or 140 days). The other method of counting elimination period days is calendar days. This means that once a person qualifies for benefits and begins to receive services, a specific number of calendar days must pass before the policy would actually pay benefits. In other words, once the insured qualifies for benefits and begins to receive services, he or she does not have to receive services on any of the remaining calendar days for those days to be counted toward the elimination or waiting period. And since you do not have to receive services each day for the day to be counted toward the elimination period, a calendar days elimination period would in almost all instances be completed sooner than a days of service elimination period. This is especially true for home care services. For this reason, premiums for a calendar days elimination period are higher than for a days of service elimination period.

Some policies follow a blended variation of the days of service and calendar days approaches. These policies count each week as seven days toward the satisfaction of the elimination period if services were received on at least one day of the week. Under this approach, the insured in the previous example would start receiving benefit payments after 60 days have elapsed from the date the first service was received, provided that services were received at least one day each week during the 60-day period.

Another variation of the elimination or waiting period found in reimbursement policies is for the insurer to start counting days toward the satisfaction of the period as soon as a physician certifies that LTC is necessary, even if services are received from someone who does not make a charge. Therefore, family members or friends could provide the services until the elimination period is satisfied, and then the insurer would start paying benefits for the services of a paid caregiver.

Companies count days on a daily, weekly, or monthly basis, so the elimination period is measured quite differently from one policy to the next. Be cautious and read the policy provisions carefully. Do not assume all policies are the same because they use the same terms. The definitions may be very different. The way a policy defines the elimination period can obviously have a dramatic impact on premiums and benefit eligibility.

One final thought about the elimination period concerns its relationship to the requirement that tax-qualified policies cannot pay LTC benefits unless the inability to perform ADLs is expected to last at least 90 days. Actually, despite what some people think, there is no relationship! This is certification, not elimination, and it is a different concept. For example, if an insured is certified as unable to perform the requisite number of ADLs (that is, two of the six ADLs) for at least 90 days, benefit payments can start immediately after the satisfaction of the elimination period, be it 0, 20, 60, or any other specified number of days. If the insured makes a full recovery after the elimination or waiting period has been satisfied but before the 90 days have elapsed, the insured is entitled to keep any benefits already received. This is because his or her inability to perform the requisite 2 out of 6 ADLs was *expected* to last at least 90 days when benefit payments actually commenced.

In some cases, an insured will not be eligible for LTC benefits because a medical practitioner will not certify that the insured is expected to need care for as long as 90 days. If, in fact, the period of necessary care continues for 90 days and the situation is reevaluated, LTC benefits can be paid retroactively to cover the period of time from the satisfaction of the elimination period until the end of the 90 day period.

Maximum Duration of Benefits—The prospect is also given a choice as to the maximum period for which benefits are paid, often referred to as the benefit period. Note that this period only begins to run when benefit payments start after the elimination period has been satisfied. It does not start when the policy is issued. In addition, the benefit period does not necessarily coincide with each separate time period in which LTC benefits are paid. Rather, it is a period that applies to the aggregate amount of time benefits are paid under the policy. When the maximum benefits are paid, the policy will terminate. However, if benefits are only partially exhausted during an episode of LTC, they may be restored under certain circumstances, as explained later. Also, as noted earlier and explained later, the length of the benefit period may actually differ from the period chosen if the policy uses the pool of money method.

Most insurers require the prospect to select the benefit period, and they make several options available. For example, one insurer offers durations of 2, 3, and 5 years as well as lifetime benefits. A few insurers extend the maximum benefit period (if it is less than a lifetime limit) by a specified number of days for each year the insured does not collect any benefit payments. Such an extension is usually subject to an aggregate limit, such as one or 2 years. There are also a few policies, usually of the indemnity (per diem) type, that do not specify a benefit period, but only specify the maximum amount of benefits that will be paid (that is, a stated dollar amount, such as $100,000). Once the maximum benefits have been paid, the policy terminates.

Some comprehensive policies have separate benefit periods for stays in a LTC facility and home health care. For example, if each of these periods is 3 years, an insured could potentially collect benefit payments for up to 6 years—3 years while receiving benefits at home and an additional 3 years after entering a LTC facility.

There are actually two ways that the benefit period is applied in the payment of benefits. Under one approach, benefit payments are made for exactly the benefit period chosen. For example, if the insured's policy has a benefit period of 4 years and he or she collects benefits for 4 years, the benefit payments cease. The other approach, which was described earlier, uses a pool of money. Under this approach, there is a pool of money from which benefit payments are made. When the pool is exhausted, the policy terminates. However, the pool of money may last well beyond the policy's specified benefit period. The exhaustion of the pool of money will only coincide with the specified benefit period if benefits are paid every single day in an amount equal to the MDB. This usually does not happen. For example, if the MDB under a reimbursement policy is $200 and the benefit period is 1,460 days (or 4 years), then the pool of money is $292,000 ($200 x 1,460). This pool will only be exhausted at the end of 4 years of benefit payments if the MDB is paid each and every day. This is unlikely to happen unless the actual LTC charges for each day equal or exceed the MDB.

Several important points about this pool of money should be mentioned:

- Benefit payments from the pool of money cannot exceed the maximum daily, weekly, or monthly limit as specified in the policy.
- Under comprehensive policies, the pool of money is typically determined by using the MDB amount for institutional care.
- If the policy has inflation protection, the pool of money is periodically increased to take this into account.

Policy Provisions

The National Association of Insurance Commissioners (NAIC) developed the Long-Term Care Insurance Model Act and the Model Regulation that will be discussed in chapter 8. The Model Act established guidelines for insurance companies to voluntarily follow regarding policy design, policy definitions, and provisions that must be offered in policies, as well as marketing procedures and important notifications that must be given to prospects and insureds. The Model Regulation was designed to help state insurance regulators control the insurance activity within their jurisdictions and to bring some standardization to the LTCI policies being offered throughout the country.

Mode of Payment—Premiums for LTCI policies are normally expressed in terms of annual premiums. Regardless of the length of the premium-payment period, the policyowner is normally given the option of paying the annual premium in semi-annual, quarterly, or monthly installments. Payroll deduction for worksite policies is another important method of payment.

Waiver of Premium—Most LTCI policies contain a waiver-of-premium provision, under which the policyowner does not have to pay premiums after the insured has begun to receive benefit payments or has received them for a period of time. While the premiums are being waived, the policy remains fully in force.

Unlike comparable provisions in life insurance and many other types of health insurance, there are a variety of requirements that might apply to the waiver-of-premium provision for LTCI:

- Some policies begin waiving premiums at the time the elimination period has been satisfied. Other policies do not waive premiums until the insured has been collecting benefits under the policy for a period of time, such as 30, 60, or 90 days. Most policies following this approach require that the period consist of consecutive days. Still a third possibility is that premiums will be waived after a specified period during which the insured has been receiving LTC, regardless of the length of the elimination period. Under this approach, it might be possible for the premium waiver to begin before the elimination period is satisfied.

- Many comprehensive policies waive premiums if the insured is receiving benefit payments for nursing home care, but some policies waive premiums if care is received in any type of institutional setting covered by the policy, such as an assisted-living facility. Other policies also waive premiums if the insured is receiving home health care. If the waiver applies to both institutional care and home health care, there may be different provisions that apply to each type of care. For example, one insurer waives premiums after the insured has been confined in a LTC facility for 90 days. Premiums are also waived after 90 days of benefits for home health care but only if the care had been received for at least 5 days per week.

- The waiver of premiums usually ceases when the insured is no longer receiving benefits under the policy. However, some policies waive the premiums forever, even if the insured recovers from the condition that resulted in the need for LTC.

- Some policies waive the premiums for both spouses if either spouse is receiving benefits, as long as each spouse is insured with the same company. A few policies also waive the premium for a surviving spouse after the other spouse dies as long as the company insured both spouses and the policy had been in force for some period of time, such as 10 years.

Here again is a lesson in policy differences in an area as seemingly uncomplicated and basic as waiver of premium. The details and definitions vary from policy to policy. Checking to see if waiver of premium is included in a policy involves more than just a yes-or-no answer. You need to read this policy feature very carefully. Questions should be asked when comparing policies being considered for purchase, or when the policy is already in-force and is being reviewed. You should be able to answer the following questions about a company's LTCI policy:

- What triggers waiver?
- How are the elimination or waiting period days counted?
- Does the waiver pertain to home care as well as facility care?
- When does the waiver end?

Incontestability—For a LTCI policy that has been in force for less than 6 months, the insurer may rescind the policy or deny an otherwise valid claim by showing that a misrepresentation was material to the acceptance of coverage. For a LTCI policy that has been in force for at least 6 months but less than 2 years, the insurer may rescind the policy by showing that a misrepresentation was both material to the acceptance of coverage and pertained to the condition for which the benefits were sought. After a LTCI policy has been in force for two years, it is not contestable on the grounds of misrepresentation alone; it may be contested only by showing that the insured knowingly and intentionally misrepresented relevant facts about his or her health.

30-day Free Look—If a policyowner has any doubts about whether the new coverage is right for him or her, he or she has the right to return the policy to the company within 30 days for a full refund. The 30-day period begins when the policy is delivered to the policyowner. This means that either the advisor physically delivers the policy or the company mails it. The delivery must take place no longer than 30 days after the date of approval.

Grace Period—Most policies have a 31-day grace period. This means that the premium can be paid any time within the 31-day period after it is due, and during this period the policy will remain in force. However, if the premium is not paid within the grace period, the policy will lapse unless an alternative premium payer has been named.

In order to prevent the inadvertent lapse of a policy, particularly by a person with physical or cognitive impairment, the NAIC model legislation requires that the policyowner be given the option of naming another person to receive notification of the cancellation of a LTCI policy for nonpayment of premium. This provision is often referred to as an alternative premium payer provision, or the third-party notification of lapse provision. It requires the insurer, after the premium is overdue by at least 30 days, to notify both the policyowner and the alternative premium payer that (1) the premium is overdue and (2) the policy will lapse 30 days after the notice is mailed (plus 5 days for mailing), unless the premium is paid prior to that time. Some insurers allow the policyowner to name two or three alternative premium payers to receive the notice.

Reinstatement—Another provision designed to protect the insured is the reinstatement provision. It requires the insurer to reinstate a lapsed policy within 5 months after the end of the grace period (6 months from the premium due date) if the insurer receives proof that the insured was cognitively impaired at the time the premium was due. The reinstatement is retroactive to the date of lapse and is made without the insured having to show any evidence of insurability. However, any overdue premiums must be paid.

If a policy lapses for any other reason, reinstatement is at the insurer's option. Most policies provide that the policy can be reinstated if the overdue premiums are accepted by the insurer without an application. However, in most cases, the insurer will require a new application, and the case will again be subject to underwriting. If the insurer decides to reinstate the policy, the reinstatement date will be the date the insurer approves the reinstatement application. Most policies also state that if no approval is received within a specified period after paying the premium, such as 45 days, the policy will be reinstated at that time unless the policyowner has been notified that the application was disapproved. After a policy is reinstated, benefits are paid only for LTC that is received on or after the date of reinstatement.

Nonforfeiture Benefits—Most companies permit a LTCI prospect to purchase a nonforfeiture benefit, and some states as well as the NAIC model legislation require that such a benefit be offered. With a nonforfeiture benefit, the policyowner will receive some value for the policy if the policy lapses because the required premium is not paid.

The most common type of nonforfeiture option, and the one almost always available in tax-qualified policies, is a shortened benefit period. With this option, coverage is continued as a paid-up policy, but the length of the benefit period (or the amount of the benefit if stated as a maximum dollar amount) is reduced. Under the typical provision, the reduced coverage is available only if the lapse is on or after the policy's third anniversary. The amount of the benefit is equal to the greater of the total premiums paid for the policy prior to lapse or 30 times the policy's daily nursing home benefit.

Two other features related to nonforfeiture benefits should be considered.

Contingent Benefit Upon Lapse—The NAIC model legislation and most states that require an insurer to offer a nonforfeiture benefit also stipulate that a policy must provide for a contingent benefit upon lapse in cases where the nonforfeiture benefit is not purchased. This benefit allows the policyowner to select certain options each time the insurer increases the premium rate to a level that results in a cumulative increase of the annual premium equal to or exceeding a specified percentage of the premium at the time of policy issue. The percentage is a sliding scale that is determined by the issue age. For example, the percentage is 130 if the policy was issued when the insured was age 45 to 49 and 110 if the issue age was 50 to 54. The percentage amount continues to drop to 70 percent for an issue age of 60, 40 percent for an issue age of 70, and 20 percent for an issue age of 80. (See Table 5-1). The options available for the policyowner to select are (1) a reduction in benefits to a level sustainable by the current premium, or (2) the conversion of the policy to a paid-up status with a shorter benefit period. The policyowner typically must be notified of the rate increase and of these options 30 days prior to the increase. However, the policyowner is not required to select either of these options and can continue the current policy benefits by paying the higher premium amount.

Return-of-Premium Rider—Some policies offer a nonforfeiture benefit in the form of a return-of-premium rider, under which a portion of the premium is returned if the policy lapses. For example, the policy of one insurer pays nothing if the policy lapses before it has been in force for 5 full years. Fifteen percent of the total premiums paid are returned if the policy was in force for 6 years, 30 percent for 7 years, 45 percent for 8 years, 60 percent for 9 years, and 80 percent for 10 or more years. Other insurers may refund as much as 100 percent of the premiums paid. There are also some policies that refund all premiums paid if the insured dies before age 65, but if the insured dies after age 65, the percentage of the premiums refunded gradually decreases to 0 over a period of time such as 10 years. Depending on the insurer, any benefits paid while coverage was in force may or may not be deducted from the refund.

This rider is typically offered with non-qualified policies where returned premiums are not considered taxable income.

TABLE 5-1
Contingent Benefit Triggers for a Substantial Premium Increase

Issue Age	Percent Increase Over Initial Premium	Issue Age	Percent Increase Over Initial Premium
29 and under	200%	72	36%
30–34	190%	73	34%
35–39	170%	74	32%
40–44	150%	75	30%
45–49	130%	76	28%
50–54	110%	77	26%
55–59	90%	78	24%
60	70%	79	22%
61	66%	80	20%
62	62%	81	19%
63	58%	82	18%
64	54%	83	17%
65	50%	84	16%
66	48%	85	15%
67	46%	86	14%
68	44%	87	13%
69	42%	88	12%
70	40%	89	11%
71	38%	90 and over	10%

Renewability—LTCI policies currently being sold are almost always *guaranteed renewable*, which means that premiums cannot be raised for a particular insured. However, premiums can and often are raised for the whole underwriting class to which the insured belongs. Some companies offer rate guarantees in the 3- to 10-year range. This feature will come at the cost of an extra premium. In the long run, a rate guarantee probably does not mean much, since it will typically be longer than this time frame when claims will come due. Consequently, it is better to look at the history of rate increases by the company and the overall appropriateness of their premiums.

A second type of renewal provision found in LTCI policies is one that makes them noncancelable by the insurer. This type of provision offers the highest level of protection for the policyowner, since the premiums are guaranteed and the contract cannot be changed. The insurer assumes all the risk concerning the actuarial assumptions used in underwriting the policy, no matter what changes subsequently take place. The NAIC LTCI Model Regulation allows only *noncancelable* policies to use the term *"level premium."* While insurers are permitted to issue policies that are noncancelable, very few policies of this type are written because of the uncertain nature of future claim costs.

Limitations and Exclusions—With some exceptions, most LTCI policies contain the exclusions permitted by the NAIC model legislation. These exclusions are listed below. One area where differences are found among insurers pertains to mental health. This is an area that insurers avoid as much as possible because of the possibility of fraudulent claims and the controversies that often arise over claim settlements. A few insurers cover mental and nervous disorders just as they cover physical disorders. However, most insurers use a typical policy exclusion: "This policy does not provide benefits for the care or treatment of mental or nervous disorders without a demonstrable organic cause." This exclusion denies benefits for conditions such as schizophrenia and depression. However, conditions such as Alzheimer's or Parkinson's disease would be covered. As a result of state law, many insurers state in their policies that Alzheimer's and Parkinson's are covered.

Some of the other areas where an insurer's exclusions might differ from the NAIC model legislation include:

- Most policies do not exclude benefits for expenses or services that are covered under another policy. Rather, the issue of other insurance is a factor taken into consideration during the underwriting process.

- Policies written on an indemnity (per diem) basis seldom exclude services or expenses that are provided under Medicare, although policyowners may have the option when purchasing such contracts to coordinate them with Medicare. Policies that coordinate with Medicare will be less expensive than policies that do not. To be tax-qualified under HIPAA (discussed later in this chapter), policies written on a reimbursement basis must coordinate their benefits with Medicare. In most cases, the exclusion is only for actual duplicate coverage. In some cases, however, the exclusion also applies to amounts that are not paid by Medicare because of its deductible and coinsurance provisions.

- While most policies do not provide benefits for services or treatment received outside the United States, some insurers provide benefits while the insured is in Canada. In addition, a few insurers provide benefits for a limited period, such as 30 or 90 days, for services or treatment received in any foreign country. Like many other LTCI benefits, there is liberalization in this area, and worldwide coverage is becoming more common.

- Some policies have a preexisting-conditions provision that specifies benefits will not be paid within the first 6 months for a condition for which treatment was recommended or received within 6 months of policy purchase. However, other policies have no such provision regarding preexisting conditions listed on the policy application. There is little need for such a provision because insurers in most states are not allowed to use post-claims underwriting. If properly underwritten at the time of application, claims within the usual preexisting-conditions period are unlikely to occur. Elimination or waiting periods for benefits often serve a similar purpose.

Under the NAIC LTCI Model Regulation, a LTCI policy may not limit or exclude coverage except for:

- preexisting conditions or disease
- mental or nervous disorders (this does not permit the exclusion of Alzheimer's disease)
- alcoholism and drug addiction

- illness, treatment, or medical condition arising out of war, participation in a felony, service in the armed forces, attempted suicide, and aviation if a person is a non-fare-paying passenger
- treatment provided in a government facility, unless required by law
- services or items available or paid under another LTCI or health policy
- services for which expenses are reimbursable under Title XVIII of the Social Security Act or would be so reimbursable but for the application of a deductible or coinsurance amount. These services include:
  - services for which benefits are available under Medicare or other governmental program, with the exception of Medicaid
  - services for which benefits are available under any workers' compensation, employer's liability, or occupational disease law
  - services available under any motor vehicle law
  - services provided by a member of the covered person's immediate family
  - services for which no charge is normally made in the absence of insurance
  - services available or paid under another LTCI or health policy

Shared or Joint Benefit—A few insurers provide for a shared benefit for a husband and wife. Under this benefit, each spouse can access the benefits of the other spouse. For example, if each spouse has a 4-year benefit period and one spouse has exhausted his or her benefits, benefit payments can continue by drawing on any unused benefits under the other spouse's policy. In effect, one spouse could have a benefit period of up to 8 years as long as the other spouse received no benefit payments. If the insurer uses the pool-of-money method, a single pool combines the benefits of both spouses, and either or both spouses can draw benefit payments from the pool. In another variation of benefit sharing, an insurer might allow the transfer of any unused benefits to a surviving spouse's policy, or an insurer might allow the spouses to purchase an extra pool of money equal to the separate pool of money on each spouse. If either or both spouses exhaust their individual pools, this extra pool can be accessed. In addition, there is at least one insurer that offers a shared benefit for family members. Based on the significant difference in money available under these three optional benefits, the total annual premiums can vary by as much as 40 percent depending on which option is selected. These optional benefits demonstrate that it is not enough to know that a policy offers some type of shared benefit. You must carefully study the exact policy language to understand the differences when comparing policies.

Survivorship Benefits—Survivorship benefits are another variation on the shared benefit theme. This type of benefit may be included in the basic coverage, or added as an optional rider when both spouses own a policy or are covered under the same policy. A typical provision states that if the coverage remains in force for a specified number of years and one spouse dies without having received any benefits, the surviving spouse would then have a paid-up policy. You could interpret this provision as a lifetime premium waiver for the survivor. Different policies require different in-force time durations, as well as whether or not the payment of a claim would terminate the benefit.

This benefit provides yet another example of how coverage variations can be found in different policies. The more generous policies provide a full survivorship benefit after the required in-force time duration regardless of whether a claim was paid. You should expect, however, that this more generous provision would also be more expensive. In addition, some companies allow this benefit to apply to committed couples of the same or different sexes, with or without a civil or religious ceremony to unite them, or to two family members living in the same household. As you can see, some policies are more liberal than others. These survivorship benefits may be best suited for situations where at least one of the spouses has a family health history where someone required LTC, or where there is a large age difference between the spouses.

Restoration of Benefits—A few companies offer a restoration-of-benefits provision with their policies that are written with less than a lifetime benefit period. Under this provision, insureds can have their full complement of benefits restored if they previously received less than full policy benefits and have not received any policy benefits for a certain time period, often 180 days. Without this provision, the benefits available for a subsequent claim would be reduced by the benefits previously paid. This type of provision may be included as part of the policy's basic coverage, or it can be added as a rider for an additional premium. The use of this benefit has been infrequent, perhaps because as the duration of chronic illness claims increases, the chance of recovery and being able to restore benefits decreases.

Inflation Protection—Most states require that a LTCI policy offer some type of automatic inflation protection. The prospect is given the choice of selecting this option, declining the option, or possibly selecting an alternative option. The cost of an automatic inflation option is usually built into the initial annual premium, and no additional premium is levied at the time of each annual increase in benefit amount. However, a few insurers increase the annual premium each year in a step-rate fashion to reflect the automatic increase in benefit amount.

As a result of the NAIC LTCI Model Act and HIPAA, the typical provision found in almost all policies is a 5-percent benefit increase that is compounded annually over the life of the policy. Under such a provision, the amount of a policy's benefits increases by 5 percent each year over the amount of benefits available in the prior year. New benefit amounts are often rounded to the nearest dollar.

A common alternative that many insurers make available is based on simple interest, with each annual automatic increase being 5 percent of the original benefit amount. Other inflation options that are occasionally found are increases (either simple or compound) based on different fixed percentage amounts, such as 3 or 4 percent.

The effect of an automatic increase in benefits can be dramatic, as shown in Table 5-2, below. However, an automatic increase provision is also accompanied by significantly higher premiums.

TABLE 5-2 Effect of an Automatic Increase on a $100 Per Day Benefit			
End of Policy Year	No Increase	5% Simple Interest	5% Compound Interest
5	$100	$125	$128
10	100	150	163
15	100	175	208
20	100	200	265
25	100	225	339
30	100	250	432

If an automatic inflation option is not selected, some insurers allow the policyowner to increase benefits without evidence of insurability on a pay-as-you-go basis at specified intervals, such as every one, 2, or 3 years. Each benefit increase is accompanied by a premium increase that is based on the attained-age rates for the additional coverage.

The amount of the periodic benefit increase under a pay-as-you-go option may be a fixed dollar amount, such as a daily benefit increase of $20, or a percentage amount based on an index, such as the CPI. Some insurers have an aggregate limit on the total amount of benefit increases or an age beyond which they are no longer available. Failure to exercise a periodic benefit increase or a series of such increases over a specified period of time typically terminates the right to purchase the additional benefits in the future.

It is important to note that increases in benefits are often inadequate to offset actual inflation in the annual cost of LTC, which has shown double-digit increases over the last decade.

Bed Reservation Benefit—Policies that provide nursing home care often provide a bed reservation benefit, which continues policy payments to a LTC facility for a limited time (such as 20 days) if the insured temporarily leaves the facility. It may be that insured needs to be hospitalized for an acute condition or wishes to take a personal leave from the nursing home to attend a family reunion or holiday activity. Without the continuation of payments to the facility, the bed may be rented to someone else and unavailable upon the insured's return. A standard requirement for this benefit to take effect is that the insured must have satisfied the elimination or waiting period and be qualified to receive benefits under the policy.

Premium-Payment Period—The majority of LTCI policies have premiums that are payable for life and determined by the age of the insured at the time of issue. For example, a policy may have an annual cost of $800 at the time of purchase. Assuming the policy is guaranteed renewable, this premium will not change unless it is raised on a class basis. However, a few insurers will not raise premiums for a specified period after a policy has been issued. In the past, guaranteed renewable policies were often advertised as being "level premium," but this is misleading because premiums may be, and in some cases have been, increased by class. As a result, the current NAIC LTCI Model Act prohibits the use of this term unless a policy is noncancelable, which means that rates cannot increase. A few companies have guaranteed renewable policies with scheduled premium increases. These increases may occur as frequently as annually or as infrequently as every 5 years.

In recent years, insurers have increasingly begun to offer accelerated premium payment periods. These shorter premium-payment periods, which result in higher annual premiums, are popular with many insureds that want to have their policies paid for prior to retirement. Some of the accelerated premium payment options include:

- a single-premium option (one-time payment)
- a paid-up-at-65 option under which the policyowner pays an annual premium until he or she reaches age 65
- a shortened payment period of 2, 5, 10, or 20 years

After all the premiums have been paid under one of the accelerated premium payment options, the policy is paid-up and no subsequent premiums are required to keep the policy in force. With premiums being paid on an accelerated basis, the policyowner has a lot to lose if the policy terminates in a short period of time—because of either lapse or death. As a result, some states require some type of return-of-premium rider to accompany an accelerated premium payment period of 10 years or less.

Spousal (or Partner) Discounts—Most policies today offer some type of spousal or (partner) discount, although they vary considerably in their scope and complexity. Depending on the requirements of the issuing company and the application state, the discounts may vary depending on whether both spouses are accepted by the same company; or only one spouse is accepted. Some states even require that a married person be given the discount whether or not the spouse applies for or is even insurable for LTCI. In fact, some companies offer the discount to unmarried couples or same-sex partners. Whatever the combination of the two adults, they typically must be from the same generation and live in the same household. However, some newer policies can cover several members of the same family who are from different generations. The variations of this benefit, like so many others in LTCI, continue to be introduced and break old design models. Living with another person tends to lower the need for LTC, so companies are gradually becoming more favorably disposed to offering these types of discounts.

Although there is a trend to somewhat higher premiums overall, the amount of the spousal (or partner) discount continues to increase. Where 10 percent for each spouse (or partner) used to be the standard discount, 15 to 20 percent is now typical, with a few companies increasing the discount to 25 percent or even to as much as 40 percent.

This is one area where you may receive many questions about the amount and type of discount, particularly from individual people who will not qualify. The reason for the discount not applying to individual people is that they are more likely to go on claim than are people with spouses or partners who can assist with and/or supervise the caregiving process and provide for companionship and support.

Care Coordination—Many policies provide for the services of a care coordinator who works with the insured, his or her family, and licensed health care practitioners. The care coordinator's function is to assess the insured's condition, identify needs, evaluate care options, and develop an individualized plan of care that provides the most appropriate services. The care coordinator may also periodically reevaluate ongoing plans of care and act as an advocate for the insured. In many cases, the care coordinator is recommended by the insurance company but is not its employee or an employee of a care provider. Care coordinators most often work for independent agencies and have social work or nursing backgrounds. They understand the admissions and qualification process for entering LTC facilities and how to place insureds with appropriate care providers. This is especially important for home and community care. Many care coordinators work for large organizations that can negotiate with care providers based on the large business volume they can bring to these providers.

This type of coverage varies greatly from company to company. Some policies require care coordination, some have no provision for it, and others may have a variety of similar provisions. If a care coordinator recommended by the insurer is used, additional benefits might be available to the

---

Care Coordination: The Prospect's Perspective

The need for LTC often presents new emotional, practical, and financial challenges for individuals and families. In reviewing policies, the family decision-makers should ask the following questions about care coordination:

- Does the policy offer care coordination? How does it work?
- What are the qualifications and experience of the care coordinators?
- Are the care coordination services local?
- Are the services a part of the basic policy or do they cost extra?
- Who decides what care is prescribed, the care coordinator or the insured?

---

insured, such as the waiving of elimination or waiting periods, increased benefit levels, or no decrease in maximum policy benefits that might otherwise occur because of the cost of using the care coordinator. Care coordination may be a part of the basic policy, or it may be an additional benefit with a separate charge. However, if the insured or his or her family selects a care coordinator that is not recommended by the insurer, there may or may not be coverage.

Alternative Plans of Care—Many policies provide benefits for alternative plans of care, even though the types of care might not be covered in the policy. For example, a policy covering nursing home care only might provide home health care benefits if these benefits are less expensive than care in a nursing home. As a general rule, the alternative plan must be acceptable to the insurer, the insured, and the insured's physician. It is intended to be mutually beneficial to both the insurer and the insured. If done properly, it can save the insurer claims money and provide the insured with more comfortable care that better meets his or her needs. The adoption of an alternative plan also interacts with the use of a care coordinator.

An alternative plans clause serves as a "catch-all" provision to accommodate changes in LTC services and coverage that will most certainly occur in the future. Today there is a constant introduction of new policy features and modifications of existing ones. There are also new types of facilities, services, and provider options that are continually being made available. Not long ago there were no adult day care centers and no assisted living facilities. Without such flexibility being built into policies, they may not be able to cover new types of services that become available in the future and, consequently, will become outdated long before they may be needed years later.

Combination Products

Today prospects can choose from several different insurance products to cover LTC expenses. Of course, the most widely recognized and utilized is the individual LTCI policy that provides benefits on either an indemnity (per diem) basis or a reimbursement basis. Additionally, there are several combination products that package other insurance coverage with LTCI. Under these package products, life insurance, disability income insurance, or an annuity is combined with LTCI to provide customized solutions to a variety of prospect needs and goals. These combination products have been referred to as *hybrid products*, *linked policies*, *blended polices*, or *packaged policies*.

There are two very compelling reasons why these combination products have been developed. First, packaging two products together can create benefits with added appeal for the right prospect. Second, because many prospects are concerned about paying a large amount of money for LTC protection that they may never use, packaging LTCI with another coverage makes for a more acceptable product than LTCI by itself. Nevertheless, sales growth for combination products has been modest because many companies market them less aggressively.

The slow sales growth of combination products is due to several factors. First, many of them were designed to take advantage of the high interest rates and the continually increasing stock market values that existed a few years ago. Now that interest rates are lower and stock market values have fallen, these products are less attractive. Second, these products combine complex LTCI policies with complex life insurance or annuity contracts. The resulting policies are quite difficult for advisors to understand and explain to their prospects. Third, many advisors view LTCI as meeting a different need than a life insurance or annuity contract, and feel that separate products should be used for each need.

Life Insurance/ LTCI Combination Products

The life insurance in a life insurance/LTCI combination product can take the form of almost any type of cash value life insurance, but most combination products that have been sold to date use universal life insurance, including variable universal life insurance. Premiums can be paid in any mode, but most sales involve the payment of a single premium. Single-premium products can work well using whole life, universal life, or variable life designs. The large single premium typically will provide for a significant death benefit, and the cash values will grow tax-deferred. Purchased with a single premium, this combination may be especially valuable if the prospect has a lump sum of money earning a low rate of interest and seeks both LTCI and life insurance protection.

Purchasers of single-premium combination products tend to be people of moderate-to-high net worth who transfer assets from traditionally low-yielding investments, such as money market accounts and certificates of deposit. They also tend to be people who feel their heirs should receive something (a death benefit) from them to the extent that they do not need their wealth for living or for LTC expenses.

Additionally, these people like to keep control of their own financial options and they like the tax-favored nature of life insurance.

Permanent (cash value) life insurance packaged with LTCI creates an appealing product that can meet multiple needs. The life insurance provides income-tax-free death protection as well as lifetime cash values that can be used if LTCI is not needed. The existence of life insurance provides an additional reason for buying this unique product. It may overcome the most common objection to buying a stand-alone LTCI policy, which is that the premium would be wasted if the LTC benefits were never needed.

Universal Life (UL) Insurance Coverage

As indicated above, the most common type of life insurance/LTCI combination product uses universal life. The following discussion dissects this combination product and focuses on each coverage separately, starting with universal life.

Universal life (UL) insurance is an interest-sensitive product that, unlike traditional cash value life insurance, divides the pure life insurance protection and the cash value accumulation into separate and distinct components. The insured is required to pay a specified initial premium for the amount of coverage desired. After a deduction to cover state premium taxes and administrative expenses, the premium is used to create a cash value account. Each month, deductions are made from this account to pay for the life insurance protection and, in the case of a combination product, for the LTCI protection. Interest is also credited monthly to this account on an ongoing basis.

The insured receives an annual statement that shows contract values and any transactions that have taken place during the year. The statement is provided on a monthly basis if the insured is receiving LTC benefits.

Characteristics of the UL insurance combination coverage include a guaranteed minimum interest rate—usually 4 percent—credited to the cash value account. Often, however, the insurer pays a higher initial interest rate, currently ranging from 5 to 6 percent. This initial interest rate remains in effect for a minimum period of time, usually one year. After that time, the insurer can adjust the rate on a monthly, quarterly, or semi-annual basis, subject to the minimum guarantee.

At the time the contract is purchased, the benefits are determined on the basis of the current interest rate being credited. If this interest rate changes, the projected cash value account may also change. If the rate decreases, the cash value account may become insufficient to pay the required insurance and expense charges. In such cases, the insured is often given the option of paying an additional premium to bring the cash value account back to its projected level so that the original contract benefits can be maintained, or to reduce the amounts of the death benefit and/or monthly LTC benefit.

Any growth in the cash value account is tax deferred. However, if the account grows beyond the total premiums paid, any deductions for the LTCI protection may represent taxable income. (Tax experts and insurers disagree on this issue, and there is no definitive IRS opinion.) If the insured is under age 59½, there is also a penalty tax if the deductions are treated as withdrawals.

- Charges for the insurance protection are usually subject to the insurer's current mortality experience for a period of time, after which they may change. As with interest rates, any changes will affect the contract's cash value account and possibly its benefits.

- The policyowner is usually allowed to take loans from the cash value account. There is an interest charge for these loans, and any loan is subtracted from the death benefit. An outstanding loan may also result in the lapse of the contract if the loan exceeds the amount in the cash value account.

- The policyowner is also usually allowed to take partial surrenders of the cash value. However, there may be a surrender charge, particularly in the early years of the contract. Any surrender reduces the amount of insurance proportionately.

- When this combination product is purchased with a single premium, there usually is a lifetime money-back guarantee. If the insured surrenders the contract for any reason, the amount received upon surrender is never less than the premiums paid, less any amounts taken as partial surrenders or loans or paid as LTC benefits. Any withdrawal from a single-premium contract—whether it is a loan, a LTCI premium, or some or all of the cash value—is subject to income taxation. This is because the contract, when purchased with a single premium, is classified as a modified endowment contract (MEC) under IRC Section 7702A. And when an insurance contract is a MEC, any distribution that represents a gain is subject to income taxation, and any taxable distribution prior to the insured's age 59½ is also subject to a 10 percent penalty.

For an insured who wishes to be more speculative, some insurers offer variable universal life (VUL) insurance/LTCI combination products. Instead of crediting the cash value account with periodic interest, the insured elects to have the cash value account invested in one or more of several different types of investment funds, which subjects the account and insurance benefits to an even greater possibility of fluctuation.

LTCI Coverage

In a combination product, LTCI is designed to be tax-qualified and is subject to most of the same HIPAA and state regulations that apply to an individual LTCI policy. However, these combination products are treated as life insurance policies that accelerate the death benefit to pay for LTC expenses, similar in concept to the accelerated death benefit rider in a stand-alone life insurance policy, so they are treated somewhat differently under state regulations than a stand-alone LTCI policy. Nevertheless, the LTCI design under a combination product is similar to that found in comprehensive policies sold on a stand-alone basis. Despite the similarities, there are still several differences between the stand-alone policies and combination products. Combination products differ as follows:

- The amount of the LTCI benefit is a function of the amount of life insurance protection purchased. Or conversely, the LTCI benefit amount dictates the amount of life insurance required to provide that benefit.
- The LTCI benefit periods are often limited to 2, 3, or 4 years. However, some insurers make lifetime benefits available.
- There is usually no choice of the elimination or waiting period. The usual period is 90 days.
- There is usually no automatic option to protect against inflation. An annual election to increase the death benefit and the LTCI benefit by 5 percent of the prior year's coverages may be available. Failure to exercise the annual option may result in the loss of the right to elect additional coverage in the future.
- There is no LTCI nonforfeiture benefit because the cash value of the life insurance serves this function.

The type of LTCI combination product described above pays daily LTC expenses in the same way as under a stand-alone LTCI policy. It also provides a death benefit that pays the remaining portion of the face amount not previously utilized for LTC expenses. However, because prospects' concern that LTCI benefits may never be used originally led to the development of this product, the amount of any death benefit that remains after paying for LTC expenses should be less of a concern.

Another type of combination product accelerates the death benefit by paying 25 percent of the face amount every 6 months if the insured is confined to a nursing home for 90 days or receives care under a home care plan. This type of contract will also accelerate the death benefit payment if the insured is diagnosed with a terminal illness, regardless of any nursing home confinement or the completion of a 90-day elimination or waiting period. A few insurers offer life insurance and LTCI in a combination product where the coverages are completely separate. In these packages, use of the LTC benefits will not reduce the death benefit as the premium for each coverage is determined separately.

The packaging of life insurance with LTCI can enhance the salability of both coverages. For example, asset repositioning allows a prospect to liquidate an asset that is not performing well or that is not committed to a particular need and invest the money in a single premium combination product that provides LTC protection during life and a lump-sum benefit at death. You can explain to the prospect how life insurance cash values increase on a tax-deferred basis. The rate of return will possibly equal or exceed the rate that was being earned by an asset that was repositioned or the rate that could have been earned from a comparable investment that is subject to current income taxation. The prospect's risk profile, suitability, and needs can be closely matched with a policy type. However, it should be remembered that these combination products are more expensive than stand-alone LTCI policies because they involve both mortality and morbidity costs, and the benefits are being provided for more than one type of coverage.

Disability income/LTCI Combinations

LTCI is a health insurance product, a catastrophic disability income policy in a sense. The combination of disability income insurance and LTCI in one package is natural since both provide protection from essentially the same risk. At least one carrier has a disability income product that can be exchanged for a LTCI policy between the ages of 60 and 70. This disability income policy also can be purchased with a rider that allows the insured to increase the amount of LTC benefits available when the exchange takes place. At least one group disability policy provides that if a disabled individual loses the ability to perform two or more ADLs, the disability benefit will be increased by a certain percentage to provide for LTC expenses. It can be anticipated that the development of new products in this area will continue to evolve over time.

Example of a Universal Life/LTCI Combination Product

This combination product uses universal life insurance and requires a single premium of at least $10,000 or, if greater, a single premium of sufficient size to purchase a minimum face amount. The contract also includes a LTCI benefit that in the aggregate is double the life insurance death benefit. The LTCI coverage provides benefits on a reimbursement basis from a pool of money, and the benefits can be used for all types of LTC services. For an additional premium, benefits can be increased by 5 percent each year to help fight inflation.

Helen has decided to purchase this contract at age 60 with 4 years of benefits at $200 per day. She needs total LTC benefits of $292,000 (1460 days times $200 per day). If Helen fits into the insurer's best underwriting classification, her lump sum premium is $52,000. For this premium, Helen also receives a $146,000 death benefit. If Helen purchases this contract and dies without needing the LTC benefit, her beneficiary will receive the $146,000 death benefit. If Helen receives up to $146,000 in LTC benefits before her death, her beneficiary will still receive a $146,000 death benefit. However, if Helen receives LTC benefits greater than $146,000, the excess amount over the death benefit will be deducted from the death benefit. For instance, if Helen receives $200,000 in LTC benefits, her death benefit will be reduced by $54,000 ($200,000 less $146,000) to $92,000. This contract, like those of many other insurers, has a minimum death benefit equal to 10 percent of the life insurance face amount. Therefore, Helen's beneficiary will always be able to receive a death benefit of at least $14,600.

Please note that these benefit amounts would be different if Helen had purchased additional benefits or if she had taken any loans or made any withdrawals. Also note that there are other variations of how the death benefit is offset or reduced by the payment of LTC benefits.

Annuity/LTCI Combinations

Annuity/LTCI combinations are a relatively new innovation, and though few such products exist today, future growth is expected. With this type of product, asset accumulation can be combined with asset protection and preservation.

For example, an annuity/LTCI combination product may be funded by a single deposit that creates a separate benefit for both needs. The deposit buys an amount of LTC protection equal to twice the value of the annuity account. The policyowner, in effect, triples his or her protection for LTC by purchasing the annuity. The annuity account grows tax-deferred to accumulate funds at a fixed rate of interest, with all the usual annuity options available. In the event of a need for LTC benefits, the first benefit payments are considered a liquidation of the annuity account. After the annuity account is liquidated, the remaining LTC benefits come from the LTCI portion of the contract. Because the policyowner is, in effect, paying for LTC expenses with his or her own money from the annuity account before any LTCI benefits start, the insurer has time before its liability begins, thus lowering costs and the underwriting time needed to issue the contract. If the insured dies before receiving any benefits from the contract, a death benefit equal to the original deposit is paid to the beneficiary.

Under the combination product of another insurer, the insured purchases a deferred variable annuity. The initial deposit is split between two accounts, one for the annuity and the other to fund the LTC benefits. The insured has the choice of several options for each account, and the final annuity and LTC benefit amounts depend on investment results. This insurer's product provides two totally separate benefits. If the insured withdraws annuity benefits, there is no effect on the LTC benefits. Similarly, if the insured uses LTC benefits, the annuity account remains unaffected. There is a guaranteed death benefit under the contract, so that the

---

A Product Innovation to Follow

"Annuity and LTC combination contracts are a product innovation you need to follow. These are annuity contracts that have embedded LTC benefits. Not many exist today, but more will debut in the face of rapidly rising demand. A definite market for the product already exists, given the huge buildup that has occurred in annuity ownership. As owners of these contracts approach retirement age and beyond, they will become less concerned with asset accumulation and increasingly concerned with asset preservation and independence."

Source: Cary Lakenbach, "Keep an eye on Annuity/LTC Combos," National Underwriter, January 15, 2001, p.16.

---

insured's beneficiary always receives an amount at least equal to the initial deposit.

A few companies have introduced innovative annuity designs that may gain more recognition and popularity as the public and the industry look for solutions to address the LTC funding problem. An *underwritten or impaired risk annuity* is medically underwritten by the insurer. Those people who have a shorter life expectancy than normal receive a higher monthly income amount. Another annuity combination product design that addresses LTC needs has two accounts: one that pays a regular interest rate and another that pays a significantly higher rate. The first account works like a traditional annuity, while the second allows withdrawals only if the person needs assistance with at least two ADLs or has cognitive impairment. Another, similar annuity combination product allows higher payments once a person demonstrates functional impairment. The LTC benefit is paid on a reimbursement basis. Monthly maximums are set. If the person does not use all of the money on LTC, the amount remaining in the cash fund will then pass at death to the beneficiary outside of probate. Whether the product is tax-qualified or non-qualified is significant, since taxes may be due on any money that is dispersed for LTC from a non-qualified product.

There are three waiver provisions found in annuity contracts that can be used in case of a need for LTC services. These waiver provisions may require that the contract be in force for a certain period of time and that an elimination or waiting period of 90 or 180 days of confinement be met before the waiver takes effect. A *nursing home waiver* is an annuity contract provision that allows for the withdrawal of cash values to help pay for nursing home expenses without applying any surrender charges. A *terminal illness waiver* works very much like a life insurance accelerated death benefit provision. If the person has a limited life expectancy as certified by a physician, the insurer will eliminate the surrender charge on the cash value. Lastly, a *disability waiver* will waive surrender charges if the person is unable to work due to injury or illness.

Annuities, either immediate or deferred, can also be used to help prepare for the LTC needs of those who are uninsurable, and who

---

Financing Alternatives

Another use of annuities, cash value life insurance, or mutual funds is to use the contract values to pay LTCI premiums. Some companies have formal programs for withdrawing money from one of these types of contracts to pay premiums on a LTC policy without company surrender charges. Any federal or state tax penalties would be applicable.

---

already have some need for services. This use of annuities is discussed elsewhere in this book.

Effect of HIPAA Legislation

The Health Insurance Portability and Accountability Act of 1996 (HIPAA) established standards for LTCI and helped to stabilize the industry, which up until that time had little uniformity. It also made the tax treatment of LTCI policies more favorable if they met prescribed standards. In most cases, the imposition of these federal standards resulted in broader coverage. Policies issued on or after January 1, 1997 generally must meet the federal standards to be considered tax-qualified, while policies in force before January 1, 1997 generally are grandfathered and automatically qualify for tax benefits.

It should be emphasized that changes brought about by HIPAA primarily relate to federal income tax law. However, states still have authority to regulate LTCI contracts and are not required to bring state regulations into conformity with federal tax law changes. Nevertheless, all states allow tax-qualified contracts so consumers can obtain the favorable tax benefits.

Eligibility for Favorable Tax Treatment

To understand whether a LTCI policy will receive favorable income tax treatment under HIPAA, it is necessary to understand the meaning of several terms.

Qualified LTCI Contract—HIPAA provides favorable income tax treatment to a qualified LTCI contract This is defined as any LTCI contract that meets all the following requirements:

- *Chronic Illness Definition*—The insured must require substantial assistance with at least 2 of 6 ADLs or be cognitively impaired.
- *Chronic Illness Certification*—A licensed health care practitioner must at least annually certify that the insured remains chronically ill.
- *No Medical Necessity Trigger*—A licensed health care practitioner's recommendation alone cannot trigger benefit payments.

- *90-day Expectation of Disability*—A licensed health care practitioner must certify that ADL dependency is expected to last at least 90 days.

- *Qualified Long-Term Care Restriction*—The insured must receive services that help him or her perform ADLs or that provide substantial supervision for cognitive impairment. The only insurance protection provided under the contract is for qualified LTC services. However, an indemnity (per diem) contract can satisfy this requirement even though payments are made without regard to the expenses incurred during the period to which the payments relate, provided the payments do not exceed $220 per day in 2003.

- *Coordination with Medicare*—The contract cannot pay for expenses that are reimbursable under Medicare or would be reimbursable except for the application of a deductible or coinsurance amount. However, this requirement does not apply to expenses that are reimbursable if (1) Medicare is a secondary payer of benefits, or (2) benefits are paid on an indemnity (per diem) or other periodic basis without regard to the expenses incurred during the period to which the benefits relate.

- *Guaranteed Renewable*—The contract must be guaranteed renewable.

- *No Cash Value*—The contract does not provide for a cash surrender value or other money that can be borrowed or paid, assigned, or pledged as collateral for a loan.

- *Treatment of Refunds and Dividends*—All refunds of premiums and all policyowner dividends must be applied as future reductions in premiums or to increase future benefits. A refund in the event of the death of the insured or a complete surrender or cancellation of the contract cannot exceed the aggregate premiums paid under the contract.

- *Consumer Protection Provisions*—The contract must comply with various consumer protection provisions. For the most part, these are the same provisions contained in the NAIC LTCI Model Act and already adopted by most states.

- *Life Insurance/LTCI Combination Product*—The act also specifies that a qualified LTCI contract can include that portion of a life insurance contract that provides LTCI coverage by a rider or as part of the life contract as long as the above criteria are satisfied.

While the term qualified LTCI contract is used in HIPAA and the Internal Revenue Code, different terminology is often used for the sake of brevity. Thus, it is common to see these contracts referred to as tax-qualified (TQ) contracts (or policies) and non-qualified (NQ) contracts (or policies).

To further complicate the issue of terminology, sometimes the reference to tax-qualified contracts is preceded by the word federally to clarify that HIPAA provides favorable income tax treatment with respect to federal tax laws, not state tax laws. However, it should be noted that most states do not tax LTCI benefits.

Qualified LTC Services—HIPAA defines qualified LTC services as necessary diagnostic, preventive, therapeutic, curing, treating, and rehabilitative services, and maintenance or personal care services that are required by a chronically ill person and are provided by a plan of care prescribed by a licensed health care practitioner.

Chronically Ill Person—A chronically ill person is one who has been certified by a licensed health care practitioner as meeting one of the following requirements:

- The person is expected to be unable to perform, without substantial assistance from another person, at least two activities of daily living (ADLs) for a period of at least 90 days due to a loss of functional capacity. HIPAA allows six ADLs: eating, bathing, dressing, transferring from bed to chair, using the toilet, and maintaining continence. A tax-qualified LTCI policy must contain at least five of the six.
- Substantial services are required to protect the person from threats to health and safety due to substantial cognitive impairment.

For purposes of certifying a person as chronically ill, a licensed health care practitioner is a physician, a registered professional nurse, licensed social worker, or other person who meets requirements prescribed by the Secretary of the Treasury. Recertification must take place at least every 12 months.

Benefit Eligibility

All tax-qualified LTCI contracts use the same two criteria, known as *benefit triggers*, for determining whether an insured is chronically ill and eligible for benefits. The insured is required to meet one of the two criteria. The first criterion or benefit trigger is that the insured is expected to be unable, without *substantial assistance* from another person, to perform at least two (out of six) ADLs for a period of at least 90 days due to a loss of functional capacity. Prior to HIPAA, these terms were undefined and left to interpretation by each company. An Internal Revenue Service notice clarified the definitions of these terms as they are used to meet the federal standards for benefits.

Substantial assistance includes either or both of the following:

- *Hands-on assistance*—The physical assistance of another person to perform ADLs.
- *Standby assistance*—The necessary presence of another person within arm's reach to prevent, by physical intervention, injury to the individual while performing ADLs. This also includes verbal cueing, which involves verbal prompting, gesturing or other demonstrations in order for the person to accomplish an ADL.

The six ADLs and their definitions under the NAIC LTCI Model Regulation (and HIPAA) are

- *bathing*—washing oneself by sponge bath; or in either a tub or shower, the task of getting into or out of the tub or shower
- *continence*—the ability to maintain control of bowel and bladder function; or, when unable to maintain control of bowel or bladder function, the ability to perform associated personal hygiene (including caring for a catheter or a colostomy bag)
- *dressing*—putting on and taking off all items of clothing and any necessary braces, fasteners, or artificial limbs
- *eating*—feeding oneself by getting food into the body from a receptacle (such as a plate, cup or table) or by a feeding tube or intravenously
- *toileting*—getting to and from the toilet, getting on and off the toilet, and performing associated personal hygiene
- *transferring*—moving into or out of a bed, chair, or wheelchair

The second criterion or benefit trigger is that substantial services are required to protect the person from threats to health and safety due to substantial cognitive impairment. Most policies use the definition of cognitive impairment that is in the NAIC LTCI Model Regulation, which is a deficiency in a person's (1) short or long-term memory, (2) orientation as to person, place, and time, (3) deductive or abstract reasoning, or (4) judgment as it relates to safety awareness.

Non-qualified LTCI contracts, on the other hand, have more liberal eligibility requirements for benefits. Many of these contracts use the same two criteria that are used in tax-qualified contracts, except there is no time period that applies to the inability to perform the ADLs. A small number of non-qualified contracts require only the inability to perform one ADL and/or use more than the six ADLs allowed by HIPAA. Finally, some non-qualified contracts make benefits available if a third criterion or benefit trigger—medical necessity—is satisfied. This generally means that a physician has certified that LTC is needed, even if neither of the other two criteria is satisfied.

Federal Income Tax Provisions

Premiums—A tax-qualified LTCI contract is treated as accident and health insurance. With some exceptions, costs for LTC services, including insurance premiums, are treated like other medical expenses. That is, people who itemize deductions can deduct unreimbursed LTC services, including insurance premiums, in excess of 7.5 percent of adjusted gross income (AGI). However, there are limits on the amount of personally paid LTCI premiums that can be claimed as medical expenses. These limits, which are based on a covered person's age and subject to cost-of-living adjustments, are shown for 2003 in Table 5-3, on the next page. Medical expense deductions cannot be taken for payments made to a spouse or relative who is not a licensed professional with respect to such LTC services.

Premiums for non-qualified contracts are not deductible.

Benefits—Under HIPAA, a LTC recipient will receive benefits income-tax-free when paid from a tax-qualified policy of the reimbursement type. Indemnity (per diem) policy benefits are also free from income taxation up to $220 per day in 2003 (this amount is increased each year by inflation) regardless of whether actual qualified LTC services were

TABLE 5-3 LTCI Deductible Premium Limits for 2003	
Age	Annual Deductible Limit per Covered Individual
40 or younger	$ 250
41–50	470
51–60	940
61–70	2,510
Over 70	3,130

received by the insured. However, any indemnity (per diem) benefits received by the insured in excess of $220 per day are not tax-free unless it can be shown that the qualified LTC services received by the insured actually equal those benefits.

There has been some controversy and uncertainty regarding the tax status of non-qualified LTCI policies. HIPAA gives no clear statement regarding the taxation of benefits provided by non-qualified policies. There is a growing consensus, however, that such policies are in fact taxable because they are not listed by HIPAA as tax-free. On the other hand, some experts have concluded that the benefits of non-qualified policies are not taxable income because they should be treated for tax purposes like any other accident and sickness insurance benefits. To add to the uncertainty, the IRS has so far not issued a ruling on this matter. Once the IRS acts, the controversy surrounding the tax status of non-qualified policies should disappear.

All LTCI claimants receive a Form 1099-LTC at the beginning of the year following their receipt of benefits. This form provides information to the claimant and IRS regarding the total amount of benefits paid in the preceding calendar year. The claimant then uses this information to complete IRS Form 8853. Form 8853 is used to determine the difference between the amount of benefits received and the cost of qualified LTC services. If the cost of qualified LTC services equals or exceeds the LTCI benefits received, the benefits are tax-free. If the LTCI benefits received from a tax-qualified policy exceed the cost of qualified LTC services, the amount in excess of $220/day in 2003 is taxable income.

LTCI and the Consumer

Consumer Attitudes and Perceptions of LTC and LTCI

Making LTCI consumer friendly is especially important because of the product's market challenge. That is, those people who are better able to afford the product tend to be younger, healthier, and more likely insurable, but are less likely to feel a need for the product to protect a risk that seems so distant. People who feel a greater need for the product tend be less able to afford the product and to obtain coverage because they are often retired, older, and less healthy or have chronic health conditions.

LTCI is a product developed to meet a real and growing risk that is gradually surfacing in the public's consciousness. Consumer attitudes toward LTCI grow out of their perceptions of the potential need for LTC and the means available to pay for it as much as their attitudes and perceptions of the products themselves. Surveys have shown that many consumers are significantly uninformed about LTC and LTCI. Unless individuals believe they are likely to need LTC sometime in their lives and to be personally responsible for the high cost associated with it, they will not seek an insurance plan to protect themselves. This is the major task and challenge in this marketplace, as discussed elsewhere in this book.

Selling this product, which is discussed in the next chapter, usually involves educating the prospect or client about the need for LTC and possible product solutions. Most prospects underestimate the costs and likelihood of needing LTC. Consumers have a limited or incorrect understanding of financing alternatives for LTC expenses. In fact, many people incorrectly believe Medicare or private medical insurance will cover most or all of their LTC costs, including nursing home and assisted living expenses. These misconceptions are changing and are slowly giving way to reality. One possible explanation for the slow growth in this market is that many people believe they have coverage when in fact they do not. Additionally, there are obvious psychological and emotional reasons why young, healthy, and independent people ignore, deny, procrastinate, and have a general reluctance to buying LTCI. Lastly, cost is a practical deterrent to purchasing coverage. Many prospects misunderstand the cost of a policy, greatly overestimating the cost, or underestimating the value of the policy relative to its cost.

Historically, LTCI buyers have tended to be older, more affluent, and better educated than their counterparts in the general population. The general trend for the average age of LTCI buyers is decreasing. They tend to be married with both spouses purchasing coverage. Their attitudes are understandably more realistic about the need for LTC and their responsibility to pay for it. They do not expect the government to pay the costs of LTC services. Protecting assets and/or leaving an estate, preserving financial independence and/or guaranteeing the affordability of needed services are their most important reasons for obtaining coverage.

Tables 5-4 to 5-7 include statistical information regarding the design characteristics of LTCI policies, including the age and income characteristics of people who bought them in 2000. As expected, prospects with higher incomes are more likely to buy higher-premium policies with more features. The exception to this rule is that they do not buy policies with short elimination or waiting periods. Instead, they prefer fairly long elimination periods because they can afford to self-insure for the initial period of LTC. Contrary to what the higher-income people buy, older people tend to buy LTCI policies with lower benefits and fewer features. This is simply the result of premiums increasing with age, and retired people having smaller incomes than younger people who are still working.

TABLE 5-4
Key Policy Design Parameters Chosen by Individual Long-Term Care Insurance Buyers, by Level of Income, 2000

Policy Features	Level of Income			
	$20,000	$20,000-$34,999	$35,000-$49,999	$50,000 and Over
Benefit Duration				
Average	3.7 years	4.6 years	4.8 years	6.2 years
1- 2 years	37%	22%	21%	9%
3- 4 years	42	45	42	33
5 years	12	11	14	18
Lifetime	10	21	24	40
Nursing Home Benefit Amount				
Average	$95	$96	$98	$117
Up to $40	5%	4%	2%	2%
$41-$50	3	7	8	2
$51-$70	8	11	11	8
$71-$90	19	10	11	10
$91 and Over	66	67	68	80
Home Care Benefit Amount				
Average	$95	$92	$98	$113
Up to $40	5%	2%	1%	2%
$41-$50	7	11	10	6
$51-$70	10	13	7	6
$71-$90	15	14	13	13
$91 and Over	64	60	68	73
Percent with Inflation Protection	31%	31%	37%	53%
Average Elimination Period	60 days	61 days	72 days	70 days
Percent with Home Care	86%	80%	79%	95%
Average Annual Premium Monthly Premiums	$1,656	$1,675	$1,619	$1,860
Up to $50	6%	7%	10%	3%
$51-$75	22	18	15	14
$76-$100	7	15	18	15
$101- $125	24	13	14	16
$126- $150	12	12	8	12
$151 and Over	29	35	35	40

Source: Health Insurance Association of America, *Who Buys Long-Term Care Insurance in 2002?* Based on 5,407 policies sold in 2000.

TABLE 5-5
Key Policy Design Parameters Chosen by Individual Long-Term Care Insurance Buyers, by Age, 2000

Policy Features	Age Category			
	55–64	65–69	70–74	75 and Over
Benefit Duration				
Average	6.4 years	5.3 years	4.8 years	3.7 years
1- 2 years	11%	18%	20%	31%
3- 4 years	29	37	44	51
5 years	15	16	14	8
Lifetime	45	29	22	10
Nursing Home Benefit Amount				
Average	$117	$96	$104	$95
Up to $40	1%	1%	2%	6%
$41-$50	2	7	9	8
$51-$70	7	11	9	11
$71-$90	8	9	14	14
$91 and Over	82	72	66	61
Home Care Benefit Amount				
Average	$113	$105	$97	$95
Up to $40	1%	2%	4%	3%
$41-$50	5	6	9	8
$51-$70	8	7	11	11
$71-$90	12	12	15	15
$91 and Over	74	73	61	63
Percent Choosing Inflation Protection	59%	46%	32%	14%
Average Elimination Period	62 days	69 days	72 days	66 days
Percent with Home Care	92%	85%	85%	77%
Average Annual Premium Monthly Premiums	$1,213	$1,487	$1,829	$2,581
Up to $50	8%	7%	4%	2%
$51-$75	28	16	10	4
$76-$100	20	19	14	5
$101- $125	19	16	12	13
$126- $150	9	14	10	10
$151 and Over	17	28	50	66

Source: Health Insurance Association of America, *Who Buys Long-Term Care Insurance in 2002?* Based on 5,407 policies sold in 2000.

TABLE 5-6
Individual Long-Term Care Insurance Policy Designs Selling in 2000, 1995, and 1990

Attributes of Policies	Percentage of 2000 Sales	Percentage of 1995 Sales	Percentage of 1990 Sales
Types of Policies Sold			
Nursing Home Only	14%	33%	63%
Comprehensive Policies	77	61	37
Home Care Only	9	6	—
Nursing Home Duration			
1–2 years	17%	24%	23%
3 years	23	20	12
4 years	14	18	15
5 years	11	6	12
6 years	5	2	5
Lifetime Benefits	30	30	33
Average Duration	5.5 years	5.1 years	5.6 years
Nursing Home Daily Benefit			
Up to $30	1%	1%	2%
$31-$59	5	12	25
$60-$89	17	40	51
$90-$119	43	38	18
$120 and Over	34	9	4
Average Daily Benefit	$109	$85	$72
Home Health Care Duration			
1 year	5%	20%	N.A.
2 years	14	31	
3 years	22	21	
4 years	13	5	
5 years	10	10	
6 years	7	1	
Lifetime Benefits	30	12	
Average Duration	5.4 years	3.4 years	
Home Health Care Daily Benefit			
Up to $30	1%	3%	25%
$31-$59	8	26	60
$60-$89	17	33	13
$90-$119	41	31	2
$120 and Over	33	8	—
Average Daily Benefit	$106	$78	$36
Elimination Period			
0 days	23%	28%	25%
15- 20 days	3	17	41
30- 60 days	16	16	12
90- 100 days	55	39	22
>100 days	3	—	—
Percent Choosing Inflation Protection	41%	33%	40%
Simple	17	14	N.A.
Compound	22	15	
Indexed to Consumer Price Index	2	4	
Total Annual Premium			
Up to $500	5%	10%	19%
$500- $999	24	29	40
$1,000- $1,499	26	23	21
$1,500- $1,999	18	15	11
$2,000- $2,499	9	9	5
Greater than $2,500	18	14	4
Average Annual Premium	$1,677	$1,505	$1,071

Source: Health Insurance Association of America, *Who Buys Long-Term Care Insurance in 2002?* Based on 5,407 policies sold in 2000, 6,446 policies sold in 1995, and 14,400 policies in 1990.

TABLE 5-7
Policy Design Characteristics in the Long-Term Care Group and Individual Markets

Policy Characteristics	Group Market	Individual Market
Policy Type		
Nursing Home Only	3%	14%
Comprehensive	97	77
(Nursing Home and Home Care)		
Home Care Only	—	9
Average Daily Benefit Amount		
Nursing Home	$124	$109
Home Care	$ 79	$106
Average Elimination Period (NH & HC)	63 days	65 days
0 days	5%	23%
30 days	36	12
60 days	3	6
90 days	56	59
Average Benefit Duration	6.3 years*	5.5 years
Nursing Home Duration		
1- 2 years	10%	17%
3- 5 years	51	48
6- 9 years	—	5
10 years to lifetime	39	30
Home Care Benefit Duration		
1- 2 years	6%	19%
3- 5 years	21	44
6- 9 years	21	7
10 years to lifetime	52	30
Percent with Inflation Protection**	88%	41%
Simple	—	17
Compound	40%	22
Future Purchase/Benefit Increase	—	2
Options	48	—
Percent with Nonforfeiture**	29%	<1%
Return of Premium	2%	
Shortened Benefit	26	
Other	1	
None	71	
Average Annual Premium	$722	$1,677

Source: Health Insurance Association of America, *Who Buys Long-Term Care Insurance in 2002?* Based on an analysis of 3,212 group market policyholders and 5,407 individual market new buyers.

 * Average benefit durations are calculated based on the total benefit cap and the chosen daily benefit amount. Because home care benefits were typically chosen as a percentage of nursing home benefits, the amount of time needed to exhaust the total benefit pool when using home care benefits is typically greater. For home care benefits, we calculate the average benefit duration to be 7.6 years.

** It is important to note that this represents the percentage of enrollees with these particular policy design features. It is not possible to make a statement about whether the employee chose these options or if they were automatically included in the basic plan design chosen by the employer.

Note: All but one of the participating employers offered long-term care plans on a voluntary basis. Thus, employees were responsible for paying the entire premium if they chose to enroll. Only employees who chose to "buy up" from the employer-funded base plan were used for comparability.

Note: For the purposes of determining average policy duration, lifetime policy durations were set to 10 years. Elimination periods for the individual market were adjusted to fit the closed categories for the group market. Therefore, for the individual market, 0 days is equal to 0 days, 30 days is equal to 1- 30 days, 60 days is equal to 31- 60 days, and 90 days is equal to 61-100 days. The average elimination period reported for the individual market is only for nursing home benefits; however, the percentages represent both nursing home and home care benefits.

Trends in LTCI

A survey taken by Broker's World revealed the following trends for 2001:

- Total 2001 premium was down by 2 percent from 2000. This was largely due to a large carrier suspending sales for a part of the year. Excluding this company, the result would have been a 7 percent increase, following a 16 percent premium increase in 2000 and a 19 percent increase the year before.
- Limited-pay and single-pay options continue to expand in availability.
- More industry giants enter the marketplace with stand-alone LTCI products. The top five LTCI companies produced 52 percent of the industry's new business in 2001. The top 10 companies produced 70 percent of new LTCI business, and the top 20 companies produced 89 percent.
- New products are being introduced, while some companies discontinued operations. One company did both in 2001.
- The tax-qualified policy form is clearly the dominant choice in the LTCI marketplace. When HIPAA first passed, TQ and NTQ policies were fairly evenly split. The trend toward TQ policies continues upward, with 90 percent of the policies sold in 2001 being TQ policies, up from 88 percent in 2000 and 84 percent the year before that. With more companies entering the market, it can be expected that production will become somewhat more diversified over the next several years.
- Many policy features once considered unique are rapidly becoming standard offerings throughout the industry. Examples include care management services, restoration of benefits, rate guarantees, caregiver training, home modification and equipment benefits, joint waiver of premium and endorsed group discounts.
- The marketing power of the large companies in the market and the expansion of LTCI advertising should continue to expand the LTCI market. This should be enhanced by the advertising and publicity of the Federal Government LTCI program. The boomer demographics and possibility of a significant tax deduction within the next few years may fuel LTCI market expansion and the entry of new companies into this market.
- There are somewhat higher prices, although spousal discounts continue to increase.
- Issue ages are clearly expanding, with lower minimum and higher maximum ages.
- Companies are offering higher MDBs going as high as $500 or no maximum stated.
- It is common for companies to offer four, five, six or more choices for benefit periods and three to five choices of elimination periods.
- The number of benefit pools reveals a continuation towards a single pool of money approach.

Source: Broker's World, *July 2002, "Fourth Annual LTCI Survey, p. 36. Fifty-two companies represented, including largest 20 LTCI insurers. Results represent 97 percent of the LTCI marketplace.*

Prospect Decisions

Prospects are faced with many decisions when purchasing LTCI. These decisions also require that their advisors possess the needed knowledge to guide them through the maze of questions that need to be answered, including:

- Is coverage appropriate?
- When should coverage be purchased?
- Is it better to purchase a tax-qualified policy or a non-qualified policy?
- Is it better to purchase an indemnity (per diem) policy or a reimbursement policy?
- What types of coverage should be purchased?
- What is the appropriate amount of coverage?
- What is the best way to plan for future inflation?
- Is a nonforfeiture option needed?
- How should policies be compared?
- What are the considerations for switching policies?
- How should premiums be paid?
- How can insurers be evaluated?

LTCI is relatively expensive, and for many prospects the final premium they will pay is an important factor. In considering the purchase of LTCI, a prospect must address the questions listed above. As you analyze the prospect's situation and propose a recommendation, you will also need to address these questions for the prospect, since you are the expert. Therefore, we will address these questions in the next chapter.

In the final analysis, however, many of these questions do not have precise answers. The manner in which they are answered depends on the personal preferences of the prospect. Although you are expected to help the prospect design the plan, always remember it is the prospect's plan.

Case History
Designing the Plan

The following case history illustrates that a prospect must often make several decisions before arriving at an optimal solution that will best meet his or her priorities and still be affordable. See the section "Designing the Plan" in chapter 6 for a continuation of this discussion.

Bruce, aged 65, has decided that he needs LTCI. Five years ago, he and his wife sold their small hobby store and were able to retire comfortably. Their plans of a leisurely life during retirement years were soon shattered when Bruce's wife had a serious stroke. For 3 years, Bruce was able to care for her at home with the assistance of professional caregivers. After she was totally paralyzed 2 years ago by a second stroke, Bruce found it necessary to put her in a nursing home where she recently died.

Having spent almost $250,000 to provide his wife with the best care possible, Bruce is fully aware of the effect that LTC can have on a family's assets. He wants to make sure that any LTC expenses he might incur will not further deplete the $500,000 in remaining assets that he and his wife spent a lifetime accumulating and intended to leave to their children and grandchildren.

Bruce has contacted a well-respected financial advisor whom he has known for several years and asked her to help him find a LTCI policy that meets his objectives. Bruce has indicated that his ideal policy would provide the following benefits:

- a nursing home MDB of $150. A top-quality nursing home in Bruce's town will cost about $250 per day, but Bruce feels he can afford to pay $100 from his Social Security and retirement income.
- a home health care MDB of $150
- a lifetime benefit period
- a 20-day elimination period
- 5 percent annual compound inflation protection

Bruce's advisor calculates that such an ideal policy will have an annual premium of $5,060. Bruce feels that this is somewhat more than he can pay without withdrawing funds from his assets and asks her what can be done to reduce the premium to about $4,000 per year. She comes up with the following alternatives:

- If the MDB for nursing homes is lowered to $130, the premium will drop to $4,380. A further decrease to $120 will result in a premium of $4,050. Bruce decides to consider this option.
- If the home health care MDB is lowered to 50 percent of the nursing home MDB, the premium will drop to $4,130. Bruce realizes how costly home health care can be and doesn't like this option.
- If a 5-year benefit period is selected, the premium will drop to $4,135. For a 4-year benefit period, the premium will be $3,800. Bruce is aware that some patients in his wife's nursing home were there for as long as 10 years and doesn't like this option either.
- If the elimination period is increased to 90 days, the premium will drop to $4,150. For a 180-day elimination period, the premium will further decrease to $3,750. Bruce is willing to think about a 90-day elimination period, but he feels that 180 days is too long.
- If the inflation protection is changed from compound interest to simple interest, the premium will drop to $4,260. Bruce hopes to live for many more years and realizes the effect that inflation can have on LTC costs. This option doesn't appeal to him.

Bruce decides to take a day or two to think about his options. He has his advisor calculate that a 90-day elimination period will increase his out-of-pocket costs by $10,500 (70 days times $150) over what they would otherwise be with his ideal policy if he needs LTC. He also has her calculate that a lower nursing home MDB of $120 will increase his annual out-of-pocket costs by $10,950 (365 days times $30). Bruce realizes that these additional out-of-pocket costs will come from his accumulated assets. He also understands that he can afford the benefits in his ideal policy if he is willing to reduce his assets by about $1,000 per year to pay the $5,060 premium.

Bruce finally decides that his ideal policy with the $5,060 premium is the best choice for him. Its benefits make it more likely that he will receive the level of care he wants if he is unable to care for himself.

Chapter Five Review

Key Terms and Concepts are explained in the Glossary. Answers to the Review Questions and Self-Test Questions are found in the back of the book in the Answers to Questions section.

Key Terms and Concepts

caregiver training
facility-only policy
comprehensive policy
maximum daily benefit (MDB)
maximum dollar amount
pool of money
indemnity or per diem basis
reimbursement basis
survivorship benefit
reinstatement
nonforfeiture benefit
renewability
guaranteed renewable
noncancelable
combination products
restoration of benefits
hospice
homemaker companion

rescind
alternative plans of care
home health care only policy
elimination period
benefit period
shared benefit
grace period
waiver of premium
spousal discounts
inflation protection
contingent benefit upon lapse
bed reservation benefit
return-of-premium rider
HIPAA
   chronic illness definition
   chronic illness certification
   benefit triggers
   substantial assistance

Review Questions

5-1. Explain why it is advisable not to emphasize price when selling LTCI.

5-2. Explain the following as they pertain to LTCI:
   a. respite care
   b. caregiving training

c. pool of money

d. bed reservation benefit

5-3. Calculate the pool of money available for Matthew's reimbursement type of LTCI policy that has a 4-year benefit period and a MDB amount of $200.

5-4. Once home health care services commence, explain how they are counted toward the elimination period.

5-5. What is the reason that most insurers offer spousal or partner discounts for LTCI policies?

5-6. What are some of the other insurance coverages that have been packaged with LTCI in combination products?

5-7. What is the definition of a chronically ill person under HIPAA?

5-8. Explain the tax treatment of non-qualified LTCI policy benefits.

Self-Test Questions

Instructions: Read chapter 5 first, then answer the following questions to test your knowledge. There are 10 questions; circle the correct answer, then check your answers with the answer key in the back of the book.

5-1. Before qualifying for benefits under a tax-qualified LTCI policy, an insured must be cognitively impaired or expected to require substantial assistance to perform two or more activities of daily living (ADLs) for a period of at least

(a) 30 days

(b) 60 days

(c) 90 days

(d) 120 days

Questions 5-2 and 5-3 are based on the following facts:

A 55-year-old man has a tax-qualified LTCI policy with an annual premium of $1,000. In 2003, the man has $4,000 in deductible medical expenses not including the LTCI premium.

5-2. How much of the man's LTCI premium can be included with the other deductible medical expenses?

(a) $250
(b) $470
(c) $940
(d) $1,000

5-3. If the man's AGI is $50,000, what amount of medical expenses is tax deductible to him?

(a) $1,190
(b) $1,250
(c) $3,750
(d) $5,000

5-4. The MDB amount under an indemnity (per diem) contract is

(a) paid regardless of the actual cost of care
(b) paid only if the actual cost of care equals the MDB
(c) coordinated with the Medicare program
(d) coordinated with the Medicaid program

5-5. The NAIC LTCI Model Regulation only allows policies to use the term "level premium" if they have which of the following type of renewal provision?

(a) guaranteed renewable
(b) noncancelable
(c) optionally renewable
(d) shortened payment period

5-6.   Which of the following statements regarding LTCI buyers is (are) correct?

   I.   The general trend for the average age of LTCI buyers is increasing.
   II. LTCI buyers tend to be married with both spouses purchasing coverage.

   (a) I only
   (b) II only
   (c) Both I and II
   (d) Neither I nor II

5-7.   Which of the following statements regarding an alternative plans clause in a LTCI policy is (are) correct?

   I.   The alternative plan of care generally must be acceptable to the insurer, the insured, and the insured's physician.
   II. This type of clause serves as a catch-all provision to accommodate changes in LTC services and coverages that may occur in the future.

   (a) I only
   (b) II only
   (c) Both I and II
   (d) Neither I nor II

5-8.   Which of the following statements regarding LTCI benefit triggers is (are) correct?

   I.   Tax-qualified contracts require the insured to meet one of two benefit triggers.
   II. Non-qualified contracts often have more stringent benefit triggers than tax-qualified contracts.

   (a) I only
   (b) II only
   (c) Both I and II
   (d) Neither I nor II

5-9.   Under the NAIC LTCI Model Regulation, a LTCI policy may limit or exclude coverage for all of the following reasons **EXCEPT**

   (a) preexisting conditions
   (b) drug addiction
   (c) attempted suicide
   (d) Alzheimer's disease

5-10. Combination life insurance/LTCI products differ from comprehensive stand-alone LTCI policies in all of the following ways **EXCEPT**:

(a) The amount of the LTCI benefit is a function of the amount of life insurance protection purchased.

(b) There is no LTCI nonforfeiture benefit because the cash value of the life insurance serves this function.

(c) The automatic inflation option provides for an increase of LTCI benefits by 5 percent of the prior year's coverage.

(d) The LTCI benefit periods are often limited to a few years, although some insurers make lifetime benefits available.

6

Analyzing the Situation and Presenting Solutions

Overview and Learning Objectives

Chapter 6 discusses how to analyze a prospect's need for LTCI, design product solutions, and present them to the prospect with a client-focused selling approach. By reading this chapter and answering the questions, you should be able to:

6-1. Explain important aspects of analyzing a prospect's need for LTCI.

6-2. Explain how to customize a LTCI policy to fit the prospect's needs and ability to pay.

6-3. Identify key components of designing a LTCI plan.

6-4. Explain strategies for presenting solution alternatives to a prospect.

6-5. Explore techniques for handling common objections and concerns.

Chapter Outline

Analyzing the Situation

In chapter 4, we discussed information gathering, the fourth step of the selling process, which results in a discovery agreement with the prospect to design a LTCI plan that will meet his or her needs. In this section, we move to the fifth step of the selling process, analyzing the situation, in which the financial advisor designs a plan or plan alternatives to present to the prospect. In examining this step of the selling process, the text focuses on piecing together the six main components of a LTCI plan in order to create a possible solution. It also includes a discussion about analyzing a competitor's product.

Plan Design Assumptions

Our discussion of the analysis and presentation of a LTC solution is based on two assumptions. First, a two-interview selling approach is used. Second, the analysis and presentation of a LTC solution is based on obtaining a complete and comprehensive fact finder.

Two-Interview Selling Approach

This book follows a two-interview selling approach in which meeting the prospect and gathering information constitute the initial interview. The interview ends with a discovery agreement and the scheduling of a follow-up appointment. Though the initial interview includes a discussion of the prospect's desired LTCI policy benefits, in-depth analysis and plan design occur after the prospect leaves, giving the advisor time to customize a sales presentation for the closing interview.

The two-interview selling approach is recommended for two reasons. First, many experienced advisors have had great success with this approach and feel that a multiple-interview sale cements the advisor-prospect relationship because it demonstrates that the advisor understands the prospect's need to process the information. As one experienced financial advisor explained, "Selling LTCI is usually a two-interview process. I'm okay with that because I want people to be comfortable with what they are doing." Second, a two-interview

> **Selling and Buying**
>
> You are not really selling as much as getting the prospects to buy. You are removing obstacles to help them get what they want.

approach gives less experienced advisors time to analyze the situation and seek the advice of experienced advisors if necessary. It also allows time to customize the presentation. As less-experienced advisors gain more experience, a one-interview approach is feasible and, depending on style and philosophy, perhaps more desirable. The key to this transition is becoming adept at designing plans, which comes only as a result of becoming familiar with different options and their impact on the premium.

Relationship to the Fact Finder

The analysis of the prospect's situation involves taking the relevant information gathered from the fact-finder and designing a plan that reflects the prospect's needs, preferences, and premium commitment. Creating a solution to meet the prospect's needs depends heavily on the quality of the information gathered during the fact-finding process. The solution must be based on the prospect's own circumstances and preferences. Thus, the importance of a thorough fact finder cannot be overemphasized.

Because fact-finding impacts your analysis of the prospect's situation, you can use the information in this section to create fact-finding questions related to plan design features. For example, you can ask the prospect if he or she is concerned about a long nursing home stay. Such a concern would mean that you should consider recommending a lifetime benefit period. Understanding the prospect's preferences and priorities will dictate which features to include in your recommended plan options.

> A quick summary of the one-interview sales approach: Let the prospects tell you what they want, give them a quote, and see if it fits within their budget.

The Secret to Selling LTCI

Here is one experienced financial advisor's advice on succeeding in the LTCI market:

Become an advocate—a "True Believer" in LTCI's ability to solve the LTC problem. Buy it for yourself. Don't sell the product. You don't need to sell the product if you sell the need. Educate prospects about the need. Don't sell based on cost, premiums, or illustrations. Help prospects to clearly understand the need and they will buy it.

Designing the Plan

Your objective is to help the prospect get the best value for his or her money through an effective plan design. Plan design is a balancing act between the prioritized coverage needs of the prospect and his or her premium commitment. One way to approach this task is to begin with the basic coverage design, creating an "ideal plan." Then, using the premium commitment and the prospect's priorities, begin adjusting the plan to create an optimal solution that will best meet his or her priorities within the specified premium commitment.

Basic Coverage Design

Your basic coverage design will answer six important questions to determine the amount of insurance and the premium for the policy:

1. When will benefits start?
2. How much will be paid?
3. How long will benefits last?
4. Where will care be given?
5. Will policy benefits periodically increase?
6. How will the policy be treated for tax purposes?

Decisions can be made about each aspect of the coverage by referring to the information gathered from the fact-finding process. For example, the fact finder will provide information about the existing and projected resources, preferences for types of care, extent of a family-and-friend support system, physical health and lifestyle, coordination with other assets, and so forth. Unfortunately, there are many variables to account for. Furthermore, there may be a long period between the purchase of the coverage and the occurrence of a claim. As a result, the advisor and prospect must make some assumptions.

Although each question below is discussed individually, keep in mind that each one will have an impact on the others and, consequently, the final plan will be the result of answers to all questions combined.

When will benefits start? (Elimination or Waiting Period)—In general, three things must happen before LTCI benefits are paid:

1. Impairment must exist, as assessed by a health care professional.
2. Services must be received for the impairment.
3. The elimination or waiting period must be satisfied.

The third item is determined by the insured/prospect when he or she selects the policy's elimination period (also known as a *waiting period* or *deductible period*). In selecting the length of the elimination period, you need to balance the prospect's ability to pay for care during the elimination period with the higher premium associated with a shorter elimination or waiting period. Start by determining how long the prospect's assets will last, based on the amount he or she is willing to use to pay for LTC expenses. Use the following steps:

1. Divide the amount of monthly fixed income (from Social Security and retirement plans) that the prospect is willing to commit to LTC expenses by 30 days.
2. Subtract this result from the daily amount needed for care in the area.
3. Divide this difference into the total amount of assets that the prospect has available to pay for LTC expenses. This determines the number of days that the prospect can self-fund.
4. Finally, subtract the number of days representing the frequency with which your company will send a reimbursement check to the prospect. Generally this is 30 days.

EXAMPLE 1: Juanita has $20,000 in assets and $1,200 in monthly retirement income that she is willing to use to pay for LTC expenses during the elimination period. Care in her area is $180 per day. Jane Advisor's company has a 30-day lag time between the end of the elimination period and the date the first payment is made.

1. $1,200 ÷ 30 days = $40/day
2. $180/day – $40/day = $140/day
3. $20,000 ÷ $140/day = 142 days
4. 142 days – 30 days = 112 days

An elimination period of 90 days would be appropriate. The 30-day lag time in step 4 above represents the delay from when Juanita would be eligible to receive care and when reimbursement would be received from the insurance company. With a 90-day elimination period, the reimbursement for days 91 to 120 would be received after day 120. Thus, Juanita should be prepared to pay for LTC expenses for days 91 through 120 as well.

As suggested by the example, the length of the elimination period that a prospect selects depends on several variables. The most important variables are the daily cost of LTC in the area or region that the prospect lives, the amount of fixed monthly retirement income that the prospect is willing to commit to LTC expenses, and the total amount of assets that the prospect has available to pay for LTC expenses. All three of these variables are based on future values (amounts that may exist if and when care is needed sometime in the future) that are difficult to determine at the time when the prospect is trying to select an appropriate elimination period. Moreover, complicating the selection even further is the fact that the daily cost of LTC is inversely correlated to the length of the elimination period. In other words, the higher the daily cost of LTC, the shorter the elimination period should be, other things being equal. Also, it should be noted that the cost of LTCI is inversely correlated to the length of the elimination period, other things being equal. This means that the prospect who is least able to afford the cost of LTC and who, consequently, needs a fairly short elimination period, will nonetheless have to pay higher premiums for LTCI if he or she selects the shorter period. In summation, the selection of the length of the elimination period is by no means an easy task.

Also keep in mind that different insurers define the qualification of elimination period days differently, as discussed in chapter 5. For example, the elimination period may be defined by the *total* number of days the insured is eligible for LTC, in which case the previous calculation would work well. Or, the elimination period may be defined by the number of *consecutive* days that the insured spent in a LTC facility or received home health care benefits. Under this definition, the longer the elimination period, the more uncertainty there is in determining the amount of LTC expenses that the prospect will need to self-insure. The reason for the greater uncertainty is obvious. For example, let us say the prospect selects a 60-day elimination period. At some point in the future, he or she needs LTC for 30 days and recovers, then needs it for another 45 days. Neither of these periods would qualify for benefits under the consecutive-days definition of an elimination period because the insured did not receive LTC for 60 *consecutive* days. In contrast, benefits would be payable for days 31 through 45 of the second time the insured needed LTC if the policy defined the elimination period by the *total* number of days the insured is eligible for LTC.

How much will be paid? (Maximum Daily Benefit)—The *maximum daily benefit (MDB)* is the maximum amount of money that a policy will pay each day once the insured has satisfied the elimination or waiting period requirement. The MDB amount should be the difference between the daily cost of care and the amount that the prospect is willing or able to pay, either from income or established assets. The prospect does not have to buy LTCI to cover the full cost of care. In order to keep the premiums down, he or she can self-insure some of the costs. A discussion with the prospect about the coordination of the MDB and the benefit period (which we will discuss next) with the availability of other assets is appropriate during the fact-finding interview.

Types of Benefit Payments—Policies are classified according to the way benefit payments are made: on either an indemnity (per diem) or reimbursement basis.

- *indemnity (per diem) policy*—this type of policy pays a predetermined dollar amount regardless of the actual cost of care. For example, if actual nursing home charges are $150 per day and the insured has a $200 MDB, then $200 will be paid.
- *reimbursement policy*—the majority of newer policies pay actual charges up to a specified policy limit. In the previous example, a reimbursement policy would only pay $150 per day to cover the actual nursing home charges. The $50 difference between the $200 MDB and the actual charge of $150 remains part of the "pool of money" for future use.

The steps for calculating the MDB amount are:

1. Determine the daily cost of nursing home care in the area.
2. Subtract the daily amount of care that can be paid from income.
3. Subtract the daily amount of care that can be paid from assets.
4. The difference represents the MDB to include in the policy.

Look at the average daily cost of nursing home care in your area, then recommend a MDB amount as high as your prospect needs or can afford. Keep in mind that your prospect may choose whether to insure the whole potential daily cost of care (which requires higher premiums) or to insure only that portion of the cost that he or she could not afford to self-insure. The decision often turns on just how risk averse (that is, avoids risk) the prospect is with respect to the potential costs of LTC.

Example 2: (from our previous example with Juanita): Juanita is willing to use $1,200 per month from her assets (over and above the $20,000 of assets she was willing to commit to LTC expenses during the elimination period) and $1,200 in monthly retirement income to pay for LTC expenses after she starts to receive benefits from her LTCI policy. Care in her area costs $180 per day.

1. Determine the daily cost of nursing home care $180
2. Subtract the daily cost of care paid from income   −40
3. Subtract the daily cost of care paid from assets   −40
4. The difference is the MDB for the policy $100

Determine the average daily cost of nursing home care in your area and recommend a MDB amount as high as your prospect needs and can afford.

How long will benefits last? (Benefit Period)—The benefit period is expressed as either an unlimited period of time when lifetime benefits are provided or as a specified number of years. When expressed in years, the benefit period effectively limits the maximum exposure of the insurance company in the contract to a total number of days of coverage or a total dollar benefit amount that the policy can pay. The total number of days of coverage is the number of years times 365. Thus, a three-year indemnity (per diem) policy would offer 1,095 days of benefits, while a reimbursement policy would provide for a total dollar benefit equivalent to 1,095 times the MDB. For example, a 3-year reimbursement policy with a $130-MDB amount would pay up to a maximum of $142,350 toward LTC (3 x 365 x $130 MDB). As previously indicated, a reimbursement policy uses the pool-of-money method to calculate its total dollar benefit amount. In other words, a reimbursement policy measures the maximum benefit in dollar terms, not in number of days, while an indemnity (per diem) policy measures the maximum benefit in terms of the total number of days of coverage.

To recommend a suitable benefit period, you may ask if longevity runs in the family, if anyone from the family has spent time in a nursing or LTC facility, or refer to statistics on the various probabilities of lengths of stay in a nursing or LTC facility at varying ages. Keep in mind that the chances of needing LTC services for more than 5 years are relatively small. For most people, a policy covering 3 to 5 years will be cost-effective. If, however, your prospect is very risk averse (that is, avoids risk), is concerned about getting Alzheimer's or a similar chronic disease, or comes from a family with a history of disorders that can lead to extended care, an unlimited period with lifetime benefits may be warranted.

Spousal (Partner) Benefits

Spousal (partner) benefits are another area of planning concern and industry innovations. If both spouses purchase coverage, there are many options and benefits that may become available. For example:

- Some companies offer a waiver of premium on the healthy spouse's policy if the other spouse becomes a claimant.
- A shared benefit period or shared pool of money allows spouses to access a larger benefit pool.
- A survivor benefit allows for a waiver of premium for the surviving spouse if one spouse dies after the policy has been in force for a minimum number of years, usually around 10.
- A spousal discount allows for a discounted premium on one or both spouses when purchasing coverage.

As an innovative option, more carriers are providing various types of *shared benefits*. Shared benefits provide spouses an opportunity to access a larger benefit pool by sharing in each other's benefit period or pool of money while paying an additional, modest premium; or for a smaller premium, they can share a single pool of money or benefit period between them. For example, a husband and wife each purchase a 3-year indemnity policy with a "shared" benefit period. They would have a total of 6 years between the two of them. If only one spouse needed LTC services, he or she could use all 6 years of benefits. This is a practical and affordable alternative to lifetime benefits. Other companies have introduced reimbursement policies that allow family members to share benefits from a single pool of money. (See page 5-25)

Where will care be given? (Comprehensive Policy or Facility Only Policy)—Most policies today offer coverage for a full range of care services and are called comprehensive or integrated policies. The services provided generally include home care, adult day care, and care at an assisted-living, skilled-nursing, or hospice facility. In contrast, the facility-only type of policy would only provide for services in a nursing home or assisted-living facility. Likewise, home-care-only policies would limit the services provided to those needed by less-than-seriously-ill people who are still somewhat independent and only need part-time care.

A prospect's circumstances and budget will dictate which type of policy he or she should buy. For example, a prospect who does not have anyone to care for him or her at home should consider facility-only coverage. Or, a prospect may have several children in the area who will assist him or her and thus the prospect anticipates only needing occasional professional assistance. In this situation, home-care-only coverage would be appropriate.

While most people would prefer to receive care in their homes, they realize that eventually it could become impractical. As a result, comprehensive policies offering coverage for a full range of care services are the most popular policies purchased today. In addition, LTC services continue to evolve at a rapid pace. For example, LTC providers are increasing the number and types of facilities that provide less-intensive care than a nursing home. People now have the choice of entering more than one type of facility to receive the care they need, and the comprehensive policy is best suited for covering these newer types of care arrangements.

Does the Prospect Want to Stay at Home?

LTCI is not just nursing home insurance. In its most comprehensive form, it is so much more because it enables people to receive care in the setting of their choice. Most people prefer to receive care in the home, but unfortunately it is the most expensive form of LTC because it is so highly individualized. LTCI allows people to choose from an array of LTC settings, including the home. In fact, most people who want to stay at home will need LTCI.

Will policy benefits periodically increase? (Inflation Protection)— LTC costs are likely to increase in the future, as demonstrated by increases in the past. The cost has doubled over the last 15 years, increasing by approximately 5 percent per year. Adding an inflation rider that provides for automatic benefit increases can help a policy keep pace with the increasing costs of LTC due to inflation. Incidentally, like so many other aspects of LTCI, different companies refer to the same concept using different terminology or use the same terminology to refer to quite different concepts. Either way, if you are not careful about how you use the terminology of LTCI, you run the risk of confusing the prospect. So be sure to clearly explain to the prospect what your policy means by terms like *inflation rider* or *future purchase option*.

During the fact-finding process, ask the prospect how much he or she thinks nursing homes and/or home health care will cost in the future when he or she might need LTC. Or, using another approach, ask the prospect if he or she would like to include a feature in the policy that enables benefits to keep pace with the rising costs of care.

If a prospect purchases a policy before age 70 or 75, inflation protection is essential to ensure that he or she will have adequate inflation-adjusted coverage years from now when he or she may file a claim. However, many advisors feel inflation protection is not as important for prospects age 70 or older because there is a much shorter time frame until services may be needed. Nevertheless, prospects age 70 or older still need to consider inflation protection because they could easily live for another 20 to 25 years as longevity continues to increase.

Many advisors insist on including inflation riders in LTCI policies, but they can be very expensive since inflation poses an additional risk for the insurer. However, there are a number of alternative ways—including inflation riders—to meet the challenge of inflation for LTC. Let us briefly review the advantages and/or disadvantages of each method so you can help the prospect make the right choice for his or her situation.

Self-insure—Self-insuring the inflation risk is fraught with many of the same problems as not purchasing LTCI in the first place.

Purchase Additional Coverage—A prospect can plan to purchase additional LTCI at a later time. However, this will entail paying an additional premium as well as facing the risk of being declined or rated. The insured can request an increase in coverage (that is, increase the MDB amount) at almost any time by submitting a new application along with evidence of insurability. However, someone who is actually receiving benefits would not be eligible, and someone whose health had declined would either have to pay a rated premium or, more likely, would not be offered the additional coverage. The extra premium charged for the additional coverage would be based on attained age rates, whereas the premium being paid for existing coverage would continue unchanged at original age rates.

Inflation Rider—A pre-funded "level premium" inflation rider is the obvious choice for a prospect who has real concerns about future increases in the cost of care and possible problems with other alternatives. This choice will increase the annual premium significantly, so the prospect must be able to afford a higher premium. In spite of its high cost, however, an inflation rider will automatically increase the benefit amount each year and provide the best protection against inflation.

Policies with inflation riders use a variety of preset interest-rate options to adjust benefits upward, although the most popular rate currently is 5 percent. Adjustments based on simple interest always use the original benefit amount for the basis of the increase, while compound interest adjustments use the previous year's benefit amount for the basis. Needless to say, compound interest adjustments increase benefits at a much faster rate than adjustments based on simple interest. A few policies use increases in the Consumer Price Index (CPI) as the adjustment trigger.

Future Purchase Options/Guaranteed Insurability Rider—Another popular choice for prospects in their fight against inflation is future purchase options. They allow an insured to periodically purchase additional insurance (that is, increase the MDB amount) without having to furnish new evidence of insurability each time. This method of protecting against inflation is considered a *pay-as-you-go* approach, because each time benefits are increased through the exercise of an option, there is a corresponding premium increase for the additional coverage. The additional premium charge is based on attained-age rates and becomes part of the policy's new annual premium.

The amount of the benefit increase under each option may be a fixed-dollar amount, such as a $20 increase in the MDB, or an amount based on a specified percentage of the MDB, or an amount based on changes in an index, such as the Consumer Price Index (CPI). The frequency with which purchase options may be exercised varies by insurer, but typically they are available every one, 2, or 3 years. Some insurers have an aggregate limit on the total amount of benefit increases that can be purchased by exercising options or an age beyond which purchase options are no longer available. Failure to exercise an option or a series of options over a specified period of time typically terminates the right to exercise any future options.

The cost of buying LTCI with future purchase options starts out much lower than the cost of buying the same amount of LTCI with an inflation rider. Over time, however, the total amount of premiums from the LTCI policy with purchase options will increase substantially as options are exercised. Eventually, the total premiums from the policy and the exercised options will surpass the level premium required to buy a LTCI policy with an inflation rider, other things being equal.

Buy "excess" coverage initially—Some prospects insist on purchasing a MDB amount that is far in excess of the actual current costs of nursing homes in their area. This approach to protecting against inflation "builds in" a cushion that, unfortunately, tends to erode over

---

Level Premium?

The premium for LTCI will not stay level. The pricing of the product is not an exact science because it is so new. The carriers just don't know yet what the "right" premium is, but this will come in time. For now, I think you can expect price increases. For this reason, I don't think advisors should present LTCI as having a level premium. Prospects should be told to expect premium increases over time.

---

time as the costs of LTC continue to rise. Eventually, LTC costs will catch up with the policy's initial benefit amount and the insured will have to purchase additional coverage if he or she wants to stay ahead of or at least keep up with inflation.

However, there is a risk that the insured will be uninsurable for LTCI when he or she needs to purchase the additional coverage. And even if the insured is insurable, the additional coverage will cost a lot more because the insured will be much older. While initially purchasing "excess" coverage seems to work fine in the short run (up to 10 years, for example) it is not a long-term solution to the inflation problem. For a more "permanent" solution to the problem, the prospect needs to purchase either an inflation rider or a guaranteed insurability rider. Nonetheless, despite its shortcomings, buying excess coverage works as an inflation strategy for prospects age 75 or older, since many of these people will not survive more than 10 years.

How will the policy be treated for tax purposes? (Tax-Qualified or Nonqualified)—As discussed in chapter 5, HIPAA provides that policies issued on or after January 1, 1997 and follow certain guidelines are classified as *tax-qualified (TQ) policies*. Policies issued on or after January 1, 1997 that do not adhere to the guidelines are called *nonqualified (NQ) policies*. Policies issued before January 1, 1997 are grandfathered and will be treated as if they are TQ policies.

An advantage of a TQ policy is that premiums may be included as a medical expense if a person itemizes deductions on his or her federal income tax return. If a person's unreimbursed medical expenses exceed 7.5 percent of his or her adjusted gross income (AGI), the excess is deductible. However, there are limits on the amount of personally paid LTCI premiums that can be claimed as medical expenses. These limits are based on the person's age and subject to cost-of-living adjustments. (See page 5-45)

Another very important advantage of TQ policies is the income tax treatment of benefits. TQ reimbursement policies receive benefits income tax free, while TQ indemnity (per diem) policies also receive benefits tax free, but only up to $220 per day in 2003 (this amount is indexed annually for inflation), unless it can be shown that any benefits received in excess of this amount are for qualified LTC services. If the excess benefits from TQ indemnity policies are for qualified LTC services, they too will be income tax free.

There is some disagreement concerning the use of NQ policies. HIPAA did not address their tax status, which has left many advisors reluctant to sell them and prospects wary of buying them. Although most advisors sell TQ policies, some advisors prefer to sell NQ policies because they do not require the 90-day certification period. In other words, NQ policies can pay benefits for care that is expected to last less than 90 days. In addition, NQ policies may include a "medically necessary" trigger that TQ policies are not allowed to have, making it potentially easier to qualify for benefits with NQ policies.

Premium Commitment

As you design a LTCI policy, it is important to work within a prospect's premium commitment as determined in the fact-finding interview. While

---

Shopping Tips for LTCI

- Ask questions.
- Check with several companies and advisors.
- Take your time and compare outlines of coverage.
- Understand the policies.
- Don't be misled by advertising.
- Don't buy more than one LTCI policy.*
- Be sure you accurately complete your application.
- Never pay in cash.
- Be sure to get the name, address and telephone number of the advisor and the company.
- If you don't get your policy within 60 days, contact the company or advisor.
- Be sure to look at your policy during the free-look period.
- Read the policy again and make sure it gives you the coverage you want.
- Think about having the premium automatically taken out of your bank account.
- Check on the financial stability of the company you're thinking of buying from.

* This is due to specific historical situations. A supplemental policy is appropriate if needed.

Source: A Shopper's Guide to Long-Term Care. *NAIC (National Association of Insurance Commissioners).*

---

a policy with a lifetime benefit period and a compound interest inflation rider is certainly desirable, if its premium is beyond what the prospect can or will pay, then pushing the policy is a formula for losing the sale. Instead, develop some alternative policy designs that reflect the prospect's priorities and fall within his or her premium commitment. You should limit the choices to just a few so that you do not confuse the prospect. You can always customize a policy further by using a few basic illustrations as the starting point and introducing modifications (within cost parameters) by adding features, benefits, and so on. You can also enrich the sales process by interjecting your personal experiences, using a rate book, and/or making sales illustrations.

The more you work with your products, the more knowledge you will accrue about them. In an interview with a prospect, you can estimate premium differences for various features and options. You should know what the cost impact is from adding, deleting, or varying one of these features or options. For example, a lifetime benefit period will cost about 30 percent more than a 5-year benefit period, or a 100-day elimination or waiting period will cost about 20 percent less than a 20-day period.

Finally, the design of a policy and its sale to a prospect should not be considered a one-time event. The planning process should be ongoing even after the sale because the client's personal situation and coverage needs will most likely change over time. Besides, many changes could occur in the often-lengthy time lapse between when the policy is sold and when a claim is filed.

Analyzing the Competition

The NAIC's *A Shopper's Guide to Long-Term Care Insurance* and many financial advisors recommend that prospects shop around for the best policy. Despite this recommendation, many successful LTCI advisors report that they do not find themselves in competitive situations with other advisors very often. While their experience may be due to their self-confidence or confidence in their company and its products, it is most likely due to their ability to build relationships and create confidence in the prospects' minds that they are the advisors with whom to do business. They present themselves as trustworthy, knowledgeable, and having the prospects' best interests in mind.

However, there are many advisors and insurers offering a broad array of policy features and options to the public, and most likely you will encounter a competitive situation at some point. In case you do, the following material is designed to help you analyze and compare companies and policies.

Evaluating LTC Insurers

There are several key areas in which the competition should be compared with your company and the products it offers.

Financial Strength—It is important for you to evaluate the financial strength and claims-paying ability of your company compared with its competitors. The real value of a contract for a policyowner is determined by whether it pays claims should they arise. The policyowner wants the peace of mind associated with knowing that the insurer will be able to pay should a claim be filed. Consequently, prospects should only buy from insurers that have strong financial reserves and are likely to be sound far into the future; have a history of stable rates for their policies; have an excellent reputation; and have a good track for policyowner service with few or no reported complaints.

Although there is no foolproof method for assessing a company's financial strength, a useful measure is the rating given by independent rating services. Prospects are urged to obtain them for the companies whose policies they are considering. Also, it is a good idea for you to know exactly how your company ranks and compares with others. Several companies provide independent ratings for insurance companies:

- *A.M. Best Company.* (800) 424-BEST or *www.ambest.com*
- *Standard and Poor's Insurance Rating Services.* (212) 208-1527 or *www.ratings.standardpoor.com*
- *Moody's Investor Services Inc.* (212) 553-0377 or at *www.moodys.com*
- *Duff & Phelps, Inc.* (312) 368-3157 or (312) 629-383, or *www.dcreo.com*
- *Fitch Investors Service, Inc.* (212) 908-0500 or *www.fitchibca.com*
- *Weiss Research, Inc.* (800) 289-9222 or *www.weissinc.com*

Reputation—The reputation of your company is an important aspect of competition. Anything that can help you present your company in a positive light will enhance its image in the prospect's eyes. For example, if you have marketing pieces and fact sheets that champion your company's positive claims paying experience, financial strength, corporate integrity, or proud history, include them in your sales presentation binder and use them in the initial interview. If your company runs an advertising campaign that employs a celebrity to endorse its products, this will give it credibility and implicitly boost its reputation. Everyone wants to do business with a company that is reputable.

Price—It is often the advisor's perception that prospects want to pay as little as possible for their coverage and that they will shop for the best price. Consequently, there is often a tendency for advisors to sell lower-premium policies because the premiums for quality products are higher. Unfortunately, in a competitive environment too much emphasis is placed on price, perhaps because it is the easiest variable to measure. Many dimensions of value other than price are just as important and should also be considered. These include your level of professional expertise, the quality of the service you provide, your company's reputation and its financial strength, and the availability of desirable policy provisions and features.

Prospects normally get what they pay for, and low premium policies marketed by shortsighted insurance carriers can lead to the following undesirable consequences:

- disappointment with the policy's benefits because it does not cover all the LTC costs that the policyowner thinks should be covered
- the need to raise the policy's premiums because the benefits cannot be supported by the current premium structure
- low policy premiums matching the company's strict claims-paying practice and/or its poor policy service

When comparing rates, use extreme caution for the following reasons:

- The underlying benefit structure can be significantly different for each company. You need to understand this and be able to explain these differences to prospects.
- Underwriting and sales styles differ significantly from company to company. You need to know your competitors' target markets and the pricing compromises they make to reach those markets.
- A competitor's low premiums today may mean rate increases later. You will need to consider the likelihood of future premium

increases by your company and its competitors, since they may be pricing aggressively, they may be new to the business of LTCI and lack pricing experience, or they may be less rigorous in their underwriting.

- Prospects will ask about past rate increases. You need to know the history of rate increases by your company and its competitors.

Consider one last point about price. Because understanding LTCI can be complicated, many advisors and prospects who do not fully understand the policies and the differences between them will be naturally inclined to compare policies almost solely on price. Decisions based on price alone can lead to wrong solutions, which is why your prospects need you to provide guidance in understanding the differences in the available products.

Rate Stability—Because most if not all policies issued today are guaranteed renewable, the right to raise premiums by class is contractual. There are many instances of rate increases in LTCI that have caused policies to lapse or the policyowner to either make financial sacrifices to maintain the coverage or to reduce benefits. A series of substantial rate increases can cast the advisor, the company, and the industry in a bad light.

As indicated previously, premiums for LTCI vary greatly, and it is difficult to say what is the "right" premium. A high premium may be exploitative, but a low premium may be inadequate, requiring a later rate increase or series of rate increases. Inadequate premiums could be the result of deliberate manipulation ("bait and switch" tactics) or simply the lack of adequate actuarial information to make pricing decisions.

In addition, a company's underwriting practices will have an affect on future price increases. On one hand, a company with liberal underwriting makes obtaining coverage fairly easy, but the tradeoff may be a series of rate increases later on. On the other hand, it may be more difficult to get coverage from a company with strict underwriting, but the risk of a rate increase may be minimal.

Service—The concept of service takes two distinct forms in the competitive search for LTCI: the service offered by the company and that offered by the advisor.

- *Company*—Customer service issues such as policy administration and claims handling can be partially facilitated with your assistance, but they are largely out of your control. The service provided by your company is part of what constitutes its reputation. A responsive service department is a great asset to tout in a competitive situation. Prospects will also want to know about such items as the resources offered by the company at claim time, just who handles claim issues, and how they are handled. These are real concerns that you should be prepared to address.

- *Advisor*—There is a value-added element to the personalized service you provide before, during, and after the sale. The demeanor you exhibit during the approach and fact-finding process allows you to establish your image as trustworthy and professional. You are performing an extremely valuable function by conducting the due diligence processes described in this book. You should not underestimate the opportunity you have to differentiate yourself from the competition. You are at least as important to prospects as the company you represent because you perform valuable financial counseling. You may personally monitor the underwriting and policy delivery process and service in-force policies. You should also review your clients' needs periodically. This will provide you with a tremendous opportunity to impact your clients' financial and emotional well being. Take this opportunity to review your clients' needs seriously.

Differences in Policies—Due to design innovations and competition for market-share, insurers offer LTCI policies that contain many different features. The NAIC's *A Shopper's Guide to Long-Term Care Insurance* contains extensive side-by-side worksheets for comparing policy features, premiums, and coverages. It also contains illustrative proposals provided by insurers. The problem is that policy comparisons are very difficult. One reason for the difficulty is that there may be calculations involved in comparing features like spousal discounts, benefit amounts, or inflation riders. Also, it is difficult, if not impossible, to understand subtle differences in policy features without a thorough understanding of the terminology being used to describe the features. Thus, the prospect is well advised to get all the information needed to allow him or her to completely evaluate these policy differences. This is where you can provide an important value-added dimension to the buying process.

Replacement

Policyowners are sometimes faced with the question of whether they should terminate an existing LTCI policy and purchase a new one. Such a replacement must be made with a careful and thorough determination that the new policy is better than the existing one. In addition, an old policy should never be terminated before a new one is actually issued. An insured must be aware of any preexisting-conditions provision in the new policy, whereby benefits otherwise payable under the old policy would be denied. The difference in premiums must also be considered because the new policy will be written at attained age rates that most likely will be higher than those used in the old policy, which was priced at a younger issue age.

Despite the reasons for not replacing an existing policy, there may be reasons to consider a new one. For example, a new policy may be the best approach for increasing the MDB amount or adding inflation protection. However, before proceeding with replacement, it is always prudent to determine if the existing insurer will raise its policy's benefits at a lower total cost than the cost of a new policy. On the other hand, lowering benefits would normally be accomplished by modifying an existing policy rather than replacing it.

While insurers continue to improve their LTCI policy offerings, it is always worth the effort to explore the possibility of supplementing an old policy with additional benefits. Because LTCI is a relatively new product, few examples of LTCI policy replacement are available. In some cases, policy replacement may be justified; in others it may not.

> **Price**
>
> Move away from price and focus more on the prospect's life situation. Be sure that the policy selected meets his or her overall needs.

Summary

It takes time to master the art of designing a LTCI policy to meet a prospect's needs within his or her premium commitment. As you continue to read policies, study company literature, and work with prospects you will develop a better feel for the LTCI product.

LTCI products have many features, benefits, and options that differ from company to company. A company's financial strength, reputation, price, and rate stability are important factors for a prospect to weigh when comparing policies, but the most important factor is the knowledge and trustworthiness of the advisor. Remember, when it comes to competition, the relationship you build with the prospect is the greatest differentiating factor.

Presenting and Implementing the Solution

After you have analyzed the prospect's situation and designed an appropriate plan, the next step is to conduct a closing interview in which you present the possible solutions to the prospect and ask for the sale. In this section we will focus on steps six and seven of the selling process: presenting solutions and implementing the solution.

Presenting Solutions

In presenting the solution, the financial advisor shares a plan with the prospect that is designed to meet his or her objectives. The advisor presents in summary form the facts and personal attitudes previously expressed by the prospect to see if there is any reason why he or she would not want to find a solution, and upon finding a reasonable solution, not want to take action. A successful presentation enables the prospect to see how your recommendations clearly support his or her objectives. It motivates but it does not manipulate or strong-arm the prospect to buy. As you present solutions, keep in mind that the prospect must make the final decision about policy options because he or she is buying the policy, not you.

Delivering a presentation that will motivate a prospect requires preparation and execution. Preparation begins with a vision of what a good presentation should cover. From this vision, you can develop an outline to

---

The Mind Rehearsal

Before you meet with the prospect to conclude the sale, visualize what will happen in your presentation. How will the prospect answer your questions? How will you reply if the prospect asks a difficult question or voices an objection that makes you hesitate? What papers will you need? How will you handle all the forms? Where will you sit when making the presentation? What will be the expression on the prospect's face when he or she signs the application?

This is a mind rehearsal for the sales interview. Sit quietly and let your imagination take over the process of making the sale. When you can see the sale in progress and visualize the prospect saying yes, then you have the necessary confidence and are prepared to meet. Visualization prepares you for the close.

---

ensure that critical points are covered. With the outline as your guide, you will be able to gather the necessary sales materials and organize your presentation. Now, you are ready to make your presentation to the prospect.

Elements of the Presentation

Although the specifics of an effective presentation will vary from advisor to advisor, there are two main components to every presentation in a two-interview sale. The first component is to reestablish the prospect's need for LTCI; the second is to present LTCI options.

Re-establish the Need—In a two-interview sale, some time will elapse between the first and second interviews. Therefore, it is important to reestablish the prospect's interest in and need for LTCI by summarizing the relevant points from the first interview. The best way to rekindle the prospect's interest is to review the gap between his or her desired outcome and the projected outcome without LTCI. Essentially, this should involve nothing more than reviewing the key points of the fact-finding interview, including how the prospect felt about them. You want the prospect not only to recognize the financial gap again, but also to feel it. Here is one method for accomplishing this goal:

Review the facts and planning assumptions—What assumptions were incorporated into planning? Has anything changed since the fact-finding interview? Would the prospect like to change any of the assumptions? In addition, review the following information from the fact-finding interview:

- *Health*—What is the prospect's health history, and how is his or her current health? What medications is the prospect taking? Is the prospect active? Does the prospect get regular exercise? Does the prospect maintain healthy nutrition and good hygiene? If the prospect shows signs of deteriorating health, point it out. In this case, the motivation for buying LTCI is obvious and it may be a lot more expensive for the prospect to wait. If the prospect has great health, congratulate him or her. Use the prospect's great health as the motivation for buying LTCI. If the prospect purchases now, he or she may qualify for a discount because of his or her good health.

- *Family history*—What is the history of longevity in the prospect's family? How long did the prospect's ancestors live? What kinds of hereditary conditions or illnesses are prevalent in the family? A family history of longevity and/or debilitating illnesses and conditions are reasons for the prospect to strongly consider buying LTCI.

- *Risk exposure*—What is the likelihood that the prospect will need LTC services, and what financial resources will the prospect have to pay for them? Statistical studies indicate that there is a fairly good chance of using a nursing home—as high as 50 percent at some point in a person's lifetime. This statistic contrasts with a 2-percent chance of being involved in a car accident and only a one-percent chance of suffering a property or liability loss. It is often very helpful in a sales presentation to present the comparative risks of several everyday exposures that a prospect would typically insure to help him or her understand and gain perspective on the LTC problem.

List the prospect's objectives—Review and confirm the prospect's objectives, concerns, and priorities. Essentially you are summarizing the prospect's answers to the following questions.

- What does the prospect want to provide for his or her benefit, and for the family?
- What does the prospect want to leave to his or her heirs and to charity?
- What priorities does the prospect have for his or her lifestyle in retirement?
- Does the prospect plan to spend time with his or her family?
- Does the prospect plan to travel, relocate, or remain involved in community and family activities?
- What is the prospect's premium commitment?

It is extremely important to match policy benefits with a prospect's objectives and priorities. These will vary for each prospect depending on his or her age and circumstances. In many cases the sales presentation will be built around a "hot button" or primary concern of the prospect. For example, an older prospect may be most concerned with asset preservation and having enough money to last through his or her retirement. He or she may also desire to pass money on to the next generation or to provide for charitable bequests. In addition, independence is often a key objective of older prospects. Thus, a lifetime income and not burdening their children are often "hot buttons."

Still other prospects may be more concerned about choosing where they will live and how they will be cared for if they need LTC. For these reasons, single people are often good prospects, as well as couples whose children live far away. People with a history of serious illnesses in their families may also have an interest in LTCI since they have experienced the need for LTC. Those who have lived through a LTC experience with a loved one will often be quite sensitive to the need for LTCI from an emotional as well as financial standpoint.

Relatively young prospects typically look ahead, plan their estates, and seek wealth protection devices. However, the younger prospects often have other demands on their financial resources, such as: funding for retirement, paying down mortgages, paying for their children's educations, and perhaps even paying for their parents' long-term care. These prospects often need help with a whole host of financial problems. Consequently, an important selling point for young prospects to consider is that paying for LTCI over many years starting at a fairly young age may be less expensive than paying for one year of nursing-home care sometime in the future. Buying a policy at a younger age also protects insurability. Should a person develop a chronic illness or debilitating injury later in life, insurability would be jeopardized. Besides, even if a person is still insurable later in life, LTCI will cost more at the older age. This fact alone should be a strong motivating force for buying the coverage when young.

Outline the expected cost of LTC—While reestablishing the prospect's need for LTCI, you should also refresh his or her understanding of just how expensive LTC can be, especially without LTCI.

Summarize the prospect's current LTC plan—This is a review of what may happen if the prospect does not buy LTCI. Recap the information from the fact-finding interview. Give the prospect your professional assessment of the current plan's ability to achieve his or her stated objectives considering his or her current situation with respect to:

- *Financial resources*—Project the funds needed by the current plan, including the prospect's fixed income that he or she committed to using for LTC, as well as other possible sources of financial assistance, such as family members.

- *Health insurance*—Review the prospect's health insurance coverages, including Medicare and Medigap insurance, that may cover some LTC needs. This will allow you to again point out just how inadequate they are for meeting LTC needs.
- *Family assistance*—Summarize the prospect's feelings about the role that family members will play in providing LTC. Note whether family members are located in the area, work outside the home, or have been spoken to about providing care.

Presenting LTCI Solutions—Once you have re-established the prospect's need for LTCI, you are now ready to present possible solutions to the prospect. Here are some suggested steps.

Summarize your observations—Summarize your observations about the current plan's inability to accomplish the prospect's objectives. These observations should paint a picture of the gaps you found in the current plan, demonstrating just how important it is that the prospect implement the recommendations you are about to make if he or she wants to achieve his or her stated objectives for meeting LTC needs.

Make your recommendations—Outline your recommendations, including both insurance and non-insurance solutions. If you are working with very affluent prospects, write your recommendations in a proposal that you give them. You should have a recommendation for each observation.

In the interview, present your recommendations beginning with the non-insurance solutions that are the easiest to implement. For example, if you notice the prospect does not have a living will, you can recommend that he or she see an attorney and have one drafted. Starting with an insurance recommendation might make the prospect cynical, raising his or her fears that you are only interested in making a sale.

During your presentation, you want to focus the discussion around the plan alternatives you are recommending. You want the prospect to pick the alternative that suits his or her needs, priorities, and budget. Discussion creates a sense of involvement on the part of the prospect and reinforces in his or her mind the selected alternative's ability to meet the objectives.

Self-Insure or Transfer the Risk?

One advisor explains how he ends the discussion on self-insuring the LTC risk:

The prospects must have a preference for LTCI to continue the sales process, so I conclude the discussion on self-insuring by asking the question: "Would you like to continue self-insuring, or would you like to transfer the LTC risk to the insurance company for pennies on the dollar?" The prospects have to decide right there. The sales process terminates if they would rather self-insure the risk; it continues if they prefer to transfer the risk.

If at this juncture your prospect still has some reservations about LTCI, you may find it necessary to review the relevant financing alternatives so you can eliminate them as possibilities. Since you do not want to muddy the waters, review only those alternatives that the prospect is considering using instead of LTCI. These alternatives are covered in chapters 3 and 4 and are briefly summarized below to show how they can be used in the presentation with the prospect. With these alternatives are questions that highlight some of the reasons why they may not be sufficient by themselves to cover the cost of LTC or may need to be part of a more comprehensive plan that includes LTCI.

- *Self-insure from savings*—Does it make sense for the prospect to work hard all his or her life, saving money just to see it all disappear to pay for LTC? How much money will be needed? Savings would have to be enormous to fund nursing-home care for any extended period of time, in which case LTCI makes more sense. How long could the prospect pay for LTC? What other needs would the prospect's savings have to satisfy?

- *Annuities*—Many deferred annuities provide for the withdrawal of funds (without any penalties or surrender charges) to pay for either retirement or long-term care expenses. Immediate annuities can also be used to fund retirement expenses, LTCI premiums, or other needs. Just how would either of these funding options impact the desire to leave a legacy to heirs?

- *Life insurance living benefits*—Life insurance cash values can be used to supplement other savings programs to fund current expenses, including LTC expenses. Will the cash values, along with other forms of savings, be sufficient if the prospect experiences a prolonged illness that is not terminal? In addition, life insurance death benefits can be paid out to the insured under an accelerated benefits provision if the insured suffers from a specified medical condition that is terminal. This enables the insured to withdraw a portion of the policy's death benefits while he or she is still living. The insured should check with his or her insurer to see whether this alternative is available because some companies will allow payment of an accelerated death benefit even when the provision is not included in the policy.

- *Viatical settlement*—Under a viatical settlement, the insured sells his or her life insurance policy for a percentage of the death benefit. The insured, often elderly or terminally ill, can use the cash to pay for medical or LTC expenses. The purchaser receives the policy death benefit on the subsequent death of the insured. Will the cash received by the insured be adequate to fund his or her LTC expenses?

- *Reverse mortgages*—Today's seniors have benefited from the housing market appreciation over the years, and now their homes are their most valuable asset. A reverse mortgage can be a source of cash for an individual to meet daily living expenses, pay for home health or nursing home care, make home improvements, or even purchase annuities or LTCI. What is the prospect's situation with regard to this possibility, and how does he or she feel about this alternative?

- *Relatives*—Family members are often called on to provide LTC because such care is preferred, no other arrangement has been made, or there is no alternative. However, this option is becoming less feasible as more and more family members become geographically dispersed and dual-income or single parent families have less time to devote to providing care. In addition, delaying the start of a family is becoming more popular. Consequently, many parents are still caring for young children at the time that their parents may need care.

   There is also a dignity issue, which is difficult to discuss but must be addressed. Many care issues involve privacy and hygiene matters that make it difficult to receive care from a close family member, a child, or other relative. Also, giving care for an extended period can be an enormous emotional, physical, and financial burden. If the parent needs to move in with the relative, resentment of the situation can affect all concerned. Even if relatives do provide care willingly, they will need a break and caregiving services will have to be provided. Has the prospect discussed this possibility with his or her family? Does the family have a realistic understanding of the burdens that caregiving can impose on them?

One Comparison of Buying LTCI versus Saving the Premium

Assumptions:

LTCI Policy	Premiums Saved
• initial $100 per day MDB amount • maximum benefit period: 1095 days (3 years) used consecutively • 5 percent compounded automatic increase in benefits each year • the prospect is aged 65 at the time of purchase • $1,500 annual premium • waiver of premium	• five percent tax-free rate of return • compounded annually • save $1,500 at the beginning of each year

Age Benefit Begins	Cumulative Premium	Assumed 1095 Days Maximum Benefits	Net Benefit	Savings at 5% Tax-Free
	(A)	(B)	(B − A)	(C)
70	$7,500	$147,095	$139,595	$8,288
75	15,000	187,610	172,610	18,867
80	22,500	239,075	216,575	32,368
85	30,000	305,505	275,505	49,599
90	37,500	389,820	352,320	71,591
95	45,000	497,130	452,130	99,658

Conclusion: Many financial decisions involve risks and rewards. In this case, the reward for someone who purchases a LTCI policy and who utilizes three full years of benefits is shown in the net benefit column. On the other hand, the risk is that one never uses the policy benefits and thus forfeits the use of the premium dollars. This risk is shown in column C. For example, assume a person purchases a policy at age 65, pays premiums for 10 years and begins receiving benefits from the policy at age 75. He or she will have received a positive benefit of $172,610. However, if the policyowner dies at age 75 without having collected any policy benefits, the economic loss is $18,867. Alternatively, if it is assumed that a person purchases a policy at age 65, pays premiums for 20 years and begins receiving benefits from the policy at age 85, he or she will have received a positive benefit of $275,505. However, if the policyowner dies at age 85 without having collected any policy benefits, the economic loss would be $49,599.

Source: United Seniors Health Council. Long-Term Care Insurance: A Professional's Guide To Selecting Policies. *Washington, D.C., 1995.*

- *Medicare/Medicaid*—Medicare is not a solution for providing LTC. It will pay for LTC only if skilled-nursing care is also medically necessary. Furthermore, there are limitations to the number of days and types of services covered. Medicare is designed to pay for acute medical expenses, not the custodial or supervisory care associated with most LTC situations.

Medicaid is the option of last resort. A person must be "indigent" to qualify for it, exhausting nearly all personal and family assets. Also, not every facility accepts Medicaid recipients, causing waiting lists and overcrowding at those that do. Is this an alternative that a person would voluntarily choose?

In the final analysis, the alternatives to LTC financing must be inferior to the purchase of a LTCI policy if a sale is to be made. By purchasing a LTCI policy, the expenses and other burdens of this problem can be transferred to an insurer. People with few assets to protect and little income after expenses probably are not good candidates for LTCI. For pennies on the dollar, wealthier prospects can shift the risk of LTC, and many elect to do so.

Outline the implementation plan—The implementation plan provides you with a way to review your recommendations while providing the prospect with the action steps necessary to complete them. It should identify who is responsible for implementing each step and establish deadlines for the implementation.

Preparing for the Presentation

The key to an effective presentation is preparation. Take the time to prepare and put together a standardized presentation for your sales presentation binder. The amount of time needed to prepare will decrease as you gain more experience, but initially you will want to create a detailed presentation outline for each closing interview. Here are some examples of ways for you to prepare for this interview:

- Analyze your prospect. What were his or her attitudes toward LTC and LTCI? Does he or she appear to recognize and accept the risk? What are the prospect's probable motives for buying? What are the barriers?
- Create a summary of the fact-finding interview that you can use as an outline when you re-establish the LTCI need. Use the outline suggested in the previous section as a start.

Presentation Checklist

Review the following items in preparing to deliver your solution presentation:

- Determine your purpose: What are the prospect's financial objectives, goals, and needs that you will help him or her solve?
- Who is your prospect, and what decision-makers will be present?
- What are the buying motives of the prospect and/or the decision-makers?
- What is the prospect's current situation?
- What is the prospect's desired situation?
- What are the specific buying conditions, such as budget (premium commitment), other resources, desired policy features, start date, parameters of coverage, and so on?
- Does the prospect agree with your assessment of the problem?
- Develop your solution and statements to support it. This may involve a few alternative plans.
- Review specific factual and feeling-finding information collected.
- Anticipate any objections or concerns and prepare responses to these.
- Rehearse your presentation and answers to objections or any other anticipated verbal exchanges.

- Check your suggested plan alternatives. How do they reflect the prospect's needs, priorities, and budget? What are the pros and cons to each alternative? Which do you feel is the best alternative and why?
- Collect any company-approved sales material you will use in the presentation. If you have a series of such items, put them in order in your sales presentation binder.
- Create policy illustrations for all of your recommendations ahead of time. Check the prospect information (name, age, and so forth) for accuracy.
- Put together any written proposals you will use with your presentation.
- Confirm the appointment time and location with the prospect.

The better prepared you are, the more you can focus on the prospect and handle any objections or concerns. Furthermore, you will present a professional image to the prospect if everything you need is right there.

Presentation Techniques and Tips

There are many complicated aspects to LTCI: underwriting concerns, financing alternatives, benefit choices, and helping the prospect to understand the need. No matter how well you have prepared, or how good your recommendations, presenting them is still the critical element. There are a few things you can do to enhance the effectiveness of your presentation.

Focus on Relevant Features and Benefits—One mistake financial advisors make is to think that the purpose of the presentation is to educate the prospect about the technical, legal, tax, and product aspects of LTCI. While an advisor should discuss these aspects, they should be discussed in light of the features and corresponding benefits that are relevant to the prospect and are the basis for your recommendations.

A product *feature* is a characteristic of the product itself—what it is and what it does. A feature is a fact about the product. On the other hand, a *benefit* is what the prospect gets as a result of the feature. It is what the product does for the prospect and usually why he or she wants it.

Features produce benefits. For example, you buy a drill because you need a hole.

When you explain a feature of a LTCI policy, stress the benefits that the prospect will receive. Prospects respond to benefits. How a feature provides a benefit is not the point. Focus your presentation on the benefits—what a feature will do for a prospect is what he or she cares about. Concentrate on the benefits that matter most to your prospect—those you uncovered in the fact-finding process. For example, if independence is valued by the prospect, show the prospect how LTCI will give him or her control over when, where, and how he or she will receive LTC services. If not burdening the prospect's children is important, demonstrate how LTCI will enable him or her to receive quality care in the setting of his or her choice without disrupting the children's lives.

When presenting a recommendation, you want to explain what it is, how it solves the LTC problem, and what it does for the prospect. The benefit aspect is very important. Is it worth the price? Is it the best option? Will it save money? How well will it work for the prospect? These and other similar questions must be addressed and answered if the prospect is to buy your solution. Thus, the benefits for the prospect must be clearly communicated.

Sample Benefit Statements

Unlimited Lifetime Benefit—"This means you can feel comfortable knowing that you can never outlive your benefits."

Inflation Protection—"This feature increases your policy's MDB amount to keep up with the increasing cost of care."

LTCI—"This coverage is a wise decision because it protects the estate you have worked so hard to create."

Keep the Prospect Involved—It is important to have the prospect's participation and involvement in the sales process for several reasons:

- It helps prospects feel responsible for solving their own problems.
- It helps you know whether you are on target with your presentation.
- It builds agreement one step at a time.
- It helps clarify any misunderstanding by either party.
- It helps lead to a logical and successful close—a conclusion to buy.
- It provides opportunities to deal with objections before asking prospects to buy.

The simplest and most effective way to keep the prospect involved is to ask questions throughout the presentation. Use questions to help the prospect express his or her feelings and to confirm that he or she understands what you are saying. For example, after explaining the unlimited lifetime benefit to the prospect you could ask, "What would a lifetime benefit mean to you?" This will reveal not only if the prospect understands the concept of a lifetime benefit, but also how he or she feels about it.

Insist on All Decision-Makers Being Present—LTC is a family issue. Many families will discuss LTC and using LTC services before any decision is reached about buying LTCI. Both spouses should be present at the interviews, but the advisor should encourage the prospects to have other family members who will be participating in the purchase decision to be there as well. Experienced advisors know they need to have all decision-makers present for a positive outcome. In fact, often the other family members, especially the children, are the "unseen decision makers" in the purchase of LTCI.

Be Alert for Buying Signals—Sometimes advisors find that they have talked themselves out of a sale. The prospect was ready to buy but the advisor kept on explaining details that confused and bored the prospect. To avoid this situation, monitor the prospect for buying signals. Many people who show a desire to fulfill their unmet needs are ready to buy long before they ever say so. From the prospect's comments, you should

Summary of Presentation Steps:

1. **Warm Up**—Begin to pre-qualify the prospect by asking about the family situation, caregivers, health history, current health, and so forth. Discuss the prospect's financial situation and personal plans.

2. **Discuss LTC Experiences**—Ask the prospect if he or she knows someone who has needed LTC services. Discuss the reasons for the care and who paid the bills. Share your own personal experience with LTC.

3. **Discuss the need for LTC**—The prospect must agree and accept that there is a real possibility that LTC services may be needed, and that the costs could be staggering.

4. **Eliminate those who will not pay**—Review the possible sources of LTC funding. Show how medical insurance, government programs and self-funding may leave the prospect without enough money to cover the costs of LTC services.

5. **Compare the Risks**—Show how the risk of needing LTC is greater than the risk of having an automobile insurance or a homeowners insurance claim.

6. **Find the Premium**—Discuss a budget amount that can be a premium commitment. Discuss types of coverage and any ability to self-fund. Discuss how any shortfall can be insured and the risk transferred.

7. **Present the Solution**—LTCI can be designed to provide the desired protection and to coincide with the prospect's premium commitment.

8. **Close the Sale**—Assume consent. Complete the application and ask the prospect to pay the initial premium.

be able to distinguish some fairly obvious verbal and nonverbal signals that indicate acceptance or rejection. Some examples are:

Verbal signals:

- "It would feel good knowing we had this kind of coverage."
- "I see what you mean."
- "Can we include that benefit with what I can afford to spend?"
- "Do you need a physical to get this insurance?"
- "I appreciate the thoroughness of your presentation."
- "When would the coverage start (if I sign an application)?"

Nonverbal Signals:

- Leaning forward
- Listening attentively
- Good eye contact

- Nodding, showing appreciation
- Speaking up, participating

Paying attention to the verbal and nonverbal clues will alert you that you should attempt to close the sale. Simply acknowledge the signal, whether verbal or nonverbal, and proceed with your close. For example, if the prospect says, "When would the coverage start?" You could reply, "It starts as soon as I have collected the first premium. We can get started with an application right now, if you would like." Or if they give you good eye contact you could say, "It looks like you might be ready to proceed with an application. Do you have any questions before we do that?"

Implementing the Solution

A successful presentation ends with step seven of the selling process, implementing the solution. Implementing the solution involves asking the prospect to buy your product and overcoming any objections or concerns you may encounter.

Closing the Sale

This portion of the sales process should not be pushy or manipulative. It may, however, require that you be firm and assertive with the prospect. How you conduct yourself will depend somewhat on the prospect's behavior and social style as discussed in chapter 4. Closing will also depend on how well the selling process has flowed to this point. For example, if you have anticipated and preempted all the prospect's objections, your close may be as simple as, "How do you spell your middle name?"

When purchasing a LTCI policy, a prospect must choose an advisor that he or she feels is trustworthy. Establishing trust begins with you showing genuine concern for the prospect's well being and a professional knowledge of LTC and LTCI. You can build on this foundation by using an educational and consultative approach with the prospect. He or she will want to make an informed decision and be treated with respect. Your job is to provide objective information and assist the prospect in making a decision that meets his or her needs in a non-combative way. As a reliable and dependable advisor, you can develop the all-important trust over a period of time.

If the sale has progressed through the process as outlined in this book, then there is no place or need for manipulation or pressure tactics in closing the sale. If the need for LTCI has been established, the alternatives discussed, the solution designed and presented clearly, and a trusting relationship has been established, then the sale should result. If not, examine what you did to determine where you went wrong. With a few changes, it is possible that this sale can still be made.

Client-focused selling does not mean that you allow a prospect's natural inclination to do nothing to go unchallenged. Closing a LTCI sale is like selling any other insurance product. Sometimes you have to be blunt and tough with the prospect to get your point across. This does not mean you should be rude or pushy, but sincerely concerned. If the prospect needs to take action to protect against a loss that could harm him or her, or harm his or her family, you need to warn about the consequences of inaction. Tell the prospect some emotional stories about people losing a lot because of the need for LTC and the disruption it had on their families. These stories are common. They can create a sense of urgency for the prospect that now is the time to take action.

The Fear of Closing—Advisors often fail to ask prospects to buy because they feel they are imposing on them, they feel they have not explained the solution adequately, or they fear rejection. There is some natural emotional tension between advisors and prospects at this point because it is "the moment of truth"—the time to make a commitment to a product, a company, and a relationship.

To move past this fear, remember that asking for the business is a natural step in the sales process. The prospect expects you to ask him or her to buy a policy. The prospect knows as well as you that the reason you have been spending time together is to obtain information so you can design a plan for him or her. You have earned the right to ask for the business because you thoroughly understand the

Essentials of Long-Term Care Insurance

prospect's situation and are recommending a solution to help him or her address an important need.

Overcoming Objections (Managing Resistance)

If the fact-finding process has allowed you to ask the right questions and the prospect has answered them candidly, most if not all of the prospect's concerns should have already been addressed. Nonetheless, a prospect may not feel comfortable or understand the process or the problems well enough to have previously disclosed all of his or her concerns, so they may emerge here. Since we have covered this topic in chapter 4, we will only review the principles here.

The first step in answering an objection is to listen to the prospect. Listening to what the prospect has to say will help you understand the objection. Encourage the prospect to fully explain his or her objection and tell you more about how he or she feels about the issue. Give yourself and the prospect the opportunity to confirm your understanding of the objection by restating or rephrasing it. This gives you an opportunity to learn more about the exact nature of the prospect's objection. This also puts you in a better position to address and overcome it.

The selling process should build logically to the inescapable conclusion that the prospect needs LTCI and there is no reason why he or she should not buy it now. Each step in the process supports the following one so that by the time you get to the point where the prospect raises issues and concerns, you should know enough about his or her personal and financial situation, attitudes, and feelings to respond directly, honestly, and convincingly.

A well-prepared presentation can reduce the number of objections you encounter by anticipating and dealing with them in advance. You can reduce the number of objections by

- developing rapport and trust
- getting agreement at each step in the presentation
- focusing on the benefits of your recommendations

> **If They Are Not Convinced of the Need, Nothing Else Matters**
>
> Price doesn't make any difference if prospects do not see the need. It is very important that they have had an experience with LTC. The sales process is one of explaining the need.
>
> The key to selling this product is for prospects to understand and accept the need. Just like in real estate the secret is "location, location, location," with this product the key is "need, need, need."

Handling Concerns and Objections—While you can reduce the number of objections, you will always encounter them. Do not take them personally. It is natural for a prospect to have objections to purchasing insurance. This is a natural reaction to the idea of spending money. People hate to spend money needlessly and waste it on something they do not need or something they perceive to be of little immediate value.

As you talk with your prospect, use *trial closes*, such as "Other than affordability, is this the product you think will best suit your needs?" Use questions to determine the prospect's agreement at each stage of your presentation:

- Does this make sense to you?
- Do you see how this benefits your family?
- Is this what you had in mind?
- Do you want to include this in your plan?
- Do you have any questions?

Because overcoming objections takes practice and experience, it is important not to get discouraged if at first you are not successful. There are many techniques at your disposal. The "feel, felt, found" and the "acknowledge, clarify, resolve" methods are two effective examples discussed in chapter 4.

The Problem-Solving Approach—In general, you should take a problem-solving approach to objections, focusing on three things:

- building trust and rapport with prospects
- dealing with the needs involved, not personalities
- instilling a sense of urgency

You can build trust and rapport by demonstrating, with your professionalism and forthrightness, that you care about answering the prospects' concerns with real answers. Be empathetic—put yourself in the prospects' shoes. Reassure the prospects that by keeping their objectives in mind and reviewing the various alternatives available, they can move toward their goals—or as far along as possible. Working together can help to resolve the issues that are causing them concern.

You can deal with needs rather than personalities by focusing on the issues rather than winning debate points, getting the upper hand, or having the last word. When prospects raise difficult objections, you should not imply that unless they buy LTCI, they do not love their families. Their real concern may be a lack of money or improper timing. In addition, avoid arguing with prospects. Pointing out to prospects that their objections are not valid is sales suicide. You may win the argument, but you will surely end up losing the sale. In other words, you should not become so focused on overcoming their objections that you forget they have a real need. If they postpone or rethink their decisions to buy LTCI, they may be risking their families' financial security needs.

Finally, remember that your prospects are making an important decision. Comments, concerns, and questions are a natural and expected part of the decision-making process. In answering their objections and even in dealing with their excuses, you provide your prospects with perspectives and information that will help them understand the need for LTCI, how your product meets the need, and the urgency of acting now to put the plan into force.

> **"I'd Like to Think It Over"**
>
> One advisor provides insight into her response to the statement, "I'd like to think it over."
>
> I know many advisors don't like to give prospects an out, but I find this approach will make the sale about 80 percent of the time. Here's what I say:
>
> "I know we've covered a lot here. You may want to review it, and answer questions like, "Can I pay for it?" (Be sure the plan can fit their budget.) Let's send an application and the first premium to the company and see if you qualify. It will take some time and this will give you a chance to think it over."

Summary

For a two-interview sales process, the gap in time between the initial and closing interviews means that the presentation will need to re-establish the need for and the motivation to buy LTCI. In addition, you will want to present a LTCI solution that reflects the prospects' needs, priorities, and budgets. Using the simple concept of features and benefits, you can effectively demonstrate how LTCI can meet the prospects' needs.

If the selling process has progressed properly, implementing the solution means nothing more than a transition to taking an application. Of course, objections can and do arise, and when they do you should be prepared to handle them in light of the prospects' circumstances and motivations. Closing the sale need not be manipulative or heavy-handed, but it should not allow prospects to escape from being told the truth about what would happen if they failed to act.

Case History

The LTCI Selling Process

The following is the selling process used by Rick DiLaurenzo, a LTC specialist with over 17 years of experience selling LTCI. In addition to LTCI brokerage sales, Rick writes articles on long-term care and authors and teaches continuing education classes for LTC. Rick generally uses the two-interview sales approach outlined below.

The First Interview

I believe in a two-interview sale. In the first interview, my goal is to qualify the prospect, demonstrate the need for LTCI, and conduct a thorough fact-finder.

1. Qualifying Period (A Warm-Up Period)—I insist that the prospects sit at a table, which sets up a good atmosphere to work. I then qualify the prospects by exploring the following questions:

- "Do you know anyone who has needed nursing or convalescent care services?"
- "What is your date of birth?"
- "Do you have children? If so, how many? What are their ages? Do they live locally?" I call the children "the unseen decision makers." I require that they be present at the second interview if their opinions count.
- "What health insurance do you have? Medicare? How is your health? Are you taking any medications? Can I see them? Have you been hospitalized in the last 5 years? Have you seen a doctor in the last 5 years?
- "Have you received any or do you expect to receive any sales proposals?" I then tell the prospects, "You should get them. I agree you should look around. Just do me a favor—please don't sign anything before you let me review it with you, OK?"

- "What savings and investments do you have? Has the value of your investments gone up, stayed the same, or gone down over the last year? Over the last 5 years?" I get an idea of their income, assets, and budget. I do not include their residence.

At this point, I decide whether to continue working with the prospects. I ask myself, "Are they qualified prospects, from both a health and financial point of view? Are they immediate prospects, or could they be future prospects if recent health issues clear up?" If they are not immediate prospects, then I stop the process. Otherwise I proceed to step two.

2. Show the "Health Care Pie"—In this step, I show the gaps in their coverage, particularly regarding LTC. The Health Care Pie (similar in concept to the Circle of Health Protection introduced in chapter 4) consists of Medicare Parts A and B, and is designed to show how convalescent care is not covered, leaving a gap that can only be filled by LTCI. I then ask, "Do you want to close these gaps?" If there is interest, I proceed to step three.

3. Family Resource Questionnaire—In step three, I use what I call the family resource questionnaire, in which I ask the following questions:

- "Like many families you have gaps in your health care coverage. How are you planning to pay for the cost of convalescent care, if one of you needs it and it costs between $50,00 and $80,000 a year?" (I then wait for their answers)
- "Suppose last month one of you (use the prospects' names) had a serious stroke requiring specialized nursing home care. How would you be paying this month's bill and the bills in the coming months?"
- "Do your children have the financial resources to support the cost of your care?"
- "Do your children have the time to care for you if your condition lasts longer than a couple of weeks?"
- "Are you hoping to someday leave your assets to your children?"
- "Is there some financial reason why you haven't already purchased LTCI?"

4. How to Choose Benefits—In this step, I help the prospects understand the available LTCI plans and benefits. I discuss the options and how to select them. I begin with the types of plans and show them a facility-only plan, a home care only plan, and a comprehensive plan. Then I ask, "What type of plan would you like?" and "What amount would you like for each benefit?" as I show them the options available for each benefit and help them make their selections.

- Daily Benefit ($40-$350 MDB)
- Benefit Period (number of years of benefit: 2, 3, 4, 5, 6, or unlimited)
- Elimination Period "deductible," number of days care is not paid initially (It can be 0, 20, 30, 60, 90, or 180 days.)
- Inflation Protection (5 percent simple, 5 percent compound, overbuy)

5. End the First Interview—I end the first interview by asking, "What is your goal in having LTCI? Do you wish to prevent spousal impoverishment or to leave money to your children?" (If you receive an affirmative answer to the latter, recommend an unlimited lifetime benefit.) This technique helps the prospects to sell themselves.

Finally, I set the appointment for the second interview for one week later and end the meeting. I do not discuss the price of the coverage.

Preparation for Second Interview

1. Choose TQ or NQ—If the prospects do not have a lot of money to self-insure, I prefer to use a NQ policy with a medically necessary trigger and a shorter benefit qualification period. If the prospects can afford to self-insure for a period of time, then I use a TQ policy with a longer elimination period and tax-free benefits. I use TQ policies about 90 percent of the time.

2. Select a Plan(s) to Recommend—Based on my fact-finding, I create a spreadsheet to compare the different companies I represent. I look for the best match based on health history, benefits, and other factors. I then select the best plan(s) to present to the prospect.

Second Interview

1. Review the First Interview—I begin the second interview by reviewing items discussed in the first interview. I emphasize the benefits they said they wanted and confirm that they have not changed their minds. If they have changed their minds, I reschedule the interview so I can redesign the plan before presenting it to them. If they have not changed their minds, I move on to step two.

2. **Present a Proposed Plan**—I go through the proposed plan step-by-step, benefit-by-benefit. I review a sales brochure and create an image for every benefit. For example, I might say, "The policy has a home health care benefit. This means you won't need to be placed in a nursing home if you can be cared for at home." I then have the prospects repeat back to me their understanding of each benefit by asking them, "What does this mean to you?" In this way, I am sure they understand the plan.

3. **Show the Premium**—Finally, I tell them the premium amount for the plan and watch their faces carefully. I look for non-verbal clues that can help me understand how they feel about the premium.

4. **My 1-2-3 Close**—If they don't show a negative reaction to the premium amount, I then close with three questions:

- "Mr. and Mrs. Prospect, can you afford this payment, or would you like to see a plan with a lower premium?" I find that about 50 percent of my prospects would like to see a lower premium plan. So I change the least important benefit to them. For example, I may change the benefit period from 5 years to 4 years or inflation protection from compound interest to simple interest, and so forth. I change one benefit at a time, adjusting the premium until an amount is reached they can afford.

- "Are the benefit amounts high enough for you or would you like to see higher benefits? Is there any benefit you would like to change?" I find that many prospects will increase the benefits here, even if we had just lowered them in response to my first question.

- "Is there anything else you would like me to go over or anything else in terms of benefits or premiums you would like to know about?" My purpose here is to identify any objections and deal with them now.

5. **Assumed Consent**—I then take out an application and tell them, "I need to get some information for the insurance company." I ask, "Do you use a middle initial?" and begin filling out the application. I find that 80 percent of my prospects respond favorably to this close.

Chapter Six Review

Key Terms and Concepts are explained in the Glossary. Answers to the Review Questions and Self-Test Questions are found in the back of the book in the Answers to Questions section.

Key Terms and Concepts

buying signals   nonverbal signals

features and benefits   nonqualified (NQ) policy

preexisting condition   tax-qualified (TQ) policy

Review Questions

6-1. What three things must happen before LTCI policy benefits can be paid?

6-2. Briefly explain the steps involved in calculating the maximum daily benefit (MDB) amount to include in a LTCI policy.

6-3. What key areas should be evaluated when comparing the competition with your company and the products it offers?

6-4. What are some funding alternatives for LTC services other than LTCI?

6-5. Explain the difference between a policy feature and a policy benefit.

6-6. Explain why it is important to have the prospect's participation and involvement in the sales process.

6-7. Give some examples of nonverbal buying signals.

6-8. What three things should be put in focus when taking a problem-solving approach to handling a prospect's objections to buying LTCI?

Self-Test Questions

Instructions: Read chapter 6 first, then answer the following questions to test your knowledge. There are 10 questions; for questions 1 through 6, match the question with the aspect of the policy to which it relates; for questions 7 through 10, circle the correct answer. When finished with the test, check your answers with the answer key in the back of the book.

Match each question below with the aspect of the policy to which it relates.

6-1. When will benefits start? ____
6-2. How much will be paid? ____
6-3. How long will benefits last? ____
6-4. Where will care be given? ____
6-5. Will policy benefits periodically increase? ____
6-6. How will the policy be treated for tax purposes? ____

   (a) tax-qualified versus non tax-qualified
   (b) premium commitment
   (c) elimination period
   (d) indemnity benefits versus reimbursement benefits
   (e) inflation protection
   (f) comprehensive versus facility only
   (g) benefit period versus pool-of-money method
   (h) spousal discounts

6-7. In a two-interview sale, the first component of the second or closing interview is to

   (a) present LTCI options
   (b) reestablish the need
   (c) establish rapport
   (d) gather relevant information

6-8. Which of the following statements regarding the role of Medicare in providing LTC coverage is (are) correct?

   I.   It is designed to cover custodial or supervisory LTC.
   II. It provides some coverage for skilled-nursing LTC.

   (a) I only
   (b) II only
   (c) Both I and II
   (d) Neither I nor II

6-9. Suggested steps for presenting possible LTCI solutions to a prospect include all of the following **EXCEPT**

    (a)   outline the implementation plan
    (b)   summarize your observations
    (c)   make your recommendations
    (d)   obtain a dollar commitment

6-10. All of the following are things that can be done to enhance the effectiveness of your solution presentation **EXCEPT**

    (a)   avoid asking the prospect questions
    (b)   focus on relevant features and benefits
    (c)   insist on all decision-makers being present
    (d)   be alert for buying signals

7

Underwriting, Delivering, and Servicing the Policy

Overview and Learning Objectives

Chapter 7 looks at the underwriting of a LTCI policy. It then examines the principles for delivering and servicing a LTCI policy effectively. Finally, the chapter ends with a discussion of the role LTCI plays in a client or prospect's overall financial plan. By reading this chapter and answering the questions, you should be able to:

7-1.   Describe the issues involved in underwriting and taking an application.

7-2.   Explain how to conduct an effective policy delivery.

7-3.   Describe methods of servicing the LTCI plan.

7-4.   Explain the claim process to a prospect or client.

7-5.   Explain the relationship of the LTC need to other financial planning needs.

Chapter Outline

Underwriting LTCI

An individual facing the uncertainty of having to pay for the cost of LTC may seek to transfer this potentially catastrophic risk to an insurer in exchange for the certainty of paying a relatively small periodic premium. However, to protect the insurer against the possibility of adverse selection, each LTC risk that is being transferred to the insurer must go through the process of underwriting to determine whether the risk is acceptable. If the risk is found to be acceptable after a thorough underwriting evaluation, the home office underwriter then determines the terms, conditions, and price at which the LTCI coverage is to be issued.

The underwriting process initially begins when an advisor meets with a LTCI prospect. If the advisor prequalifies the prospect in the course of the interview, the next step is for the advisor to complete an application.

Completing the LTCI Application

The advisor is responsible for completing the application, obtaining all the required information, including signatures, and providing all disclosure information to the applicant. The application, with the advisor and applicant's signatures, becomes part of the policy, which is a legal contract. In signing the application the advisor and applicant represent that all the information in the application is true.

When completing the application, the advisor should focus on the following objectives:

- Obtaining all the information requested, leaving no questions unanswered. Unanswered and/or incomplete questions slow down the underwriting process considerably.
- Completing the application in the applicant's presence.
- Recording accurately all information as provided by the applicant.
- Obtaining necessary signatures.
- Completing a suitability statement.

- Providing the applicant with an outline of coverage, a shopper's guide to LTCI, and all receipts and documentation according to the laws of the state and the requirements of the insurer. A few states also require that a guide explaining Medicare supplement policies be provided to applicants over age 64.

When fully and legibly completed, the application provides the underwriter with a comprehensive picture of the applicant. Every piece of information requested on the application is vital to properly evaluate and process that application and comply with state regulations.

Most states prohibit advisors from making any changes on an application once the applicant has signed it. If an error is discovered, arrangements must be made to return the application to the applicant for any needed changes. Never use whiteout; errors must be crossed out and initialed by the applicant, or a new application must be taken. Changing or adding information by anyone other than the applicant is a misdemeanor in most states. Any information the advisor wishes to provide the company can be entered in the advisor's statement.

Proper Disclosure

State and NAIC Regulations—The National Association of Insurance Commissioners (NAIC) developed and promulgated a Long-Term Care Insurance Model Act and a Model Regulation to help regulate the industry. The Model Act is designed to be incorporated into a state's insurance law and the Model Regulation is designed to be adopted for use in implementing the law. The portion of this model legislation that pertains to suitability and marketing is briefly outlined below, but is also covered in chapter 8 in more detail.

Company Requirements—Insurers adopt their own requirements relating to the application and delivery process. Delivery receipts, disclosure notices, privacy disclosures, and other forms may have to be distributed and signatures obtained. Be sure you are familiar with the underwriting and delivery requirements of your company.

NAIC Suitability Guidelines—Suitability means determining whether LTCI is appropriate for meeting an applicant's needs. The NAIC LTCI Model Regulation requires any insurer marketing LTCI to develop and use suitability standards and to train its advisors to use the standards. These standards must take the following into account:

- the applicant's ability to pay for the coverage and other financial information appropriate to its purchase
- the applicant's goals or needs with respect to LTCI and the advantages and disadvantages of LTCI in meeting those goals or needs
- the values, benefits, and costs of any of the applicant's existing LTCI compared to the values, benefits, and costs of the recommended purchase or replacement

The insurer or advisor must make a reasonable effort to obtain the information. This requires the development of a personal worksheet with information about the proposed premium, the insurer's right to increase the premium, and the insurer's history of premium increases. The worksheet also must contains a questionnaire that requires the applicant to answer the following questions:

- How will you pay each year's premium—from income, from savings and investments, or with family help?
- Have you considered whether you can afford to keep the policy if the premium goes up by 20 percent?
- What is your annual income?
- How do you expect your income to change over the next 10 years—increase, decrease, or not change?
- Will you buy inflation protection? If not, have you considered how you will pay the difference between future costs and your MDB amount?
- What elimination period are you considering, and how do you plan to pay for your care during this period?
- Other than your home, what is the approximate value of your assets?
- How do you expect your assets to change over the next 10 years?

The applicant must sign a statement that the insurer or advisor has reviewed the personal worksheet with him or her. In addition, the applicant must indicate that the completed questionnaire describes his or her financial situation or that he or she chooses not to provide the information.

The insurer then compares the applicant's financial information with its suitability standards. If the applicant does not meet the insurer's suitability standards or does not choose to provide financial information, the insurer may decline the application or send the applicant a letter stating that the insurer has suspended the final review of the application. However, if the applicant believes the policy is what he or she wants, the applicant should check the appropriate box on the letter and return it to the insurer within 60 days. The insurer may then continue to review the application and issue a LTCI policy if the applicant meets its underwriting standards.

Suitability standards focus on determining minimum standards for the appropriateness of LTCI. A state may adopt the standards promulgated by the NAIC, or it may develop its own standards. An insurer can either adopt the state's standards or develop its own set of higher standards. Suitability standards typically include such threshold numbers as the minimum level of an applicant's income, the percentage of the applicant's income that premiums should not exceed, and possibly even the minimum amount of assets the applicant should own (excluding a home and automobile).

NAIC Marketing Guidelines—Some of the provisions of the NAIC model legislation that pertain to marketing LTCI include:

- *Outline of Coverage*—This is an important tool for explaining a policy's features to a prospect. It must be delivered to the prospect at the time of the initial solicitation and includes a brief description of the policy's most important features.
- *Shopper's Guide*—A shopper's guide must be delivered to a prospect prior to completing an application. The guide must either be in the format developed by the NAIC or one developed by the state. A shopper's guide is a good source of information and a great educational tool for the advisor and the prospect, plus it has the benefit of being a "neutral" piece from a third-party.
- *30-day Free Look*—The policyowner has 30 days after the policy's delivery to return it, without explanation, for a full refund of premium.
- *Standards for Appropriateness of Coverage*—In marketing LTCI it is necessary to determine whether such coverage is appropriate for meeting an applicant's needs. From the standpoint of the insurer and advisor, this process is referred to as suitability and is

Essentials of Long-Term Care Insurance

more fully explained in the previous section on NAIC suitability guidelines.

- *Limitations on Post-Claims Underwriting*—An issue of concern to many in the financial services industry is post-claims underwriting. This practice occurs when the insurer does little underwriting at the time of the initial application. Then, after a claim is filed, the insurer obtains medical information that could have been obtained earlier. Based on this new information, the insurer either rescinds the policy or denies the claim. To control this practice, the LTCI application must be clear and unambiguous so that the applicant's health condition can be properly ascertained. Language in the application must make it clear that the payment of any subsequent claims are dependent on the applicant providing true and complete answers to questions in the application.

- *Third Party Notification of Pending Policy Lapse*—The applicant is given the option of naming one or more persons to receive notice of a pending policy lapse because of nonpayment of premium. The notice is sent at the end of the grace period and is designed to protect against lapse because a senile or otherwise mentally impaired person or a person with a loss of functional capacity fails to pay the premium.

- *Policy Replacement*—If it is determined that a sale of LTCI involves a policy replacement, either the new insurer or its advisor must furnish the applicant with a notice regarding the replacement and its potential disadvantages. In addition, the new insurer must notify the old insurer of the proposed replacement as well as waive any time periods pertaining to preexisting conditions and probationary periods for benefits comparable to those in the old policy if the old policy has such provisions.

Communicating the Underwriting Process to the Applicant

Communicating the underwriting process to an applicant is an excellent opportunity for you to reinforce the relationship you are developing with the applicant. Once the application is complete and the first premium collected, it is important to inform the applicant what to expect over the next few weeks and to explain each step in the underwriting process. The applicant may have many questions and uncertainties about LTCI coverage and the process of obtaining it. By being forthright and communicating clearly what to expect, the advisor builds trust and solidifies the advisor-client relationship through professional behavior. This can prevent unexpected surprises that may upset the applicant and cause him or her to change his or her mind about the purchase of LTCI. You want the applicant to feel good about the decision to buy LTCI by reassuring him or her that the buy decision was the right one.

The advisor should review and explain the underwriting process to the applicant. Explain that ordering Attending Physician Statements (APSs) can add a great deal of time to the normal underwriting process. The advisor may ask the applicant to call his or her physician to explain the importance of completing and returning the insurer's request for medical information promptly.

The advisor should also explain the personal history interview, which is usually handled by telephone, and the face-to-face assessment interview, if applicable. The applicant will be more at ease and comfortable with these procedures and the overall underwriting process if he or she understands why certain procedures are done and their importance to the process. The face-to-face assessment interview typically raises the most concerns, so be sure to explain this completely. The underwriter uses all of these sources of information routinely. If a discrepancy exists between any of these sources, or if new information is uncovered that was not disclosed earlier in the process, this can cause a significant delay in what is already a lengthy process. All of these sources of information will be discussed at length later in this chapter.

Advisor Follow-up of the Underwriting Process

Review the Application—Check the application for completeness and accuracy. Ask a staff member or other person neutral to the case to review it. A "fresh" set of eyes may discover missing information or errors in the application. Process the application and follow up on any additional requirements promptly.

Ongoing Communication with the Applicant—Keep the applicant informed of the application's progress through the underwriting process. This increases trust and builds the relationship. It also reduces buyer's remorse and avoids unclaimed policies. Always be positive when communicating with the prospect. Complaining or criticizing any department in your company only creates doubt about you and your company's ability to deliver on promises. If there are delays in the process, explain the situation simply and honestly. By staying in touch, you demonstrate your commitment to service and your personal interest in the prospect.

Create a Client File—Keep a file with complete and accurate records, including copies of forms, correspondence, fact-finders, phone contacts, review sessions, and a summary of what was discussed or done in any conversations or follow-up activities. The file should also include copies of sales literature and illustrations showing the amount of coverage, the plan, and the premium. A thank-you note should also be sent in a timely manner.

Home Office Underwriting

Underwriting can be defined broadly as the insurer's process for selecting and classifying insurance applicants. Selection implies there are both acceptances and rejections, since not all applicants are accepted for insurance. Classification recognizes the differences in the applicants who are accepted.

Underwriting enables the insurance company to provide its services to insureds (including the payment of claims) and to make a profit. Without underwriting, the insurer would be vulnerable to financial loss caused by *adverse selection*, the tendency for those with a higher than average probability of loss to seek or continue insurance to a greater extent than those with an average or below average probability of loss. In other words, the people most susceptible to loss are those most likely to purchase insurance to cover that loss. The underwriter's responsibility is to minimize the impact of adverse selection so the company can insure a group of applicants whose overall claims experience approximates that expected for the rate classification.

It would seem that the best way to avoid adverse selection in underwriting for LTCI is to accept only the best applicants as standard. However, this would likely result in an excessive number of rejections and rated cases and could eventually undermine the morale of advisors. Moreover, if a company's underwriting is too restrictive, many advisors may decide to direct their prospects to other insurers, making it difficult for the company's underwriters to perform their function of selecting and classifying applicants. Consequently, the standard class should be broad enough to encompass most applicants for insurance. Underwriters must balance this standard class so that every applicant accepted with a higher than average claims expectation is offset by one with a lower than average claims expectation. This process typically results in most applicants being accepted as standard, although some applicants will still be rejected while others will be accepted but placed in a rated class that may involve benefit restrictions. Still other applicants may be placed in a preferred class if their expected claims experience justifies this status.

Appraisal of an applicant's expected claims experience cannot be exact in any case. Underwriting for LTCI is still more of an art than a science. Insurers do not yet have significant LTCI claims data available. In fact, most insurers have not sold enough LTCI to make truly accurate predictions of their LTC risk exposure. However, this situation is rapidly changing. According to the NAIC's ninth annual national study about LTCI experience, insurers writing LTCI reported that actual cumulative claims paid through the end of 2000 exceeded $11 billion going back to the inception of LTCI. Likewise, the number of covered lives nearly reached 4.5 million for the same time frame. Underwriting the LTC risk focuses on situations that may cause claims far into the future. On policies being written today, the claims experience will not be known for many years. Consequently, it will take time for the claims experience of these policies to be properly reflected in product pricing.

The Advisor and the Home Office Underwriter

It has been said that an advisor's job is to convince prospects that they need LTCI, and the underwriter's job is to tell them that they cannot get it. This is truly one dilemma of being an advisor. The advisor must convince the prospect that the risk of loss is real and then present him or her to the underwriter as an acceptable risk. For this process to work, the relationship between the advisor and the underwriter must be founded on a high degree of trust and a large amount of communication.

Data collection about prospects is primarily accomplished with questionnaires rather than physical examinations. Prominent in underwriting for LTCI is the attention paid to medical conditions such as osteoporosis or diabetes that might be an indication of a future LTCI claim.

Underwriting tends to become more restrictive as the age of the applicant increases. Not only is a future claim more likely to occur sooner, but also adverse selection can be more pronounced. The underwriting department determines the underwriting rules to be followed by its advisors and company personnel. Advisors receive instructions about the kinds of applicants who should be rejected, those who should be rated, and those who the company would like to insure.

Insurers train their advisors to seek prospects who will likely meet their underwriting criteria. In filling out applications, insurers regularly stress to their advisors that it is the advisors' responsibility to obtain complete and accurate information, especially with respect to medical conditions. Advisors are required to obtain all relevant information about applicants. Insurers encourage the advisors to identify special circumstances and clarify questionable situations. Extra efforts in these areas bolster the home office underwriter's confidence in the advisor and facilitate the approval of applicants.

In turn, the underwriter owes the advisor timely processing of applications, and prompt communication about the status of applicants. When an underwriter declines an application, the advisor needs to receive as much background information regarding the decision as can legally be divulged. Assisting the advisor to deal sensitively and effectively with applicants is an essential aspect of maintaining good field force morale.

The home office underwriter, however, is not totally dependent on the advisor for information about applicants. Without diminishing the importance of the advisor's role as a field underwriter, the home office underwriter may access information about an applicant directly through a variety of sources, such as the MIB, a follow-up telephone interview, or even a face-to-face assessment interview. The use of these direct sources of applicant information varies significantly among insurers. The underwriter's sources of information are more fully discussed later in this chapter.

A team effort involving the home office underwriter and the advisor is essential to make underwriting and product pricing work. Good risk selection is important to all parties involved and forms the basis for creating competitively priced products.

Medical Underwriting Guidelines

Remember that LTCI is a form of health insurance and underwriting it is substantially different than underwriting life insurance. Life insurance underwriting focuses on the likelihood of death of the applicant (mortality). LTCI underwriting focuses on illness (morbidity) and the probability that the applicant will become either cognitively impaired or unable to perform ADLs. Although related, these two types of insurance can be quite different in what causes favorable and unfavorable claim results.

Differences with Life Underwriting

Advisors should strive to become familiar with the underwriting procedures, guidelines, and rules regarding LTCI. As a health insurance product, unlike life insurance, multiple claims can arise for the same insured. These claims can be very costly to the insurer. As a result, underwriting tends to involve somewhat more scrutiny than in life insurance, especially with regard to the applicant's medical history. Familiarity with the guidelines the insurer uses to determine what medical conditions will disqualify a prospect or result in a rated policy is essential.

The introduction of the 2001 Commissioner's Standard Ordinary (CSO) Mortality Table has captured the attention of LTCI underwriters. Although the tables are more directly related to life insurance underwriting, the clear message is that people are living longer. What impact will this trend have on LTC? Some LTC insurers have concluded that the new tables will not have much bearing on their products. So far, results have shown that morbidity is improving along with life expectancy, and that the quality of those longer lives has improved because individuals are paying more attention to living healthy lives. Although increasing longevity could mean more and longer LTC claims, this has not proven to be the case yet, because improved morbidity appears to be offsetting this possibility. Generally, the LTCI industry is seeing fewer claims than expected, and insurers are pricing their products expecting the trend of increasing life expectancy and improved morbidity to continue at least for the short run.

Underwriting Older Ages

Age is an important factor in determining rates for LTCI for two reasons. First, the older an applicant is, the sooner LTCI is likely to be needed. Hence there is less time to collect premiums before money is paid out for claims. Second, the younger an applicant is, the longer the insurer is likely to collect premiums before a claim begins. This would allow more premiums to be collected and to earn interest before being needed to pay claims.

Significant variations exist among insurers with respect to the age at which they will issue LTCI policies. At a minimum, a person between the ages of 55 and 75 is eligible for LTCI from most insurers. Most insurers, however, have an upper age in the range of 84 to 89, beyond which LTCI is not issued. Coverage written at age 85 or older, when available to someone who qualifies, is often accompanied by restrictive policy provisions and very high premiums. Prohibitive cost and decreased insurability are two reasons why procrastinating to buy LTCI until much older is an undesirable decision.

Medical Rating Predictor

Each insurer has one or more underwriting classes. A few insurers have a single class and all applicants are either accepted and charged the rate for that class, or declined for coverage. Most insurers have a series of underwriting classes that have different rate structures. The applicant's medical condition determines the class into which he or she falls. Even with several underwriting classes, some applicants will be unacceptable risks to an insurer.

The advisor must have an understanding of the applicant's health status and consult the underwriting guide provided by the insurer. An underwriting guide lists medical conditions for which the insurer requests that the advisor not submit applications. It may also identify certain medical conditions along with a possible preliminary prediction of the underwriting class in which the applicant may fall.

In some cases, when multiple medical conditions affect an applicant's insurability, the underwriting guide instructs the advisor to contact the insurer's underwriting department before submitting the application. The combination of two or more medical conditions can complicate the underwriting picture. Often a medical condition may not be of great significance, yet when present with another condition can signal a considerable risk for needing LTC services. These are known as co-morbid factors and they can make an already existing condition worse. For example, cigarette smoking, excessive weight, or high blood pressure could exacerbate heart disease and diabetes.

There are also differences in how certain conditions are underwritten by different insurers. Depending on the condition or combination of conditions, underwriting could range from an applicant being declined to the issuance of the policy with an extra premium rating. You may want to become familiar with the differences in insurers' underwriting for

---

Advisor's Underwriting Guide—An Example

One insurer has four LTCI underwriting classes, with class 1 having the lowest premium and class 4 the highest. The insurer's lengthy underwriting guide lists many conditions that make an applicant unacceptable for LTCI, as well as common medical conditions and probable underwriting treatment. Some conditions are acceptable under different classifications, depending on severity and treatment. A few of the conditions on the list include cerebral palsy, personality disorders, Down's syndrome, continuous use of oxygen, senility, and active tuberculosis. The guide also details information for the advisor about the underwriting process. It offers underwriting guidelines such as periods of recovery, medications, height and weight charts, and much more.

---

different medical conditions. Experienced advisors know which insurer is most likely to issue a policy to an applicant with a specific health problem, and thus send the application to the appropriate company.

Sources of Information

The underwriter must select those applicants who are within the insurer's range of acceptability, as determined by its underwriting objectives for the type of policies issued and the claims experience anticipated. In the process of determining acceptability, the underwriter relies on many sources of information. These fall into the following five categories: the application, attending physicians' statements (APSs), the MIB, a personal history interview by telephone, and a face-to-face assessment interview.

The Application—The application is the basis for an underwriter's initial review of an applicant. If the applicant appears insurable, the underwriter analyzes all necessary sources of information to determine whether the company should approve the coverage as applied for, modify it, obtain more information, or reject it entirely. Consequently, the application form requires careful drafting to elicit truthful and complete answers from the applicant as well as the accurate recording of all information by the advisor.

While application forms vary from insurer to insurer, the typical application form contains all of the following types of information to assist the underwriter in the selection process:

- *Personal information*—The data in this section serve primarily to identify the applicant and provide basic information, such as age, gender, birth date, address, phone number, social security number, height and weight, and address and phone number of his or her primary care physician.
- *Coverage selection*—The applicant selects among the benefit options available under the policy and any available riders. Premium mode and initial premium are indicated.
- *Prequalification questions*—Most applications contain four to 10 questions designed to prequalify an applicant for coverage. If an applicant answers yes to any of these questions, the applicant is not eligible for coverage.
- *Medical information*—This section asks questions concerning specific medical conditions. A yes answer to any of the questions

requires further information about hospitals, physicians, treatments and medications, and prompts the insurer to request medical records for the past several years.

A typical advisor's underwriting guide directs the advisor to avoid soliciting or taking applications on persons who have medical conditions that would make them uninsurable or that would require special underwriting. Applications from uninsurable individuals require the company to initiate underwriting procedures that are both costly and wasteful of valuable resources. The underwriting guide also alerts the advisor to the probable underwriting class to which the applicant would be assigned so that a realistic premium quotation can be made. This initial underwriting classification is subject to a final decision by the underwriter.

- *Medications*—Insurers want to know about medications taken. Medication type and treatment specifics indicate the type and nature of the disorder. If an applicant is taking certain medications, he or she may not be eligible for coverage.

- *Authorization to release medical information*—The applicant authorizes a blanket release of information from health care providers, other insurance companies, and other organizations that have relevant personal and medical information that may be needed because of his or her response to certain questions on the application.

- *The advisor's statement*—Although not a part of the application formally, the advisor's statement provides the advisor an opportunity to make a personal statement and answer questions about the applicant, and to verify that the advisor followed company procedures.

Attending Physicians' Statements (APSs)—Typically this is the primary source of medical information for underwriting LTCI. An APS from each physician who treated the applicant provides the underwriter with detailed medical information about the applicant.

The MIB, Inc. (formerly the Medical Information Bureau)—The MIB is a not-for-profit association of insurance companies that exchanges information among its members relevant to the underwriting of life, health, disability income, and LTCI. Its purpose is the protection of insurers, and ultimately their policyowners, from losses by facilitating the detection and deterrence of fraud by applicants who may omit or try to conceal facts relevant to their selection and/or classification for insurance purposes. Not all LTC insurers use the MIB, but there is a trend toward more insurers participating, as special coding for LTCI underwriting is now available.

Personal History Interview (Telephone)—After the application is received in the home office, the applicant may be contacted for a telephone interview. The interviews are conducted by specialized agencies under contract, or by specially trained company personnel. Telephone interviews provide an independent verification of information on the application, and they afford an opportunity to clarify responses. Additional questions may also be asked, such as about lifestyle matters and to assess cognitive ability.

It is critical that you inform the applicant that a telephone interview may take place. Since people are hesitant to take phone calls from persons or companies with whom they are not familiar, knowing about a possible call ahead of time will put them at ease and facilitate the process if they receive such a call.

Face-to-Face Assessment Interview—An underwriter may order a face-to-face assessment interview of the applicant, either at the underwriter's discretion or because underwriting guidelines call for such an assessment interview if the applicant has reached a certain age or has a particular medical condition. A paramedical company or case-management company normally performs the assessment interview in the applicant's home.

A face-to-face assessment interview may be used to determine or clarify an applicant's medical history. It may also be used to determine an applicant's ability to perform ADLs or IADLs. For example, an insurer routinely uses such an assessment interview to evaluate an applicant who has had a stroke, a limb removed, or a joint replacement. Finally, a face-to-face assessment interview may be used to evaluate an applicant's cognitive ability through the administration of various tests that have been developed for this purpose.

Selection Factors

The following factors are used in accepting or rejecting applicants for LTCI coverage.

> **When we first started selling LTCI, we did not understand underwriting. We had a lot of declinations until we figured it out.**

Medical Condition—Medical condition is the single most important factor in underwriting LTCI. Medical history and current physical status are basic indicators of the probability of future problems that may require LTC services. They determine the basis on which LTCI is offered or refused. Underwriters evaluate an applicant's potential for incurring LTC services by estimating the probable influence of previous medical history and current impairments on future claims. This is accomplished by a thorough review of the applicant's personal medical history provided by the attending physician's statement (APS).

```
Know Your Underwriting

I go to different insurers for different types of
underwriting problems. If I have a prospect
that has a history of heart disease or some
other disorder that can complicate the
underwriting, I have learned which insurer to
approach depending on the condition. I know
each insurer's underwriting rules and which
insurer will accept or reject certain ailments.
So I place the prospect with the insurer where
I can get the best offer.
```

Medical evaluation of an applicant requires a great deal of underwriting skill and judgment. Evaluation begins with the applicant and advisor's statements on the application form. The evaluation may continue in one of several ways depending on the information in the application.

It is also important to point out that since LTCI is a relatively new type of coverage, many potential claims from existing policies have yet to occur. Therefore, the underwriter must use a greater degree of subjectivity and conservatism than is used with many other types of insurance for which decades of claims experience exist. Consequently there are significant differences in the underwriting standards of LTC insurers with respect to the evaluation of specific medical conditions. As a field underwriter, you should be aware of these differences and learn more about them. You may even request a preliminary underwriting viewpoint from an insurer so that you will know its position on a specific medical condition before you submit an application.

Insured's Lifestyle—There are certain lifestyle factors that tend to have a bearing on the frequency and severity of LTCI claims. Two of these—marital status and tobacco use—can help determine into which underwriting class the applicant will be placed as well as the premium rate that he or she will be charged. Other factors are more subjective. For example, an underwriter may want to know if an applicant owns and lives in his or her own home. Such people are less likely to move to a LTC facility than are people who rent an apartment if they are living independently and have a support system of family and/or friends. The same is true of single and/or widowed people who have support from family and/or friends. Evidence indicates that people who work, drive, have hobbies, or participate in social, recreation, or volunteer activities are less likely to need LTC than people who lead much less active lifestyles. For example, a retiree who sits on the couch all day watching television, drinking alcohol, and smoking cigarettes is not making choices that are likely to result in a long, healthy retirement. On the other hand, a retiree who volunteers at the blood center or church, travels extensively, is socially active, eats healthy meals, plays tennis, and walks a couple of miles per day is more likely to enjoy a long, healthy retirement. The latter scenario describes the type of applicant that a LTC underwriter likes to accept.

Duplicate Coverage—The NAIC model legislation requires an insurer to obtain information about any LTCI in force during the prior 12 months. In addition, the applicant must state whether a new policy is intended to replace one currently in force.

Classification Factors

Classification involves determining which rate category is appropriate for an applicant once he or she is accepted. The insurance company's actuaries determine the rate and premium for each category, with input from underwriters. Federal and state laws prohibit classifications based on race, ethnic origin, and religion. Rate categories are based on age, medical condition, marital status, and tobacco use.

Risk selection performed by underwriting will impact claims experience for years, possibly decades into the future. Claims experience will, in turn, dramatically affect profitability. If an insurer underwrites carelessly and classifies risks improperly, its policyowners are the ultimate victims because the company has only two choices: raise premiums, or sell the block of business.

Age—As noted previously, age is a critical factor in underwriting for LTCI.

Medical Condition—As also noted previously, an applicant's medical condition helps determine the underwriting class into which he or she will be placed. Each class's rate structure reflects the degree of risk for the insurer.

Marital Status—Most insurers offer some type of spousal discount, although the exact nature of this feature is subject to regulation in each state. Experience shows that claims from married people are less frequent and of a shorter duration than claims from single or widowed persons. This favorable claims experience results from many married couples taking care of each other for as long as possible before LTC services are needed. Some insurers give a spousal discount only if they insure both spouses; others give a discount even if they insure only one spouse; still others give a discount to unmarried couples who live together.

Tobacco Use Versus Nonuse—Tobacco use in any form poses a significant health risk. Consequently, some insurers offer lower rates to people who do not use tobacco to reflect anticipated differences in claims or the timing of claims. Because an applicant who uses tobacco may state that he or she does not, it may take a review of medical reports or a paramedical examination to determine the truth.

Declinations

A very important goal for advisors is the elimination of declinations (that is, the rejection of applications), since the time and effort of advisors, applicants and their families, and insurers are costly, both financially and professionally. Avoiding the declination or rejection of an applicant is in the interest of all parties involved.

If you should receive a declination from your company, the first rule is to be honest with the applicant about his or her rejection. You may want to suggest to the applicant that his or her personal physician be consulted to see if there is a remedy.

One of the best ways to prevent taking an application on someone who is not insurable is to adhere to a prequalification process, as was discussed in chapter 4. Consult your advisor's underwriting manual when initially interviewing a prospect to see if he or she has a

---

A Review of the Types of Questions to Ask as Part of the Prequalifying Process

1. Do you know anyone who has needed nursing or convalescent services?
2. What is your date of birth?
3. Do you have children? If so, how many? What are their ages? Are they local?
4. What health insurance do you have? Medicare? How is your health? Are you taking any medications? May I see them? Have you stayed in a hospital in the last 5 years? Have you been seeing a doctor in last 5 years?
5. Have you received or do you expect to receive any LTCI sales proposals?
6. Let's discuss your savings and investments. How would you define your income, assets, and budget? (Do not include the residence.) Have their values risen, stayed the same, or decreased over the last year? How about over the last 5 years?

medical condition that makes him or her uninsurable. Any doubts regarding the prospect's condition should be referred to your company's underwriting department for clarification. Advisors have become more aware of the necessity to prequalify applicants and have become quite proficient at it. Knowing that a prospect is uninsurable allows the sales process to transition to products and solutions other than LTCI. Knowing that a prospect is insurable but has a medical condition that may be rated allows the advisor to prepare the prospect for the potential underwriting outcome, and also place the coverage with an insurer that may be more liberal in underwriting the condition. Declinations today result more often when the applicant appears healthier than he or she really is, or fails to disclose all information in the initial prequalification process. Also, a small minority of advisors are unwilling and/or unable to field underwrite. These advisors should rethink their position and either do or learn to do field underwriting if they ever hope to be successful selling LTCI.

Advisors must be proactive as field underwriters. They need to observe the applicant and ask him or her several questions. Observe the applicant to see if he or she can walk normally and steadily. Look to see if there are any signs of physical aids (canes, walkers, and so on) that may indicate ambulatory problems. Determine if the applicant is unable to get up from a sitting position. Ask the applicant to see his or her medications, then record the types and dosages for underwriting purposes. Use common sense to determine if the applicant appears to be a good LTCI risk.

Underwriting Results

According to a Blue Cross/Blue Shield study of the Rochester, New York area in the Winter of 2000/2001 (Inquiry—Blue Cross/Blue Shield Association; Chicago, Vol. 37, issue 4), at least 15 percent of the eligible population aged 65 to 79 may be uninsurable for LTCI. This finding is consistent with other industry surveys.

The reasons cited in the study for rejecting LTCI applications follow closely those published by insurers in their advisor underwriting guides. For example, a prospect who has one or more of the following conditions would be uninsurable for LTCI:

- suffers from cognitive impairment (all types)
- requires prompting, supervision, or physical assistance to perform routine activities

- is unable to walk around without assistance
- has been recommended for surgery or diagnostic testing
- did not meet the recovery time for a particular condition
- answered yes to any part of the health statement section of the application
- uses a wheel chair, quad cane, or oxygen
- requires assistance from another person to perform one or ADLs
- is unable to perform IADLs
- is taking medication(s) that can potentially indicate a poor risk selection

The same Blue Cross/Blue Shield study also indicated that accepted applications were classified for underwriting purposes as follows:

- 65 percent accepted at preferred rates with a 15 percent premium discount (risk factor = .85)
- 30 percent accepted at standard rates (risk factor = 1.00)
- 4.5 percent accepted at impaired rates with a 30 percent extra premium charge (risk factor = 1.30)

The risk factor relates to a percentage of standard issue. A standard risk factor equals 1.00. A risk factor of less than 1.00 is more favorable than a standard risk. A risk factor greater than 1.00 is less favorable than standard.

Another survey revealed that LTC insurers are generally reluctant to discuss the percentage of applications not approved by underwriting. In fact, 20 of the 35 insurers surveyed refused to provide any information at all, even after being assured that only summary statistics would be published. Of those providing data, the statistics showed that, on average, about 15 percent of applicants are rejected by insurers for health reasons, with most insurers' rejection rate falling in the range of 13 percent to 20 percent. (*National Underwriter*, Life and Health/Financial Services edition, November 16, 1998). The survey also showed that, on average, insurers accepted 47 percent of LTCI applicants at a preferred rate, but the range for the 15 responding insurers was from a low of 3 percent to a high of 74 percent. These widely divergent results show just how much underwriting decisions vary from insurer to insurer. For example, the survey pointed out that in underwriting diabetics, some insurers reject all insulin-dependent diabetics, while others reject only those diabetics who require large dosages of insulin or those who already suffer diabetic-related complications. In contrast, a few insurers have no automatic rejection rules for diabetes.

Underwriting practices obviously affect claim costs. "Loose" or very liberal underwriting insurers seldom do face-to-face interviews and might not ask applicants for medical records. Insurers with "tight" or very stringent underwriting require interviews and ask for records, and their tight underwriting results in lower claim costs. For all LTCI policies in force for 3 years, the average claims ratio is 38 percent. For policies in force between 5 and 9 years, the overall claims ratio is 57 percent, but loose underwriters have a claims ratio of 77 percent, while tight underwriters have a claims ratio of only 49 percent. (Allison Bell, "'Tight' LTC Writers Have Lower Claims Rates," *National Underwriter,* Life and Health/Financial Services edition, October 9, 2000).

The LTCI market is changing rapidly, because of advances in medical research and technology. Underwriting manuals may need to be rewritten and updated based on these changes. Medical advancements are prompting LTC insurers to rethink how they underwrite impaired risks. The industry is liberalizing its underwriting of serious illnesses such as cancer, heart disease, stroke, depression, hypertension and others. Consequently, the LTCI market is expanding as these underwriting changes are being made. On the other hand, these same advances in medical research and technology are responsible for increases in the length of time that LTC services may be needed and used. If advances in medicine and technology prolong life for the impaired, but do not proportionately increase life expectancy for the non-impaired, then LTCI policies sold today may turn out to be under-priced. This bears close watching because, as noted earlier in this chapter, results have shown thus far that morbidity is improving along with life expectancy, and that the quality of those longer lives has improved since people are paying more attention to living healthy lives. Nonetheless, the potentially greater need for LTC today, compared to a couple generations ago, is precisely because of the advances in medicine and technology that have prolonged life and allowed those with serious medical conditions to survive longer than they would have survived otherwise.

Lapses—Lapses may have a significant effect on the profitability and claims-paying ability of an insurer. Lapse rates (that is, the number of policies lapsing each year) have been lower than expected for LTCI. This means that insurers are retaining more of the risk, which may hurt their claims experience years later. In the meantime, however, they are collecting more premiums than were anticipated when the rate structure was devised.

In the case of LTCI policies without nonforfeiture benefits, a lapse rate higher than expected is favorable to an insurer's claims-paying ability. This is because when insureds lapse their coverage and they have no nonforfeiture benefits, they forfeit the premium dollars paid into the insurer up to that point in time. Those premium reserves are then released and used to cover costs for other insureds that stay in the risk pool and do not lapse their coverage. Generally, a lapse in the later years of a policy has a more favorable impact on an insurer's claims-paying ability than a lapse in the early years of the contract, when reserves are still small and policy acquisition costs (such as the cost of agent commissions, APSs, medical reports, and underwriting expenses) have not yet been recovered.

Most insurers, however, offer LTCI policies with some type of nonforfeiture benefit. In fact, some states and the NAIC model legislation require that nonforfeiture benefits be offered. With nonforfeiture benefits, policyowners receive some value back if they lapse their coverage. The nature of what they receive back depends on the type of nonforfeiture benefit in their policies. (See page 5-20 for a discussion of the types of nonforfeiture benefits found in LTCI policies.)

Summary

Underwriting is a critical component of the insurance equation. Determining who qualifies for coverage (selection) and on what terms and conditions and at what price (classification) is what underwriting is all about. If these two functions of underwriting are not performed properly, the insurer may stand to lose money. This becomes quite evident when the relationship of underwriting to the rate-making, sales, and claims settlement activities of the insurer are considered. For example, if rate makers include a low or inadequate margin in premiums to cover for possible variations from expected losses, it may be necessary for the home office underwriters to become "tighter" or more restrictive in their acceptance and classification of LTCI risks. Yet if underwriters are too "tight" in their treatment of LTCI applicants, the insurer may be viewed as uncompetitive with business being lost to competitors, much to the chagrin of the sales force. On the other hand, if underwriters are too "loose" in the selection of LTCI risks, the insurer may be exposed to adverse selection causing problems for the claims department, which may have to become stricter in settling claims in order to avert rate inadequacy. As can be seen, the goals of the various departments of the insurer are not necessarily consistent nor in consonance. Therefore, good cooperation and communication among everyone involved in the insurance equation is mandatory in order to achieve success. Central to this success is a well-balanced and smooth underwriting process.

In addition, advisor responsibility and compliance with sound underwriting principles is also essential for the success of the underwriting process. An advisor who has a reputation for submitting "clean" LTC risks may receive more liberal, or at least less scrutinous, underwriting treatment for his or her applicants than for those submitted by other advisors. This would not be considered a reward for the advisor but rather recognition that he or she is performing proper field underwriting on the risks that he or she submits.

Delivering the Policy

Now that you have received the issued LTCI policy, it is time to visit your new client and perform some very important functions that will help you build your LTCI practice. This step in the sales process must not be taken lightly, for it offers an occasion to strengthen the sale and the advisor-client relationship and to build future sales opportunities.

Preparing for the Delivery

A small amount of time spent preparing for the policy delivery enables the advisor to reinforce his or her commitment to the client. This also greatly enhances the advisor's professional image in the eyes of the client. When delivering the policy, the advisor should take the necessary time to educate the client about the policy. This can help avoid embarrassing and potentially costly misunderstandings regarding future claims.

So when you receive the policy, check it over for complete accuracy to be sure that no mistakes have been made. Mistakes can happen and they should be caught before you deliver the policy. However, mistakes are not the only reason why a policy may be issued that is different than requested in the application. The underwriter may have made changes to policy benefits because of medical history, current health conditions, or eligibility. Any changes made by the underwriter should be understood by you so that you can fully explain them to your client.

Prepare the policy for delivery by including with it any approved brochure, sales literature, or other material that supports you, your company, or the client's decision to buy LTCI. Presenting this information and the policy in a handsome yet inexpensive policy wallet can enhance the value and image of the policy and you. HIPAA requires that the policy be delivered to the insured within 30 days of the advisor's receipt of the policy.

Conducting the Delivery Interview

The delivery interview has several objectives:

Reinforce the buying decision—It is common for buyers to feel that they made a mistake in a purchase or that there are other product options that may be better solutions for them. This is known as buyer's remorse. It is critical that you answer any questions your client may have and reinforce his or her decision to buy the LTCI policy. If this is not done and the client has concerns, there is a danger that the client will lapse the policy, exercise the policy's free-look provision, or succumb to the competition's attempts to replace the policy.

Review the policy—The advisor is required by law in most states to fully explain the policy. This is in the best interest of the advisor since most people have very little knowledge of insurance and appreciate a clear explanation of the policy.

Build the advisor-client relationship—Continued contact helps to build trust. You want to be viewed by the client as his or her financial advisor, a relationship that is ideally based on a deep feeling of respect and trust. Commit yourself to serving and servicing your clients.

Obtain Required Forms—In today's environment of disclosure and sensitivity to compliance, there are a number of forms that you either need to complete or have the client sign or both. In addition, a delivery receipt and an outline of coverage must be delivered to the policyowner. Failure to comply with these requirements can lead to the policy not being put in force and the client not being properly protected. It is critical to deliver all required documents and obtain completed forms with signatures at the time of delivery.

Develop Other Sales Opportunities—There may be other sales opportunities that were uncovered in the fact-finding process that you can now revisit. The client may have an interest in and need for other insurance products, investments, retirement planning, or estate planning that you can provide. You should also ask for referrals. If you have done a professional job, you have earned the right

---

Policy Delivery Letter

One advisor sends a letter to new policyowners, saying:

"You have made one of the best financial decisions of your life. When you make good decisions and realize their value, you need to share that with other people you know, like family and friends, co-workers, and people at church. Think about whom you might want me to talk to and I'll call you next week to get their names.

P.S. Do a friend a favor and tell them about LTCI."

to ask the client if you could speak with people that he or she knows who may benefit from your products and services.

Rated Case Delivery

There is one last type of policy delivery that needs to be reviewed and that is delivering a rated case. You may feel uneasy because the policy does not carry a standard premium and you are bringing bad news to the applicant about his or her health. In truth, most applicants know in advance that they may have a problem getting standard rates. Usually, they have already discussed their health problems with their doctors. Nonetheless, you should have discussed the difference between standard and substandard ratings earlier in the interview process, when you filled out the medical history section of the application or when you finished the prequalifying interview, especially if a negative underwriting issue emerged. Since underwriting LTCI is so thorough, it is essential that a conversation about the probable outcome of underwriting be discussed before an application is taken. Possible outcome, premium charge, and alternatives should be reviewed to prepare the applicant for what may result from the underwriting process. Some advisors say this type of delivery is actually easier than many of their other deliveries. The applicant often feels grateful to be able to buy any LTCI.

It is not unusual to have a rated case now and then. Standard issue is only available to those who can qualify. You may not have many rated clients, but it stands to reason that every advisor will have some applicants that have more difficulty qualifying than others. Companies are issuing rated policies and people are taking them and paying for them.

The best way to deliver a rated policy is to resell the need. The need is even greater in view of the increased risk. Acceptance of the policy transfers the risk from the applicant and his or her family to the insurance company where it belongs.

Let the applicant know that you feel the company's action was correct. Do not sympathize. Have confidence in your home office underwriting department that the applicant was properly classified. Keep in mind that the applicant is still insurable, and the company is offering to provide the coverage.

Servicing the LTCI Policyowner

Maintaining Records

Many companies today have file inspection and maintenance requirements as a routine part of the compliance process. In all cases follow your company procedures, which may require that you keep records of such things as the following:

- fact-finding forms
- written notes describing basic events and discussions with the client
- contact log with dates and topics discussed
- copies of quotes or illustrations
- copies of applications and related materials
- copies of correspondence with the client

Normally no original documents or blank signed documents should be in a file. Original documents should have been submitted to the company and blank signed documents are strictly forbidden.

Periodic Reviews

The periodic review covers many objectives of the advisor-client relationship. Relationship building is fostered by regular contact, which should lead to policy persistency, cross-selling, networking, and referral opportunities. Proper servicing is based on timely reviews and contacts, and prompt responses to client requests. Any changes in coverage should be made to conform to changes in the client's situation. Although the traditional review period is annually, a mutually agreed-upon interval should be established based on the client's circumstances and needs.

Keeping in touch by various methods is an important part of this process. Newsletters, birthday or anniversary phone calls, and periodic mailings about topics of interest continue to put you in front of the client, build prestige, and foster the advisor-client relationship.

Retaining clients can have a huge effect on your bottom line. Research shows that profits can grow by 100 percent from a 10 percent increase in retention. U.S. businesses lose from 10 to 30 percent of their customers each year, yet most of those customers would not have changed if they encountered a more helpful and friendly attitude along with a passion to make things right. How can you sustain significant growth when you have to replace 20 percent of your customers each year just to stay even? The cost of acquiring a new client is five to seven times higher than retaining a current one. It is cheaper and easier to sell more to existing clients than it is to cultivate new ones. Here are some tips for conserving your existing clients:

- *Relate one-to-one*—All business is personal and no relationship is static
- *Reinforce relationships*—Seize every opportunity to learn about your client's needs, dreams, and realities. Communicate and reinforce the reason your client chose you. People do business with people, not companies.
- *Exceed expectations*—Meeting clients' expectations is the price of admission into today's market. Strive to exceed expectations to create client commitment and loyalty. Expect to lose business if you only deliver what the client needs, since he or she probably has many avenues to get it. Instead, discover and deliver what the client wants. If you do not add value, you are no longer necessary.
- *Be an expert listener*—Demonstrate your knowledge and gain client loyalty by asking the right questions and listening closely to the answers.
- *Differentiate yourself*—Do not compete on price, but rather on the value of your expertise and products. Differentiate your services in clients' minds by providing choice, research, responsiveness, and superior knowledge. Most clients do not buy on price alone. Your job is to offer the best overall value, not the lowest price. Educate clients about the value of your LTCI products and service.
- *Establish strategic alliances*—Look to all of your clients and even competitors for joint opportunities that will add value to your clients. Introduce your clients to your other clients who can build value in their situations.
- *Become referable*—To get referrals you need to be referable. This means you must offer more than a product. You have to offer a process and even better, a memorable experience. ***You have to earn the trust of your clients.***

The Claims Process

At some point, many insureds will file claims under their LTCI policies. The policy spells out the procedures that must be followed. Failure of the insured to follow the procedures may jeopardize the receipt of benefit payments and the ability to bring legal actions against the insurer if disputes should arise. Claim provisions fall into several categories, including notification of loss, proof of loss, and the payment of benefits. In the following discussion the term insured is used. In many cases, however, the insured will be incapacitated and the necessary duties of complying with claim provisions will fall to the insured's legal representative.

Notification of Loss

The insured or his or her representatitve must initially notify the insurer that a LTCI claim is being made. Policies often specify that this be within 180 days after a covered service starts or as soon as reasonably possible. In most cases, the notification will be by telephone, and policies often contain the telephone number to call. However, many insurers will also want a written notification of a claim. Some insurers initially do little other than send the claim forms to the insured with instructions to have them completed and returned to the insurer. However, many insurers are very proactive and work with the insured to see that all necessary paperwork is properly completed. At this time, the insurer may provide the services of a care coordinator to help evaluate the needs of the insured and determine the best setting for care.

Proof of Loss

The insurer will require a written proof of loss. Most policies state that no claim will be paid unless this form is filed within a specified time—often one year after the start of covered services—unless the insured is legally unable to do so. The proof of loss requires a physician to certify that the insured meets the conditions to qualify for benefits. In the case of a TQ policy, this means that the insured meets the

---

The Claims Process

People expect "instant" service on claims. They think they can call you and act like they want you to bring a check right over. Sometimes they get irritated to see all the forms and the drawn out process that filing a claim entails. The process is not often as smooth as you would like, but this is the way insurance companies work. At first people get unnerved, but once the claim is filed and worked out, they are generally satisfied. Often the problem is that the people do not understand what is covered and expect to be reimbursed on a claim that is clearly not covered. I try to remind them that this is LTCI for the chronically ill. It is not major medical insurance. Even though I carefully explain this, they either forget, are not listening, or simply do not understand.

HIPAA definition for being chronically ill.

At various times during the claim-paying period, the insurer may require verification that the insured still satisfies the criteria for benefits. The insurer also reserves the right, at its own expense, to have the insured examined as may be reasonably necessary during the course of the claim.

Payment of Benefits

Benefits are payable as soon as the required proof of loss is received by the insurance company. The insured is entitled to the benefit payments, but they can generally be assigned to others, such as providers of care. However, benefit payments cannot be paid, assigned, or pledged as collateral for a loan.

Typical Forms for Submitting a LTCI Claim

1. Claimant's Statement—to be completed by the insured or his or her representative.
2. Authorization Clause—gives permission for release of medical records.
3. Plan of Care—to be completed by a physician and/or a licensed health care practitioner. Be aware of the terms on TQ policies, such as "substantial assistance, 2 of 6 ADLs, a period of 90 days, and substantial supervision."
4. Provider's statement—-to be completed by the nursing facility or home health care agency.

The Claims Process

The assistance policyowners receive from their insurance companies provides a major benefit and advantage to owning a LTCI policy. As insureds begin to experience the inability to perform ADLs, they may have access to care managers. The care manager helps them navigate the health delivery system at precisely the time when the average family is unprepared to deal with the issues of LTC. Sometimes a care manager's advice, such as an alternative plan of care, allows an insured to stay in his or her own home longer than anticipated. Understanding the claims process equips the advisor to be a better LTC advocate and ensures a continuum of care for the client.

Care Coordinators—Care coordinators occupy pivotal positions in some LTC programs, though their use varies by both company and policy. Some policies require the use of a care coordinator. In others it is optional and in still others it is not available, particularly in older policies. Care coordinators' responsibilities include screening insureds, determining eligibility for services, conducting provider

---

Claims-Paying Ability

Insurers are coming out with more liberal policies. These policies are perhaps too generous. Liberal policy definitions and provisions may eventually harm a company's claims-paying ability or force it to increase premiums.

---

referrals, monitoring outcomes, and counseling families. The coordinator develops a plan of care based on a comprehensive assessment of the insured's physical and cognitive needs, social situation, health condition, and other factors. Case management, through a collaborative process, directs and coordinates LTC services between the insured, his or her family, healthcare professionals, service providers, and others who may need to be involved. Care coordinators assess, plan, implement, advocate, coordinate, educate, monitor, and evaluate options and delivery of health services and community resources.

When a claim is submitted, a care coordinator is assigned, an assessment is completed, and a plan of care developed. This is a customized, comprehensive plan designed to meet the care needs of the insured. The physician, insured and his or her family participate in its development. The plan not only addresses care needs, it also identifies associated issues that may affect family stability and require the use of community services as well. Much of the planning revolves around the use of home care versus community care services and which are best for all involved. In some policies, the use of a care coordinator may waive the elimination period for certain services.

The care coordinator informs the insured and his or her family about available benefits and appropriate providers and how they may best meet the objectives of the approved care plan. The insured can be an active participant, helping to make informed decisions. Having an informed care coordinator available, at no charge, to coordinate and explain care choices can be of significant value to everyone. The care coordinator becomes an advocate and ally of the insured, not a gatekeeper like in managed care. Typically, insurers contract with care coordination firms to provide the service to their policyowners.

Summary

The delivery and service aspects of the sales process is where the advisor proves his or her worth to the client. These two functions provide the advisor with many opportunities to develop the advisor-client relationship and to cultivate future sales opportunities. If the functions are performed properly, the advisor earns the right to be referred to the client's personal and business contacts.

Summary of the Sales and Underwriting Process

1. **Initial Interview**—The advisor explains the risks of LTC and the financing alternatives for LTC services. He or she gathers information about the prospect's needs, health, and financial and human resources.
2. **Analyze the Situation**—The advisor, using facts gathered in the interview, designs a LTC plan that fits the client's needs and budget.
3. **Second Interview**—A second appointment is usually required, during which the advisor makes his or her recommendations.
4. **Application and required forms**—The advisor must furnish the applicant with an outline of coverage prior to accepting a signed application, or in some states at the time of delivery. The application must be completed accurately and in its entirety. Other forms such as a privacy notice, suitability, and replacement disclosures must be delivered. The advisor must furnish the insurer with a statement about the applicant.
5. **Premium deposit and receipt**—If a premium deposit is made with the application, coverage will be effective from that moment if the applicant is determined, through underwriting, to be insurable under the risk classification for which he or she is applying. This is explained in the receipt, which must be given to any prospect that makes a premium deposit with the application.
6. **Explanation of the underwriting process**—Advisors can alleviate any concerns or misunderstandings that applicants may have in the initial stage of policy issuance by explaining the purpose and process of underwriting.
7. **Application submission to the insurer**—After reviewing the application for accuracy, the advisor is legally obligated to forward the application and premium deposit (if one was paid) to the home office without delay.
8. **Underwriting verification**—Some insurers will telephone applicants to verify the accuracy of information provided in the application. In some cases, especially when the applicant is of an advanced age, a face-to-face assessment interview may be requested to help the underwriter determine cognitive alertness.
9. **Attending physician's statement (APS)**—If a preexisting condition is identified through the application, the underwriter will request an APS from the physician who treated the applicant.
10. **Underwriting decision**—On the basis of information gathered through the application, personal interviews, medical reports, and APS forms, the insurer makes an underwriting decision. If the applicant is insurable, a risk classification is assigned.
11. **Policy issue**—If the applicant is insurable, the policy is issued and sent to the advisor for personal delivery to the new client.
12. **Policy Delivery**—The advisor must schedule a delivery appointment, during which the entire policy is explained, including any substandard ratings, restrictions, and special provisions such as the 30-day free look period. If a premium deposit was not paid with the application, a premium must be paid when the policy is delivered. All required delivery receipts and disclosure forms must be signed by the advisor and client and returned to the insurer.
13. **Policy Service**—Regular communications with the client should be made in order to maintain and build the professional relationship. Annual or other periodic reviews should be performed to see that coverage reflects the current and possibly changing needs of the client. Any claims processing should be assisted and monitored by the advisor.

LTC and Financial Planning

Relationship of the LTC Need to Comprehensive Financial Needs

Comprehensive financial planning involves examining a prospect's overall financial affairs, not just his or her potential need for LTC. As part of the fact-finding process, you need to ask the prospect questions about his or her overall financial and personal situation as it exists now and into the future, considering goals and likely outcomes. Depending on the extent to which the prospect has already planned for his or her current and future financial needs, you may find opportunities to educate the prospect beyond the need for LTCI. This could lead to cross-selling opportunities and building a stronger advisor-client relationship. The following overview of related finanical planning topics includes concepts you will want to learn if you hope to be successful in the broader financial services market.

To participate in the broader market, you must be properly licensed to advise about and/or sell products other than LTCI. However, you need to be careful not to go beyond the bounds of your authority, because some of the planning requirements of this broader market need the counsel and drafting expertise of an attorney. This advice should be put in proper perspective; it is not meant to discourage you from being an active financial advisor to your clients. Also, it is important for you to keep in mind that other financial services professionals are now aware of insurance products. In some cases they may even be advising about and/or selling them. Be prepared to work with these other professionals as part of a financial planning team should the opportunity and/or need arise.

The Role of LTC in Retirement Planning

The tremendous financial and personal risk exposure that LTC poses must be a serious consideration in every retirement plan. A retirement plan that does not address this issue would have to be considered incomplete. To fail to take into account circumstances that could leave a person and his or her family impoverished would be a breach of your professional duties. It is insufficient to plan for financial security in retirement by focusing solely on income and investments. A secure retirement depends not only on accumulating sufficient assets, but also on protecting those assets from the potentially devastating effects of LTC.

Somewhere in your discussions with prospects and clients, you should mention the topic of LTC. One appropriate time to do this is after you have agreed on a funding strategy for the retirement plan. The following demonstrates one way to introduce LTC into the retirement plan discussion: "We have taken great care in planning your retirement. As with any plan, we should talk about possible obstacles that may interfere with the plan and what we can do to be prepared for them. One such obstacle is the need for LTC. Do you have any friends, neighbors, or family members who have needed care in a nursing home? Tell me about it."

Another logical time to initiate this discussion is when you are calculating monthly expenses. As you address the issue of health insurance, you will need to discuss the various possibilities. You can point out what Medicare, Medicaid, Medicare supplemental insurance, and major medical insurance cover and what they do not cover. You should then ask how the prospect plans to cover the cost of LTC and what financial alternatives he or she may have. Paying for LTC can quickly deplete a person's retirement nest egg and adversely affect retirement income. The average person does not know much about LTC or how it is financed. As noted throughout this book, many people incorrectly believe that government programs or private health insurance will cover the costs. Dealing with both the costs and emotional

---

The Best Time to Sell LTCI

Many financial advisors feel the best time to sell LTCI is when clients are in their late 50's. One reason for this is that these prospects have recently gone through or are going through the experience of dealing with the LTC needs of their elderly parents. LTCI premiums are also more easily handled by this age group compared to those who are in their mid- to late 60's. Of course, the best time to purchase coverage is always "now." The younger you are, the more choices you have, because costs are more reasonable and a positive underwriting outcome is more likely.

---

decisions involved in LTC is a major step towards facing a potentially overwhelming situation. You need to eliminate the uncertainty of who will pay for this care.

The central issue in the sale of LTCI is one of educating the prospect about its need. Once the prospect understands the need for it, he or she is much more likely to do something about it. It appears that people who buy LTCI understand its need and accept responsibility for taking care of the need. Those who have not bought LTCI or have no plans to buy it appear to lack an understanding of its value and the role it plays in retirement planning. Studies show that buyers of LTCI understand that their coverage is an integral part of their retirement plans. Buying LTCI to help secure retirement plans is increasing in popularity among those under the age of 65.

Take time to explore the prospect's reason for buying LTCI. Although each prospect has his or her own reason, there are some common ones. For example, the most often cited reason for buying LTCI among those over the age of 65 is to avoid dependency. These people typically want to preserve their assets so that they can take care of themselves and yet still have something left to leave to their heirs. Men are more likely to buy LTCI to protect their assets, while women are more likely to buy it to avoid becoming a burden on others. As previously noted, LTCI buyers under the age of 65 are more likely motivated by a desire to secure their retirement assets and protect their retirement lifestyle.

The Role of LTC in Estate Planning

There is much more to estate planning than just saving transfer taxes, although that sometimes appears to be the primary or only focus. Estate planning considers many issues, but the disposition of property during life and at death is a key issue. LTC and estate concerns are inextricably intertwined, as both are concerned with the preservation of assets. Because of the enormous potential costs of LTC, everything a person owns may be lost. The ultimate goal of estate planning is to fulfill the wishes of the individual regarding the disposition of his or her property at death. LTC planning is an important part of this process, because one can

---

LTCI and Estate Planning

Since LTC planning is an important part of the estate planning process, many attorneys recommend their clients buy LTCI. If the clients do not want the coverage, these attorneys ask them to sign disclaimers stating that LTCI was discussed and recommended, but they decided against buying it.

---

protect assets that might otherwise be used to pay for LTC.

The following material briefly looks at some of the more important estate planning concepts and documents that might come into play in a discussion of LTC planning. Your job as a financial advisor is to make your clients aware of these concepts and documents and how they may impact their lives. Since you cannot practice law (unless your are a licensed attorney), you are prohibited from giving specific legal advice or drafting documents. Nonetheless, you can make your clients aware of the need to periodically review their estate plans and the corresponding documents. These should be reviewed every 3 to 5 years, or when important changes occur that would impact their contents and purpose.

Will—A will is a legal document that specifies how an individual wishes his or her property to be distributed at death. Wills are governed by state law, which determine their validity. State law also determines what happens if a person dies without having a valid will. In these cases property is distributed under state intestacy laws, which distribute the property according to family relationships. State intestacy laws typically do not reflect the way an individual would want his or her property distributed at death.

A will names an executor who is responsible for administering the estate under the jurisdiction of the probate (or surrogate) court in the county where the deceased was residing at the time of death. Normally, it is recommended that either a bank or an individual who is both trustworthy and younger than the testator be named as the executor. A well drafted will can serve to reduce or even eliminate family squabbles and disagreements over the deceased's assets.

Trusts—A trust is a legal vehicle with four key components: a corpus, a grantor, a trustee, and a beneficiary or beneficiaries. The property transferred into a trust is called the corpus. The person who transfers the property into the trust is called the grantor. The person or persons for whom the trust assets are to be used is the beneficiary or beneficiaries. The trustee both holds and manages the corpus for the benefit of the beneficiary or beneficiaries, according to a trust agreement. The trust agreement is a contract between the grantor and trustee, who is the legal owner of the trust corpus (that is, the cash or property in the trust). The trust agreement contains the provisions that act as the instructions to the trustee from the grantor regarding what can and cannot be done with the trust property. Following are several examples of trusts used in estate planning, including planning for potentially needing LTC.

Revocable Living Trust—A revocable living trust is a trust created when the grantor transfers the trust property to the trustee but reserves the power to alter or terminate the arrangement and reclaim the trust property. The property transfer to the trust does not change the federal estate, gift, and income tax picture of the grantor. Consequently, there must be nontax reasons to create the revocable living trust. These can include decisions about what the grantor wishes to take place in the case of his or her disability, need for LTC, or death. In these instances, the grantor typically names the same person as trustee who he or she also names as the attorney-in-fact (that is, decision maker) for his or her power of attorney.

A-B Trust—Under one variation of the A-B trust, the grantor's will sets up two trusts: a marital (spouse's) trust (the A or marital deduction trust) and a nonmarital (family) trust (the B or bypass trust). The marital A trust is designed to hold assets that qualify for the marital deduction. The surviving spouse is entitled to all of the income from the A trust and also has the power to appoint the trust corpus to anyone including himself or herself. This income right along with the power to appoint the corpus can enable the surviving spouse to either pay for LTC expenses or pay for LTCI premiums if the income is sufficient and he or she qualifies for the coverage. The nonmarital B trust can also be used to provide the surviving spouse with additional income and even limited amounts of principal to meet LTC expenses, without causing the trust corpus to be included in the surviving spouse's estate. However, the real purpose of the B trust is to preserve the full estate tax credit for the grantor spouse.

The choice of an estate plan depends on the client's financial status, family situation, and personal preferences. While the use of an A-B trust arrangement can save estate taxes, a client and his or her family may reject the notion of any limits being placed on the surviving spouse's access to property.

Qualified Terminal Interest Property (QTIP)—A QTIP trust permits a spouse to provide for a surviving spouse by transferring assets to a trust that qualifies for the marital deduction and yet permits the transferor spouse to retain control over the ultimate disposition of the assets. To qualify for the martial deduction, assets transferred to a QTIP trust must meet certain conditions. These conditions are that the surviving spouse be given the right to all the income for life, that no one can direct assets to anyone other than the surviving spouse as long as the surviving spouse lives, and that the transferor spouse's executor must make an irrevocable election on the transferor spouse's estate tax return that any remaining assets at the surviving spouse's death be included in the surviving spouse's estate. A QTIP trust is one way for a spouse (the transferor spouse) to protect the interests of other heirs (perhaps children from a prior marriage) while also providing for the surviving spouse. If a sufficient amount of income is being paid to the surviving spouse, it can be used to pay for LTC expenses, or better yet, it can be used to pay for LTCI premiums, provided the surviving spouse qualifies for the coverage.

Irrevocable Life Insurance Trust (ILIT)—An ILIT can be of particular benefit for estate planning purposes. In fact, it is generally perceived as the most beneficial and flexible estate planning technique currently available. In an ILIT, a life insurance policy covering the grantor spouse's life is purchased and owned by the irrevocable trust established for this purpose. Properly designed, the ILIT allows the grantor spouse an opportunity to provide support benefits for the surviving spouse, including funds to pay for LTCI premiums and/or cover LTC expenses, while avoiding inclusion of the insurance proceeds in the estate of either spouse.

To accomplish this goal, the ILIT's dispositive terminology must be carefully designed. The surviving spouse must not be given a general power of appointment or unlimited invasion rights over the trust assets. However, the surviving spouse can be given all income from the trust for the remainder of his or her life as well as a noncumulative right to withdraw the greater of 5 percent or $5,000 of the trust corpus each year. In addition, the surviving spouse can be given the power to consume or invade the trust corpus subject to an ascertainable standard relating to his or her health, education, support, or maintenance. A standard is ascertainable if the power holder's duty to exercise the power is reasonably measurable in terms of his or her health, education, support, or maintenance needs. Paying for the costs of LTC falls into this category.

A Power of Attorney—A power of attorney is a document legally signed by one person (the principal) authorizing another person (the attorney-in-fact) to act on behalf of the signer. An exmaple of its use is where an adult child helps his or her elderly parent manage day-to-day affairs, or make decisions regarding LTC options and/or the purchase of LTCI.

There are three types of powers of attorney: a general power, a durable power, and a springing durable power. A general power is effective as long as the person granting the power remains in good health. Failing health, however, is often a reason for using a power of attorney, but a general power becomes legally ineffective in cases of mental incompetence or medical incapacity. A durable power of attorney solves this problem by remaining valid and operative despite any subsequent incapacity of the principal. It permits the designated family member or decision maker to step in and manage the incapacitated person's financial affairs, including the making of decisions regarding the need for LTC. A springing durable power of attorney becomes operative only when a specified event occurs, such as the physical or mental incapacity of the principal. It is designed for an individual reluctant to grant broad powers to another person while he or she is still capable of making decisions. All three types of powers are useful legal instruments that enable family members or decision makers to get involved in planning ahead for the probability of needing LTC and/or making LTC decisions.

Advance Medical Directives—Either a durable power of attorney for health care or a living will is referred to as an advance medical directive. These documents are receiving more attention, because advances in medical technology that prolong life have increased fears of lengthy artificial life support and family financial disaster. Modern medicine can keep a person alive by artificial mechanisms even though the individual is unconscious and essentially nonfunctional. Life-sustaining procedures are used in cases of accident or terminal illness where death is imminent and recovery highly improbable. Advance medical directives have evolved in response to these situations. By executing an advance medical directive, such as a living will and/or a durable power of attorney for health care, individuals may make arrangements and give authority to others to carry out their health care instructions. Usually, directives will go into effect only in the event that a person cannot make and communicate his or her own health care decisions. Preparing an advance directive lets the physician and other health care providers know the kind of medical care an individual wants, or does not want, if he or she becomes incapacitated. A directive is a signed and witnessed legal document that names the person the individual wishes to make medical decisions about his or her care. Other than the person named, it relieves family and friends of the responsibility of making decisions regarding life-prolonging actions. Advance medical directives are an important part of any LTC plan.

The Role of LTC in Income Tax Planning

There are many tax issues that are of real concern to seniors, the primary market segment needing LTC. Knowledge of these issues will help you to enhance both your image and value to this market segment. While you should not be preparing to give tax advice (unless you are qualified and your contract or practice permits it), you may, nonetheless, have an opportunity to inform older prospects and clients that they could benefit from such advice and that you can help them obtain it.

Here are several tax areas you may want to be familiar with:

- Gains from the sale of a principal residence
- Capital gain rules on the sale of capital assets (stocks, bonds, and mutual funds)
- Tax advantages and distribution rules for IRAs, pensions, and other qualified retirement plans
- Social Security rules on the taxation of benefits
- Tax breaks on premiums and benefits from buying a TQ LTCI policy

The Role of LTC in Life Planning

Life planning is viewed as a new and innovative model in retirement and financial planning. Life planning adds a "holistic" element to the process of financial planning by considering the non-financial needs of retirement. This model seeks to develop a balanced and meaningful retirement experience by attending to multiple areas of life, including finances, work, leisure, relationships, physical health, mental health, housing, and personal growth. Life planning emphasizes identifying personal lifestyle goals based on one's values and priorities. It focuses on personal goals and then assigns a financial cost to satisfying those goals and wants. Its emphasis is away from product and towards process, from economic values to human values, linking financial assets with the values in our lives.

Summary

As LTC becomes a more visible and common concern in the American financial planning landscape, it will naturally become a more integral part of the retirement, estate, and income tax planning process. Clearly, because of the risk exposure LTC poses, it cannot be ignored or put off in doing serious financial planning. Because you are aware of this, you can become a part of the solution by integrating LTC planning into your practice.

Life Planning

"Life planning is a comprehensive approach to retirement planning that is appropriate and useful at all ages, young adults as well as those approaching retirement. It is based on the philosophy that life is a continuum, and that the most successful and satisfying retirement experiences are based on a series of thoughtful, future-focused decisions made throughout one's life. Skills, values, attitudes, resources, and relationships developed and honed during one stage of life all contribute to meeting the challenges and recognizing the opportunities of the next stage of life."

(Life Planning: An Effective Model for Retirement Education, by Joyce Cohen and Carol Anderson)

Life planning is the process of helping people focus on the true values and motivations in their lives, determining the goals and objectives they have as they see their lives develop, and using these values, motivations, goals and objectives to guide the planning process and provide a framework for making choices and decisions in life that have financial and non-financial implications or consequences.

(Journal of Financial Planning, "Experts Examine Emerging Concept of 'Life Planning," by William L. Anthes and Shelly Lee)

Case History
Something is Better than Nothing

When I first began writing LTCI, I lost many sales because the prospect felt that the proposed solution was unaffordable. Such was the case for a couple who had been clients of mine for a number of years. During one of our annual reviews, I discussed LTCI with them. They eagerly applied for the coverage and were approved; however, one of them was rated. The higher premium was unaffordable and the couple decided not to buy the policies.

About 5 years later, the husband called and asked me if I still sold LTCI. The couple wanted to review their situation again. Naturally, I was a little suspicious.

The day of their appointment was a brisk, fall afternoon. I stood in my office looking out the window when they drove up in a new PT Cruiser. The passenger-side door opened and the wife got out of the car with her purse. She appeared to be fumbling with things and carrying an oxygen bottle. The driver's side door opened and the husband got out of the car. He was walking but dragging his foot noticeably. It turned out that the wife had fibroid tumors in her lungs and the husband had suffered a mini-stroke. Both of them were uninsurable.

I felt sick. Afterward, I reflected on the situation and realized that I should have been more forceful and flexible in explaining the coverage. I should have insisted that some amount of coverage was better than none and designed a plan that fit into the couple's budget by lowering the MDB or shortening the benefit period. This experience helped me adopt the philosophy that it is always better to get something in force, even if it is not the ideal plan. My recommendation to other advisors is to begin the sales process with the ideal plan, then make any necessary adjustments to fit it into the prospect's budget. Having something in force is better than having nothing in force.

In the past, I have had difficulty placing coverage when one spouse is healthy and the other one is not. I remember one case where the wife's application was approved but the husband's application was declined.

Instead of obtaining coverage for the wife, the couple decided to wait and apply again, together, after the husband's medical condition had stabilized. Unfortunately, when they reapplied, his application was accepted but hers was declined. Again, I realized that I should have been more forceful about selling LTCI to the healthy spouse at the time.

Now, in situations where one spouse has a medical history that could result in a declination, I warn the couple about it. I help them understand the importance of the healthy spouse buying a policy regardless of the underwriting decision on the other spouse. I tell them, "If you are declined, let's still purchase the policy for your spouse. Depending on the feedback we receive from underwriting, we can investigate other insurance companies who specialize in these types of risks, or we can wait and try again at some point in the future. It's important, however, that you buy the coverage for your spouse while he or she is insurable at standard rates. Something is better than nothing."

My advice to other advisors is to have a plan for handling these situations. By adopting a philosophy that something is better than nothing, you will help more of your prospects and clients protect themselves from the potential devastation of LTC expenses.

Case History
A Fork in the Road

Robert Whitaker has been an advisor for over 14 years—over 10 of those years as a branch manager.

Mrs. Smith was about 75 years old and living in a South Florida condominium. She had approximately $300,000 in CDs and received about $30,000 in income. When we completed the fact finder and I had given my recommendation, Mrs. Smith told me that she was one of those people who never made a decision the same day and that she wanted to think about it.

I wasn't surprised because "I want to think about it" is the most common objection I encounter. Statistically in these situations, I know that I am going to get back into a household about 11 percent of the time. If the prospect does not make a decision today, chances are that he or she will never make a decision. For my conscience's sake, I ask for a decision: yes or no.

I told Mrs. Smith that her answer was not an acceptable choice. I explained, "The fact of the matter is that it would be easy for me to accept, 'I want to think about it' and walk out. However, if 3 weeks from now you have a stroke, and your children come into town and find this LTCI brochure along with my business card, the first thing they will do is call and ask me if you bought the policy. I would then have to explain to them that I allowed you to tell me, 'I want to think about it.' I would rather tell them that you told me, 'No.'" After thinking for a few more minutes, Mrs. Smith decided to purchase the policy.

About 9 weeks after Mrs. Smith received the policy, her daughter called me. It was the identical scenario that I had described to Mrs. Smith during the sales interview. She went on claim for a little over a year. She then came off claim, and shortly after went back on claim again. Just recently, when I spoke with her daughter I said, "Do you remember how mad you were because I really pushed your mother to make a decision when I sold her the policy?" She said, "Yes, I know. Now you're a hero in the family. You have saved us approximately $80,000 so far."

Advisors need to understand the importance of a decision to purchase LTCI. We are the only thing that stands between a person's life savings going to his or her heirs or going to a nursing home or home care agency. It is our responsibility to make recommendations as a professional, conveying that we are the expert. If you go into a doctor's office, he tells you, "This is the problem and this is what you need to do to correct the problem." That is what advisors need to do. We have a responsibility to help people understand the exact risk they are taking by not purchasing LTCI and to recommend that they take action. We need to be a fork in the road—a decision point that makes people choose: yes or no.

Chapter Seven Review

Key Terms and Concepts are explained in the Glossary. Answers to the Review Questions and Self-Test Questions are found in the back of the book in the Answers to Questions section.

Key Terms and Concepts

NAIC Shopper's Guide
30-day free look
post-claims underwriting
third party notification
lapse
suitability
outline of coverage
MIB, Inc.
APS
adverse selection
field underwriting
personal history interview
face-to-face assessment interview
underwriting
    selection
    classification

trust
    revocable living trust
    A-B trust
    QTIP trust
    irrevocable life insurance trust
       (ILIT)
general power of attorney
durable power of attorney
springing durable power of attorney
advance medical directive
    durable power of attorney for
       health care
    living will

Review Questions

7-1. What steps must the advisor take in completing the application?

7-2. The NAIC LTCI Model Regulation requires insurers marketing LTCI to develop and use suitability standards. Explain what these standards must take into account.

7-3. What sources of information does an underwriter rely on to help in the selection and classification of LTCI applicants?

7-4. What factors are used to classify LTCI applicants into rate categories?

7-5.   What are the objectives of the delivery interview?

7-6. Briefly explain why the possibility of needing LTC has to be considered in:
   a.   retirement planning
   b.   estate planning

Self-Test Questions

Instructions: Read chapter 7 first, then answer the following questions to test your knowledge. There are 10 questions; circle the correct answer, then check your answers with the answer key in the back of the book.

7-1. An organization that exchanges medical information among its members relevant to the underwriting of LTCI applicants is the

   (a) AMA
   (b) MIB
   (c) ACLU
   (d) GAO

7-2. The LTCI Model Act and Model Regulation were developed by the

   (a) Health Care Financing Administration (HCFA)
   (b) National Association of Insurance Commissioners (NAIC)
   (c) U.S. Department of Health and Human Services (DHHS)
   (d) American Association of Retired Persons (AARP)

7-3. The document that must be delivered to a LTCI prospect at the time of initial solicitation and that contains a brief description of the policy's most important features is called the

   (a) outline of coverage
   (b) shopper's guide
   (c) advisor's statement
   (d) application

7-4. A legal document signed by one person authorizing another person to act on behalf of the signer if he or she becomes incapacitated is a

(a) revocable living trust
(b) QTIP trust
(c) durable power of attorney
(d) will

7-5. The tendency for those with a higher than average probability of loss to seek or continue insurance to a greater extent than those with an average or below average probability of loss is known as

(a) adverse selection
(b) post claims underwriting
(c) suitability
(d) classification

7-6. Which of the following statements regarding LTCI underwriting is (are) correct?

    I.   Classification determines who qualifies for coverage.
    II. Selection determines the terms and conditions of coverage.

(a) I only
(b) II only
(c) Both I and II
(d) Neither I nor II

7-7. LTCI underwriting differs from life underwriting in which of the following ways?

    I.   Multiple LTC claims can arise for the same insured.
    II. LTCI underwriting tends to involve less scrutiny.

(a) I only
(b) II only
(c) Both I and II
(d) Neither I nor II

7-8. The home office underwriter may access information about an applicant through all of the following sources **EXCEPT**

(a) a personal history telephone interview
(b) an attending physician's statement
(c) the NAIC shopper's guide
(d) a face-to-face assessment interview

7-9. The typical application form contains all of the following types of information to assist in the selection process **EXCEPT**

(a) prequalification questions
(b) an authorization to release medical information
(c) coverage selection
(d) an authorization for the IRS to release official tax records

7-10. A trust is a legal vehicle with all of the following key components **EXCEPT** a

(a) trustee
(b) prospect
(c) corpus
(d) beneficiary

8

Miscellaneous Markets, Products, and Your Professional Practice

Overview and Learning Objectives

Chapter 8 explores LTCI marketing opportunities that exist within the worksite environment. In addition, there is a discussion of state LTCI partnership plans and the federal LTCI program. Also, the relationship of compliance to the regulations that govern LTCI sales practices is explored. Finally, integration of LTCI marketing into a professional financial services practice is examined. By reading this chapter and answering the questions, you should be able to:

8-1.   Describe several LTCI products that are currently being marketed at the worksite.

8-2.   Explain how the state partnership programs work.

8-3.   Describe the features of the federal LTCI program.

8-4.   Describe how ethics and compliance relate to the LTC market.

8-5.   Describe the regulations that affect LTC sales.

8-6.   Identify the components of professionalism in building a LTC practice.

8-7.   Identify strategies for working effectively with other professional financial service advisors.

8-8.   Identify your own career educational development needs.

Chapter Outline

Business Markets and Miscellaneous Products

The sale of LTCI today exists predominantly in the individual market. This is evidenced by the fact that 73 percent (nearly 2.5 million) of the approximately 3.4 million policies in force in 2000 were individual policies. Also, 88 percent of the existing premiums being spent for LTCI are spent on individual policies. Nevertheless, according to the American Council of Life Insurers 2001 Fact Book, more than 900,000 group certificates and over 5,000 master policies were in force in 2000. Premiums for group in-force business totaled $534 million in 2000, which is an increase of 23 percent over 1999. This represents only 12 percent of the total in-force LTCI premiums.

However, due in part to the changing demographic landscape that is present in the American workplace today, there is increasing pressure on employers to offer LTCI as an employee benefit. Because of the increased longevity of aged parents and relatives, many employers find their employees preoccupied with having to care for them. Also, baby boomers who represent about half of the adult full-time workforce are increasingly finding themselves burdened with the exhausting responsibilities of caregiving for their older family members. As a result, many workers are experiencing increased absences from work, greater emotional stress from having to care for relatives, and lower productivity at the worksite. In response to these factors, there is an increasing trend toward the wholesale marketing of LTCI products in the business market.

Group LTCI

Types of Products

While LTCI products marketed at the worksite are often referred to in a generic sense as group insurance, there are actually two types of group products: traditional group contracts and mass-marketed individual policies. Insurers that offer other types of group life and health insurance tend to issue group insurance contracts. Insurers that specialize in the individual market tend to write mass-marketed individual policies. Some insurers that have historically written both group and individual products may offer both types of LTCI. Large employer groups with several thousand employees are more likely to use group insurance contracts, whereas very small employers are more likely to use mass-marketed individual policies. Between these two extremes, both types of products are commonly used. For the most part, the coverage available under either type of product is similar.

Group Insurance—The first type of group product is group insurance, which is a method of providing insurance protection to members of a group. It is characterized by a master group contract with individual certificates, group underwriting, and possibly experience rating.

Group Contract—A group insurance contract provides coverage to a number of persons under a single insurance contract issued to someone other than the insured persons. The contract, referred to as a master contract, provides benefits to a group of individuals who have a specific relationship to the policyowner—such as employees or association members. Although these individuals are not actual parties to the master contract, they can legally enforce their rights and are often referred to as third-party beneficiaries of the insurance contract.

Insureds covered under a group contract receives certificates of insurance as evidence of coverage. Each certificate is a summary of the coverage provided under the master contract rather than an actual insurance contract itself.

In individual insurance, the coverage of the insured normally begins with the inception of the contract and ceases with its termination. With group insurance, individual members of the group may become eligible for coverage long after the inception of the contract, or they may lose their eligibility status long before the contract terminates. However, the right to continue coverage on an individual basis accompanies the loss of group coverage.

Group Underwriting—Group insurance is accompanied by some degree of underwriting of the group itself. The degree of group underwriting (and possibly premium rates) will vary to the extent members of the group are also subject to individual underwriting. If members of the group are individually subject to full underwriting, there is minimum underwriting of the group as a whole. At the other extreme, the group is underwritten much more closely if members can obtain coverage on a guaranteed-issue basis. Underwriting of group products is covered in more depth later in this chapter.

Experience Rating—If a group is sufficiently large, the actual experience of the group may be a factor in determining the premium rates that are charged. However, without experience rating, experience is determined on a class basis and applies to all insured groups within the class. With the newness of LTCI and the long time needed to obtain meaningful claims data, experience rating typically is not used for group LTCI. Rather, premiums are determined based on the experience of all the groups in a class.

Mass-Marketed Individual Insurance—The second type of group product is not true group insurance but individual polices of insurance sold through a sponsoring organization, such as an employer or association. Generically, this type of coverage is referred to as mass-marketed individual insurance, because the insureds receive individual policies of insurance. It is also referred to by other names such as worksite marketing, because coverage is made available as part of an employer-employee relationship, or a voluntary benefit plan, because in some situations the insured pays the entire premium.

Types of Groups—Almost 90 percent of the LTCI coverage under group arrangements is obtained through employer-sponsored plans that employers make available to their employees. The remainder of the coverage is obtained under plans of affinity groups or associations that make coverage available as a member benefit. Examples of these types of groups include the U.S. Chamber of Commerce, AARP, banks, service clubs, and alumni associations.

Comparisons with Individual Products

The following comparison of group and individual LTCI products focuses primarily on plans sponsored by employers, since employer groups are by far the most common type of organization that uses group products.

For the most part, the coverage available under group products is quite similar to the coverage under policies sold in the individual marketplace. However, there are some differences with respect to who purchases coverage and the types of coverage they purchase. In addition, there are some variations and unique features of group products. These differences are discussed with respect to tax qualification, eligibility, premium payments, cost, benefits, underwriting, and portability. Before proceeding, however, you must realize that group products—particularly those written for large groups—may be designed as a result of negotiation between an employer and an insurer. In addition, collective bargaining may have also had a significant influence. Consequently, numerous variations are possible.

Purchasers of Group Products

Purchasers of coverage under employer-sponsored plans tend to have an average age about 25 years younger than those purchasing coverage in the individual market. This was an unexpected and surprising phenomenon to insurers when they started selling coverage in the group market. The lower average age naturally results in a significantly lower annual premium for these insureds. In addition, they also tend to select a somewhat higher level of benefits than do purchasers in the individual market. The average MDB amount is higher and the average duration of benefits is longer. There is also a greater likelihood that the group insureds under employer-sponsored plans have inflation protection and nonforfeiture benefits.

Two reasons probably account for these benefit differences. First, since purchasers of employer-sponsored coverage as a group are younger, pay lower premiums, and will probably continue working for several more years, they are better able to afford a higher level of benefits. Second, since there typically are fewer options available to group members, these plans tend to be structured to include certain types of coverage. For example, an employer's plan may automatically include inflation protection and/or nonforfeiture benefits.

Tax Qualification—Group products are tax-qualified and as such must meet all the requirements imposed by HIPAA. They are also subject to the provisions of the NAIC LTCI Model Act and Model Regulation.

Eligibility—An employer-sponsored plan may be available to all employees who meet specified employment criteria, such as working full-time, being actively at work, and having worked for the employer for a minimum period of time. Eligibility may also be limited to certain

> Purchasers of coverage under employer-sponsored plans tend to have an average age about 25 years younger than those purchasing coverage in the individual market.

classifications of employees, such as management, salaried personnel, or employees with more than 3 years of service.

As long as an employee falls within an eligible classification, group coverage is available for the employee and/or spouse. Many plans also extend eligibility to retirees and other family members, such as children, parents, grandparents, or siblings.

Plans vary as to when an eligible person may apply for coverage. When a group plan is first installed, eligible persons must usually elect coverage within a defined enrollment period. To minimize adverse selection, eligible persons who initially declined coverage are often unable to enroll until the next open enrollment period, which typically occurs once every year or as infrequently as every 2 or 3 years. However, under some plans that use individual underwriting, an eligible person may be allowed to enroll anytime. A newly hired employee and any eligible relatives will be allowed to enroll as soon as the employee satisfies the eligibility requirements; otherwise they will have to wait until the next open enrollment period.

Premium Payments—The majority of group programs are voluntary benefit plans with the employee (and other covered persons) paying the full cost of coverage. Depending on the plan, premiums may be payable for the life of the employee or over the employee's working years.

In some programs, employers pay a portion of the cost but usually only for an employee's coverage, not for that of eligible relatives. The employer's contribution may be a percentage of the cost (such as 25 or 50 percent) or a specified dollar amount (such as $200 per year). However, the more likely approach has the employer paying for a base amount of coverage with the employee being able to purchase additional benefits by paying the full cost of the added coverage. This arrangement is often referred to as a buy-up plan.

EXAMPLE: Carmella's employer recently installed a group LTCI plan. The employer pays the full cost of a base amount of comprehensive coverage for all eligible employees, which are defined to include anyone who works full-time and has at least 3 years of service with the employer. The MDB amount is $75 after a 90-day elimination period, and the benefit duration is 2 years. Employees are given an option to increase the MDB amount to $100, $125, or $150. They can also increase the benefit duration to 5 years or their lifetime. Employees who elect the higher benefits must pay the full cost of the additional coverage through payroll deduction.

Cost—The cost of employer-sponsored plans tends to be at least 5 to 15 percent less expensive than coverage purchased in the individual market. Two factors account for this lower cost. First, employers often provide, or at least assist with, many administrative services that would otherwise be the responsibility of the insurer. These typically include some or all of the following: communicating the plan to employees, handling the enrollment procedure, collecting premiums on a payroll-deduction basis, and maintaining certain records. Second, commission rates tend to be lower for group products than for individual products. This is a result of the typically larger dollar amount of premium for group plans and the assistance provided by the employer and company representatives to encourage enrollment.

Just because the cost of coverage for group plans may be less than the cost of individually purchased coverage, it should not be assumed that group coverage is always the best buy for a consumer. There are significant price variations among insurers. If a high-cost insurer provides the group coverage, it may be possible for a person to find less expensive coverage in the individual market. Moreover, the person may be able to design a benefit package that better fits his or her needs by purchasing an individual policy.

Benefits—Some employer-sponsored plans offer as wide an array of benefit choices as are found in the individual market. However, most group plans simplify the decision process by limiting the available options from which an employee may choose. This simplification may be in the form of allowing choice with respect to several specific benefit options or allowing choice among a limited number of pre-designed benefit packages. Regardless of which approach is taken, the available options are usually determined by negotiation between the employer and the insurer.

Benefit Options—An employee may have to make several benefit choices. However, the options for each choice are limited. The following are some of the choices that employees often face:

- Type of coverage. Most employer-sponsored plans provide comprehensive coverage. However, an employee may occasionally be allowed to select either comprehensive coverage or facility-only coverage. Home health care only policies are seldom offered in the group market. Policies in the group market also tend to provide benefits on a reimbursement basis.

- Elimination period. Many plans offer only one elimination period, most commonly 90 days. A few plans offer additional choices, but elimination periods of fewer than 30 days or more than 180 days are infrequently used.
- Benefit amount. Most plans offer at least two or three MDB amounts, such as $100, $150, or $200. The amount selected should approximate the cost of nursing home care where an employee resides.
- Benefit duration. Again, most plans offer two or three options, such as 2 years, 5 years, and lifetime.
- Inflation protection. An insurer must offer inflation protection to the employer who may decide to (1) not make it available under the plan, (2) require that it be part of any benefit package an employee designs, or (3) allow individual employees to make the decision whether to purchase the coverage. In most cases, the employer selects one of the latter two alternatives.
- Non-forfeiture benefits. Like inflation protection, the employer decides whether to make this coverage available to the employees. In most cases, the benefit is either not made available or the choice is passed on to the employees.

Underwriting—There are several levels of underwriting that may apply to employer-sponsored groups. These include guaranteed issue, modified guaranteed issue, simplified issue, and full underwriting. From the standpoint of applicants, employees are often subject to less stringent underwriting than their family members. Adverse selection tends to be less of a problem with employees, because they tend to be healthier since they are actively at work.

Guaranteed Issue—Insurers occasionally use guaranteed-issue underwriting for employees in employer-sponsored groups. This means that coverage is provided for all employees who apply for it. While this is the most liberal underwriting from the standpoint of employees, it also means that the insurer underwrites the group much more stringently than when it uses the other underwriting methods discussed below.

The insurer will generally use guaranteed-issue underwriting only if the group meets certain criteria that minimize adverse selection. These criteria, which are also common to group underwriting for other types of insurance, typically include several or all of the following:

- The group is large in size.
- A high minimum number or percentage of employees applies for benefits.
- Eligibility is limited to full-time employees, possibly with a minimum length of service with the employer.
- The employer pays some or all of the premium costs.
- The employee has minimal choice in picking the level of benefits.
- The group has a stable employment history.
- The group is in an industry that is not considered high risk for claims.
- The employer is able to handle some of the plan administration.

Guaranteed-issue underwriting is seldom used for applicants other than employees. In addition, it is often accompanied by a higher premium than when other underwriting methods are used.

Modified Guaranteed Issue—With modified guaranteed-issue underwriting, the insurer will accept most applicants. However, some medical questions will be asked on the application, and the answers to these questions may result in an application being declined. These questions are often aimed at determining whether the applicant has recently received LTC services or requires assistance with any ADLs. The questions may also ask whether the applicant has certain specified medical conditions such as Parkinson's disease, multiple sclerosis, cancer, or AIDS. As long as there are no unsatisfactory answers to these questions, no further medical information is requested and coverage is issued.

There may also be some underwriting of the group itself, but on a less stringent basis than when guaranteed-issue underwriting is used. Modified guaranteed-issue underwriting may also be limited to employees.

Simplified Issue—With simplified-issue underwriting, the insurer tends to ask more medically related questions than when modified guarantee-issue underwriting is used. If the answers to these questions are unsatisfactory, only then does the insurer request further medical information—such as an attending physician's statement (APS)—or request further medical assessments.

Simplified-issue underwriting might be used for all applicants, or it might be used for all applicants other than employees when the employees are subject to less stringent underwriting.

Full Individual Underwriting—In some cases, a group LTCI plan will use the same underwriting that is found in the individual market. This type of underwriting is most likely to be used in the group market when the size of the group is very small and for persons other than employees.

Portability—If an insured is no longer eligible for employer-sponsored LTCI coverage, he or she can elect to continue coverage. If the insured's coverage is in the form of an individual LTCI policy paid for through payroll deduction, the insured only needs to make arrangements with the insurer to pay the premiums on a direct-bill basis. If the coverage is under a group policy, the NAIC Model Regulation requires that the insurer provide the insured with a basis for continuation or conversion of his or her coverage. Under a continuation of coverage, the insured retains coverage under the group contract but pays premiums directly to the insurer. Under a conversion of coverage, the insured is issued an individual LTCI policy that must be identical or substantially equivalent to the group coverage. The attained age premium for the converted policy is based on the individual policy rates in existence when the insured initially obtained coverage under the group plan.

Key Employee/Group Carve-out LTCI Plans

A recent phenomenon that is emerging in the worksite marketing of LTCI is for employers to selectively provide individual policies to its key employees and executives. In order to attract and retain quality key employees some employers, as part of their benefit package, will carve-out selected employees and owner-executives from the group, and pay for their individual LTCI coverage using the company's funds. This works similarly to a group carve-out plan of life insurance for key employees in that it avoids one of the drawbacks of ordinary group LTCI, which is that the benefit choices for the rank and file employees may be minimal and restrictive. Furthermore, just as some employers have done in disability income salary continuation plans, corporations will write a resolution into their corporate minutes that states the existence of the plan. The resolution also outlines the criteria for employee selection and their qualifications that entitle them to participate in the plan. For example, the resolution could say that this coverage will be made available to all employees earning in excess of $75,000 and having 5 or more years of service.

Federal Income Tax Advantages—This type of benefit strategy is perfectly legal and federally income-tax favorable to both the company and the employee. The Internal Revenue Code (IRC) clearly states that any plan an employer institutes to provide coverage under a tax-qualified (TQ) LTCI contract is generally treated as an accident and health plan with respect to such coverage. Consequently, the following tax advantages exist for both employers and employees alike:

- Premiums for LTCI coverage paid for by a C corporation employer are not includable in the gross income of employees.
- The benefits received by both C corporation employees and self-employed individuals from TQ LTCI policies of the reimbursement type (provided by the employer) are tax-free just as they are under personally owned policies. However, under contracts written on an indemnity (per diem) basis, the benefits are only excludible from income up to $220 per day in 2003. (This figure is indexed annually.) Amounts in excess of $220 per day are also excludible from income if they represent actual costs incurred for qualified LTC services for the insured.
- Because LTCI is regarded as accident and health insurance, the monies spent by a C corporation employer on premiums for TQ LTCI contracts for its employees, their spouses, and their dependents are income tax deductible by the employer as a legitimate business expense.
- The situation is different if the employer is a sole proprietorship, partnership, or S corporation. Any LTCI premiums paid by the business on behalf of a sole proprietor are included in the sole proprietor's income. Premiums paid on behalf of a partner or an S corporation shareholder who owns more than 2 percent of the stock are included in the partner's or shareholder's gross income.
  However, self-employed sole proprietors, partners, and S corporation shareholders are eligible to deduct LTCI premiums

as a business expense, subject to limitations. Specifically, during the taxable year 2003, the *smaller* of the annual age-based LTC deductible limits (shown in the example below and in table 5-3 on page 5-45) or the actual amount paid for LTCI (for the self-employed individual, his or her spouse, and his or her dependents) may be deducted as a business expense along with other medical expense premiums in determining adjusted gross income (AGI) on Form 1040. In other words, these self-employed individuals may subtract LTCI premiums (along with other health insurance premiums) from their gross incomes in determining their AGIs. These deductions are referred to as above-the-line deductions, and they typically are more favorable than below-the-line deductions for medical expenses (including LTCI premiums), which are subject to the 7.5 percent limitation.

An example will help to illustrate the tax benefits to a self-employed sole proprietor, partner, or S-corporation shareholder. For illustration purposes, suppose that:

- Steve is a married sole proprietor, age 55.
- He paid a total of $4,000 in premiums in 2003 for LTCI for himself and his spouse.
- Besides the LTCI premiums, he has no other health insurance premiums in 2003.

For federal income tax purposes, Steve's deduction in determining his AGI is calculated as follows:

For coverage under a TQ LTCI policy, enter the smaller of:

a) Total LTCI premium payments made by Steve during 2003 ($4,000); or
b) The amount shown below using Steve's age at the end of the year.

$250 if the person is age 40 or younger
$470 if age 41 to 50
$940 if age 51 to 60
$2,510 if age 61 to 70
$3,130 if over age 70

Since Steve is age 55, the smaller of $4,000 or $940 is obviously $940. Assuming Steve is in a 30 percent tax bracket, the $940 above-the-line deduction from gross income actually ends up saving Steve $282 in income taxes ($940 x .30 = $282). However, if Steve elects to use the $940 as an above-the line deduction, he cannot then include it as part of his medical expenses if he "itemizes."

Alternatively, Steve may choose to use the $940 as an itemized or below-the-line deduction. This deduction would only be available to Steve if his deductible medical expenses (including the $940) exceed 7.5 percent of his AGI. And then only the amount in excess of 7.5 percent would be deductible. For this reason, above-the-line deductions typically are more valuable than below-the-line deductions.

It is also important to note that LTCI coverage cannot be offered through a cafeteria plan (IRC Section 125) on a tax-favored basis. In addition, if an employee has a flexible spending account for unreimbursed medical expenses, which is a typical component of cafeteria plans, any reimbursements for LTC expenses (other than medical expenses) must be included in the employee's income.

Summary

A wide variety of opportunities exist for marketing and selling LTCI at the work-site. LTCI can be sold as discounted group insurance coverage for employees, it can be sold voluntarily as individual policies to interested employees, or it can be sold at the executive level selectively for key executives.

Partnership Programs for LTC

The partnership programs for LTC are alliances between state governments and insurance companies to encourage the sale of approved LTCI policies. The goals of these programs are to protect people from being impoverished by LTC expenses and to prevent them from becoming immediately dependent on Medicaid. These programs also provide further evidence of government's advocacy of LTCI. Indeed, the states that have partnership programs make a concerted effort to inform and counsel their residents about the value of purchasing LTCI.

Many middle-class people in nursing homes qualify for Medicaid by spending virtually all of their assets on LTC or by transferring the assets to relatives to place themselves in a state of poverty. The result has been a staggering financial burden on Medicaid that endangers its mission to care for the poor in many states. The cycle of spending down to Medicaid dependence can be broken if more middle-class Americans—

especially those of more modest means who are likely to spend down to qualify for Medicaid—could be broadly encouraged to purchase LTCI.

The cost savings to the Medicaid program are obvious. If the policy's benefits prove sufficient to meet the cost of care, a person with LTCI may not rely on Medicaid at all. Moreover, a comprehensive policy provides resources to care for someone at a much lower cost at home. If the person were on Medicaid, higher nursing home costs might be incurred.

In return for the potential cost savings generated by reducing Medicaid dependence, states are willing to provide an incentive for the purchase of LTCI. Policymakers agreed that an effective incentive from the state is to allow people that purchase LTCI to qualify for Medicaid while maintaining a higher-than-usual personal asset level should they exhaust their insurance benefits. As a result, purchasers of LTCI with significant assets can still qualify for Medicaid without having to spend those assets.

Program Development

In 1987, a Robert Wood Johnson Foundation-funded study by the state of Connecticut concluded that collaboration between insurers and the state could help reduce the burden on the Medicaid program through the use of private LTCI. The foundation subsequently awarded program development grants to four states: California, Connecticut, Indiana, and New York. The resulting and continuing programs in these four states that became operational in the early 1990s became known as the partnership programs. The Department of Health and Human Services granted the required approval or waivers that permitted these states to change the Medicaid asset spend-down requirements. Purchasers of policies under these programs could then maintain some or all of their assets and still qualify for Medicaid if they exhausted the benefits from their LTCI policies.

Twenty-four insurers participate in the partnership programs in the original four states with almost half of them offering partnership policies in more than one state. Since the inception of these programs, the combined sales of partnership approved policies in the original four states exceed 100,000 with sales of more than 13,000 policies in a recent year. Premiums for partnership policies averaged approximately $2,000, slightly less than the average of other LTCI policies sold.

State Requirements

Insurers participating in the partnership programs are required to meet the states' requirements for qualified policies and reporting.

Requirements for Qualified Policies—Insurance companies participating in these programs must develop special products to qualify for approval in each state. The products meet HIPAA standards for TQ policies and may be individual or employer-sponsored. Nevertheless, the state's approval boosts consumer confidence in purchasing the product. The policy requirements of most partnership programs were considered innovative a decade ago when they were first introduced. These requirements include:

- availability of both facility-only and comprehensive policies
- minimum and maximum benefit amounts and duration
- inflation protection
- single lifetime elimination period
- a care coordinator or consultant, often from a state-approved or state-required agency, to assist in planning for care and obtaining appropriate services
- protection against a policy lapse due to nonpayment of premium through waiver of premium, and notification of a specially identified third party in the event of the insured's failure to pay the premium
- the state having a role in the claims process to assure prompt payment of claims and review of denials
- advisor training in partnership policies

Some states require insurers to offer upgraded partnership products when new products are available in the non-partnership market. At least one state (California) requires any new policy enhancements to also be offered to current partnership policyowners.

An important objective of partnership programs is to encourage the purchase of LTCI by individuals of modest means. In order to keep the cost of partnership policies affordable, the state programs may allow shorter coverage durations. For example, California and Indiana allow the sale of policies with a benefit duration of one year, and Connecticut allows policies with a 2-year benefit duration. Purchase of these policies has ranged from 30 percent to more than 50 percent of partnership policies sold in some years.

Program Types

Two basic partnership models were developed: the total assets model and the dollar-for-dollar model. Both models have minimum requirements on the amount of coverage that a consumer is required to purchase. As with all Medicaid recipients, insureds that become eligible for Medicaid must contribute their income toward the cost of care.

Total Assets Model—The total assets model adopted by the state of New York requires that participants purchase a minimum of 3 years of nursing home and 6 years of home care coverage, or some combination of the two. After these insurance benefits are exhausted, none of the insured's assets are considered in the determination of Medicaid eligibility, although the insured must contribute his or her income toward the cost of care.

Dollar-for-Dollar Model—The dollar-for-dollar model allows consumers to purchase an amount of private coverage equal to the amount of assets that they wish to protect. In general, the minimum policy must cover at least one year in a nursing home. If and when the private LTCI benefits are utilized, an amount of assets equal to the LTCI benefits that were paid for LTC services is disregarded in determining eligibility for Medicaid. Three states, California, Connecticut, and Indiana initially adopted this model. Indiana later changed its model to a total assets model for coverage amounts above a threshold level that increases annually and a dollar-for-dollar model for coverage levels below the threshold amount.

Limitations

A person with a partnership policy has all the advantages of LTCI discussed throughout this book. The limitations of the program occur if those with partnership policies exhaust their LTCI benefits and qualify for Medicaid under the program. Although assets are protected as they turn to Medicaid to pay for their care, enrollees must keep in mind all the standard Medicaid concerns discussed in chapter 3. Not the least of these concerns is that Medicaid's LTC services are typically for nursing home care and either exclude or provide limited benefits for home care and assisted living.

In addition, as mentioned previously, although assets are protected, income is not. So the program beneficiaries must spend essentially all of their income, allowing certain limited amounts for the support of a spouse who continues to live at home. This standard Medicaid requirement effectively eliminates participation in partnership programs by high-income persons.

Although insureds under these programs may receive LTCI benefits in any state, their assets are protected only in the state where they purchased their partnership-program-eligible policies. This is certainly a major drawback as many people relocate at or during retirement for leisure living or to be near family. However, with the approval of the Department of Health and Human Services, Connecticut and Indiana have established reciprocity of program benefits between them, whereby residents with partnership policies in one state who relocate to the other are eligible for asset protection in the determination of Medicaid eligibility. If partnership programs are implemented by many states, reciprocity between them would be a significant advantage creating a further incentive to purchase coverage under a program.

Pending Federal Legislation

According to an industry survey, the most important government reforms that would lead non-buyers to consider buying LTCI include the ability to deduct premiums from personal income tax and the knowledge that if they used up their policy benefits the government would help pay for their future expenses. Pending federal legislation would grant improved tax-preferred status to LTCI and allow expanded partnership programs to directly address both of these areas. Because these proposals continue to receive serious consideration in both houses of Congress, eventual passage in some form is considered likely. The proposals evidence legislative support for the growth of LTCI by giving individuals further incentives to purchase these programs and for employers to sponsor them.

Improved Tax-Preferred Status

While HIPAA allowed qualified LTC policies to enjoy tax-preferred status for the first time, that tax treatment fell short of what was accorded other accident and health insurance policies. Specifically, as mentioned earlier in this chapter, LTC coverage cannot be offered through a cafeteria plan on a tax-preferred basis, and any reimbursement drawn from an employee's flexible spending account for unreimbursed LTC expenses (other than medical expenses) must be included in an employee's income. The pending proposals would eliminate these exceptions, thereby affording LTC expenses and LTCI premiums and benefits the same tax preferences as medical expenses and premiums for medical expense insurance.

Indeed, some proposals would make premiums paid for LTCI directly deductible in whole or in part from gross income. This deduction, which could be taken without itemizing, is known as an "above the line" tax deduction. Supporters of such proposals point out that currently there is little actual tax benefit for premium payments because most people do not have medical expenses, even with LTCI premiums added, that exceed the 7.5 percent of adjusted gross income (AGI). Other proposals feature a tax credit for premiums and for caregiver expenses to help families pay for supplies, home improvements, and other services to keep a family member at home.

Expanded Partnership Programs

Proposed legislation would allow states to use discretion in seeking estate recovery under their Medicaid programs. The legislation would repeal the law that prevents states from waiving the estate recovery requirement for persons with LTCI policies purchased under approved state partnership programs. If passed, this legislation would enable the many states that have drafted partnership authorization statutes or regulations to implement them.

The Federal Long-Term Care Insurance Program

In December of 2001, the federal government's Office of Personnel Management (OPM) negotiated a contract with two large insurance companies to offer all federal employees and retirees LTCI through a newly formed limited liability partnership called Long Term Care Partners, LLC. Unlike many other LTCI programs, the federal long-term care insurance program (FLTCIP) has comprehensive coverage that makes payments toward several types of LTC (including but not limited to nursing home care, assisted living facility care, formal and informal care in your home, hospice care, and respite care). It also offers a variety of choices for MDB, policy duration, elimination period, and inflation protection. The program, which is overseen by the OPM, is expected to provide for care coordination and tax-deductibility of premiums in many states where such legislation has been passed. It is anticipated that the program will evolve with the market to adjust for technological advancements in the LTC industry.

Eligibility

The FLTCIP provides coverage on a voluntary basis with participants paying 100 percent of the premium. Those eligible for coverage include federal and postal employees and annuitants, members and retired members of the uniformed services, and qualified relatives. Qualified relatives include spouses, children (at least 18 years old), parents, parents-in-law, and stepparents. Each eligible person individually has the right to enroll in the program. Consequently, a federal employee's spouse may enroll even if the employee does not. OPM projects enrollment of 300,000 to 500,000 in the early years of the program, although the core of the eligible population (that is, active federal employees, postal workers, and members of the uniformed services; retirees; and spouses of both active and retired members of the federal family) totals about 8 million persons.

Enrollment and Underwriting

Eligible members of the federal family may apply for coverage at any time by completing one of two forms, an abbreviated underwriting application or a full underwriting application. Use of the abbreviated underwriting application is now quite limited. Currently, only newly hired or newly eligible federal or postal employees and those who have recently joined the uniformed services and their spouses may use it. The main advantage of the abbreviated form is that it allows applicants to obtain coverage at a less stringent level of underwriting that is equivalent to a modified guaranteed-issue basis. Spouses are required to answer slightly more questions than are employees or uniformed service members. However, if these applicants select the lifetime benefit option, more medically related questions must be answered and simplified-issue underwriting is used.

In addition, under the abbreviated form, those applicants who are unable to qualify for the coverage requested may apply for an alternative benefit plan that provides facility-only coverage with a 180-day elimination period, a 2-year benefit period, and a higher premium. If these applicants are denied coverage as initially requested or through the alternative plan, they may purchase a noninsurance service package. The service package provides access to a care coordinator, general information and referral services, and access to discounted networks of LTC providers and services. The alternative benefit plan is unavailable to applicants required to use the full underwriting form who do not qualify for coverage, although they may purchase the noninsurance service package.

Benefit Design

The standard benefit program provides reimbursement benefits up to the selected MDB amounts. There is a choice of two types of tax-qualified options: facility-only coverage or comprehensive coverage. The coverage is also fully portable. If an insured leaves federal employment, is no longer a member of the uniformed services, or gets divorced, the policy may be maintained at the same premium as long as premium payments continue.

MDB Amount—All enrollees must select a MDB amount within the range $50 to $300 (at $25 increments). This amount is also a factor in determining the weekly benefit, if selected, and the maximum lifetime benefit.

Benefits for Covered Services—The facility-only option and the comprehensive option each provide reimbursement of actual charges incurred for covered LTC services as indicated in table 8-1.

TABLE 8-1 FLTCIP Covered Services Under the Facility-Only Option or the Comprehensive Option	
Services	**Daily Reimbursement**
Nursing home, assisted-living facility, or hospice facility	100 percent of the MDB amount
Bed reservation benefit	100 percent of the MDB amount—limited to 30 days per calendar year
Caregiver training	100 percent of the MDB amount—lifetime limit of 7 times the MDB amount
Respite services	100 percent of the MDB amount—limited to 30 times the MDB amount per calendar year

Enrollees selecting the comprehensive option also receive the benefits for covered LTC services indicated in table 8-2.

TABLE 8-2
Additional FLTCIP Covered Services Under the Comprehensive Option

Services	Daily Reimbursement
Home health care services by formal caregivers	75 percent of the MDB amount
Home health care services by informal caregivers	75 percent of the MDB amount—lifetime benefits limited to 365 days for family members or other informal caregivers who do not normally live in the enrollees home at the time of benefit eligibility
Hospice care at home	100 percent of the MDB amount
Adult day care	75 percent of the MDB amount—limited to 30 times the MDB amount per calendar year

Weekly Benefits—Enrollees selecting the comprehensive option may also select a weekly benefit amount equal to seven times the MDB amount selected. Thus, the reimbursement levels in tables 8-1 and 8-2 would provide a weekly benefit amount in place of the MDB amount indicated in each instance. Weekly benefit levels are encouraged because they adapt to varying expense levels that may be incurred over the course of a week.

Benefit Period—Enrollees may choose a 3-year, 5-year, or lifetime benefit period. Together, the benefit period and the MDB amount form a pool of money (that is, the benefit period times the MDB amount equals the pool of money) that determines the lifetime maximum benefit amount that can be used for covered services. As explained in chapter 5, under this approach the policy pays benefits until the pool of money is exhausted. This process may take longer than the 3-year or 5-year benefit period if the insured does not receive covered services every day or if benefits paid are less than the daily or weekly benefit amount. Benefits paid reduce the pool of money, dollar for dollar. When the pool is gone, the LTCI ends. If the lifetime benefit period is selected, the pool of money never ends.

Elimination Period—Enrollees must select either a 30-day or 90-day elimination period. Because the elimination period consists of only the days when care is actually received, a 90-day elimination period typically lasts longer than 90 calendar days unless care is received every day. However, the elimination period needs to be satisfied only once in a lifetime, and it does not apply to hospice care, respite services, or caregiver training.

Inflation Protection—Enrollees may choose one of two inflation protection features:

- *automatic-increase option*—The MDB amount and the remaining portion of the pool of money automatically increase by 5 percent each year over the benefit levels available in the prior year (compounded annually). Premiums are designed (but not guaranteed) to remain level for life, even when benefits increase. The automatic increase inflation option is recommended for purchasers who are not likely to need benefits for many years.
- *future purchase option*—The MDB amount and the remaining portion of the pool of money increase every other year based on the consumer price index (CPI) for medical care or another agreed upon inflation index. However, unlike the automatic increase option, premiums increase as benefits increase. The policyowner may decline to accept the benefit increase, but three refusals to accept the every-other-year increase will cause any subsequent increase to be based on satisfactory evidence of insurability.

In addition, within the limits of the program's design and subject to applicable underwriting and rating requirements, benefits may be upgraded (or downgraded).

Prepackaged Plans—While enrollees may customize their benefit packages, there are also four alternative prepackaged plans to assist enrollees in making their choices among the program's many options. One prepackaged plan provides facility-only coverage with a $100 MDB amount, a 3-year benefit period, and a 90-day elimination period. The other prepackaged plans are comprehensive programs with various combinations of MDB amounts that are either $100 or $150, benefits periods of 3 or 5 years, and a 90-day elimination period.

Other Plan Features—Other plan features include a care coordinator, alternative plan of care, care abroad, contingent nonforfeiture benefit, limitations and exclusions, and third-party review of disputed claims.

Program Premiums—The law requires that the participants pay 100 percent of the premiums and that premiums reflect the cost of benefits provided. Premiums do not differ by enrollee class, such as active employee or member of the military, spouse, or parent. Premiums are based on age when the coverage is purchased and the benefits selected. There are no spouse or family discounts.

Comparison with Other Policies—LTCI policies issued under the FLTCIP may appear similar to policies purchased ouside the program. However, there is a fundamental difference: FLTCIP policies are governed by federal law and are exempt from any state or local laws, including insurance regulation. This difference has several important implications:

- Coverage, benefits, and other policy provisions available under the FLTCIP are identical, in whatever location an applicant purchases a policy.
- Binding arbitration is required for disputed claims.
- The rate stability and financial solvency of the program are protected by OPM, not the state insurance commissioners.

OPM is also responsible for monitoring FLTCIP performance, auditing the program, and anticipating financial problems. OPM and LTC Partners must agree on any rate increases. The General Accounting Office must evaluate the program and may audit it as well. The program's funds can only be used for program expenses, including administration. These funds must be maintained and accounted for separately from any other funds of the LTC Partners, including those from their other lines of business.

By law the premiums must reflect the cost of benefits provided. OPM estimates these to be as much as 20 percent lower than other available policies. Additional reasons that OPM cites for keeping premiums low include its negotiating role, economies of scale, and direct purchase that eliminates the advisor/broker system distribution costs (no commissions). Nevertheless, other policies can be quite competitive based on a premium comparison.

Several characteristics of the FLTCIP might make the policies of other insurers competitive from a cost standpoint. Among them are the FLTCIP's absence of preferred rates, the lack of spousal or family discounts, and a rich package that includes expensive benefits that many buyers may not want, such as caregiver training and payment to informal caregivers. In addition, the absence of substandard ratings may deny coverage to those who would otherwise qualify outside of the FLTCIP.

Summary

The federal government is launching a major educational campaign to explain LTCI to its employees. Therefore, free marketing about the need for LTCI is being targeted to an audience of over 20 million people in the "federal family." Studies have shown that while most Americans worry about their LTC needs, two-thirds of the general public admit they will not have enough funds available should they become disabled. Clearly the government is acknowledging that people need to be prepared for their LTC needs and that Americans need to confront this issue.

Before you contact prospects who are federal employees, familiarize yourself with the FLTCIP. You can find information at www.ltcfeds.com, including a primer, a sample proposal, and an outline of coverage. Additional information about these plans can also be found by calling 1-800-LTC-FEDS. You could even use the information to educate non-federal employees about the need for LTCI as well. After all, if the government is making a federal case out of LTC, LTCI must be important!

Making a Federal Case Out of LTC

One advisor interviewed for this book related the following story:

"I have a client who retired from the federal government and is now active with a group of retirees. She asked me about my company's LTCI policy. To prepare for the interview, I did a lot of research on the federal government's program so I could compare it with my company's LTCI policy. The research paid off. When we met, my client figured out quickly that my company's LTCI plan was much better than the one that the federal government offered. After I had made the sale, she turned to me and said, "There are a lot of retired federal employees in our group and many of them do not have LTCI. Can you come explain this product at one of our meetings?"

Ethics and Compliance in Selling LTCI

Your career choice carries with it a tremendous responsibility. As a financial advisor, you approach others, both friends and strangers, and ask them for the opportunity to help protect them and plan for the future. You ask them to accept your advice and to trust your recommendations. In doing so, you have an absolute obligation to maintain the highest possible ethical standards.

You assume responsibility for helping prospects and clients meet their financial needs. It is this responsibility, combined with your training, specialized knowledge in areas that are difficult to understand, and the promise of service, that raises insurance sales to the professional level.

What must you do to live up to this responsibility? Certainly you must comply with all applicable laws and regulations. Compliance means following the laws and regulations, including company rules regarding the sale of insurance products. These are the minimum standards. State and federal laws regulate the insurance industry to protect consumers from unfair sales practices. Company rules are developed to make certain that the company and its advisors meet state and federal requirements. They are also designed to make sure that the company has complete and accurate information on which to base its underwriting and claims decisions.

However, professionalism and ethical conduct demand more than mere compliance. We will explore these two concepts later in this chapter. For now, an examination of the following regulations and rules is necessary for you to understand the financial services industry's business conduct guidelines for selling LTCI.

> What lies behind us and what lies before us are tiny compared to what lies within us.
>
> —*Oliver Wendall Holmes*

NAIC Model Legislation

Background and Purpose—The LTCI policies in existence in the early 1980s were primarily designed to provide care during the recovery period following an acute illness. They seldom met the needs of persons who required LTC for chronic conditions. In addition, due to improper sales practices, consumers were led to believe that policies were more comprehensive then they actually were. In effect, policyowners felt that they were purchasing "nursing home" insurance that would cover them anytime nursing home care was needed. At claim time, many people came to realize that their coverage was very limited. Few of the early policies had a "free look" provision that allowed the return of the initial premium within the first 10 to 30 days of the policy. Finally, there was no favorable tax treatment given to LTCI. Premiums were not deductible, and benefits and employer-paid premiums under group plans resulted in taxation to employees.

These symptoms in the LTCI marketing environment led to the adoption of positive changes that have enhanced the product and the sales practices surrounding it. Despite the call for federal regulation of the sale of LTCI, the changes resulted from the actions of state insurance regulators, and the insurance companies themselves. The negative publicity surrounding early policies led many insurers to modify their existing policies and new companies entering the business tended to offer more comprehensive policies. The National Association of Insurance Commissioners (NAIC) promulgated the Long Term Care Insurance Model Act in 1987, and in 1988, the Model Regulation was issued to enable state jurisdictions to implement the Model Act. This important legislation established guidelines for insurance companies to follow regarding policy design, policy definitions, and provisions that should be offered in policies, as well as marketing procedures and important notifications that should be provided to prospects before taking their applications and to insureds after their coverage takes effect.

Because of its widespread adoption by the states, it is important to discuss the NAIC model legislation regarding LTCI. The legislation consists of a Model Act that is designed to be incorporated into a state's insurance law and a Model Regulation that is designed to be adopted for use in implementing the law. This discussion is based on the latest version of the model legislation, which is amended almost annually. Even though most states have adopted the NAIC legislation, some states may not have adopted the latest version. However, the importance of the model legislation should not be overlooked. With most insurers writing coverage in more than one state, it is likely that the latest provisions have been adopted by one or more states where an insurer's coverage is sold. Because most insurance companies sell essentially the same LTCI product everywhere they do business, the NAIC guidelines are often, in effect, being adhered to in states that have not adopted the legislation.

Before proceeding with a summary of the major provisions of the NAIC model legislation, it is important to make two points. First, the model legislation establishes guidelines, but insurance companies still have significant latitude in many aspects of product design. Second, many older policies still in force were written prior to the state's adoption of a recent version of the model legislation.

LTCI

The model legislation states that LTCI is any insurance policy or rider that is advertised, marketed, offered, or designed to provide coverage for not less than 12 consecutive months for each covered person in a setting other than an acute care unit of a hospital for one or more of the following: necessary or medically necessary diagnostic, preventive, therapeutic, rehabilitative, maintenance, or personal care services. This definition is broad enough to include policies or riders that provide coverage for LTC in a single setting such as the home, or a variety of alternative settings that range from the home to a skilled-nursing facility. The 12-month period has been the source of considerable controversy because, in effect, it allows policies to provide benefits for periods as short as one year. Many critics of LTCI argue that coverage should not be allowed unless benefits are provided for at least 2 or 3 years. Statistics would seem to support their views. Approximately 55 percent of all persons currently in nursing homes have been there in excess of one year. The figure drops to about 30 percent for stays of 3 years or longer. The average length of stay for persons currently in nursing homes is about 2.5 years.

The Model Act specifically states that the term LTCI also includes group and individual annuities and life insurance policies or riders that provide directly or supplement LTCI. LTCI does not include an insurance policy that is offered primarily to provide any of the following:

- medicare supplement coverage
- basic hospital expense coverage
- basic medical-surgical expense coverage

- hospital confinement indemnity coverage
- major medical expense coverage
- disability income or related asset protection coverage
- accident only coverage
- specific disease or specified accident coverage
- limited benefit coverage

In addition, LTCI does not include life insurance policies (1) that accelerate the death benefit specifically for one or more of the qualifying events of terminal illness, medical conditions requiring extraordinary medical intervention, or permanent institutional confinement, or (2) that provide the option of a lump-sum payment for the previous benefits if neither the benefits nor the eligibility for benefits is conditional upon the receipt of LTC. However, the act specifies that any product advertised, marketed, or offered as LTCI is subject to the act's provisions, even if it is included in the previous list of policies or riders otherwise excluded from the definition of LTCI.

The model legislation focuses on two major areas: policy provisions and marketing.

Policy Provisions

Many of the criteria for policy provisions pertain to definitions, renewal provisions, limitations and exclusions, preexisting conditions, prior levels of care, incontestability, inflation protection, and non-forfeiture benefits.

Definitions—Many words or terms cannot be used in a policy unless they are specifically defined in the policy and conform with the model legislation. Examples include activities of daily living (ADLs), adult day care, cognitive impairment, home health care services, mental or nervous disorders, personal care, and skilled-nursing care.

Renewal Provisions—No policy can contain renewal provisions other than guaranteed renewable or noncancelable. Under neither type of provision can the insurance company make any unilateral changes in any coverage provision or refuse to renew the coverage. Under a noncancelable provision, premiums are established in advance and the insured has a right to continue the coverage in force by the timely payment of premiums. Under a guaranteed renewable provision, coverage is also continued by the timely payment of premiums, but the insurance company is allowed to revise premiums on a class basis.

The term level premium can be used only when the insurance company does not have the right to change the premium. Thus, a noncancelable policy can be called a level premium contract, a guaranteed renewable policy cannot.

Limitations and Exclusions—Limitations and exclusions by type of illness, treatment, medical condition, or accident are prohibited, except in the following cases:

- preexisting conditions or disease
- mental or nervous disorders (but this does not permit the exclusion of Alzheimer's disease)
- alcoholism and drug addiction
- illness, treatment, or medical condition arising out of war, participation in a felony, service in the armed forces, attempted suicide, and aviation if a person is a non-fare-paying passenger
- treatment provided in a government facility, unless required by law
- services for which benefits are available under Medicare or other governmental program, with the exception of Medicaid
- services for which benefits are available under any workers' compensation, employer's liability, or occupational disease law
- services available under any motor vehicle law
- services provided by a member of the covered person's immediate family
- services for which no charge is normally made in the absence of insurance
- expenses for services or items available or paid under another LTCI or health policy.

In addition, the model legislation permits exclusions and limitations for services provided outside the United States and for legitimate variations in benefit levels to reflect differences in provider rates.

Preexisting Conditions—The definition of preexisting conditions can be no more restrictive than to exclude a condition for which treatment was recommended or received within 6 months prior to the effective date of coverage. In addition, coverage can be excluded for a confinement for this condition only if it begins within 6 months of the effective date of coverage.

Prior Levels of Care—No policy can provide coverage for skilled-nursing care only or provide significantly more coverage for skilled care in a facility than for lower levels of care. Eligibility for benefits cannot be based on a prior hospital requirement and eligibility for benefits provided in an institutional care setting cannot be based on the prior receipt of a higher level of institutional care. A policy that conditions eligibility for non-institutional benefits on a prior receipt of institutional care cannot require a prior institutional stay of more than 30 days.

Incontestability—A policy must contain a provision that makes it incontestable after 2 years on the grounds of misrepresentation alone. However, the insurer can still contest the policy on the basis that the applicant knowingly and intentionally misrepresented relevant facts pertaining to the insured's health. If the policy has been in force for less than 6 months, the insurer can rescind the policy or deny an otherwise valid claim upon showing that a misrepresentation was material to the acceptance of coverage. If the policy has been in force for at least 6 months but less than 2 years, the insurer can rescind the policy or deny an otherwise valid claim upon showing that a misrepresentation was both material to the acceptance of coverage and pertains to the condition for which benefits are sought. Any benefits paid under a policy prior to the time a policy is rescinded cannot be recovered by the insurer.

Inflation Protection—Insurers must offer their clients protection from inflation. In such policies, benefits increase along with reasonably anticipated increases in the cost of services covered by the policy. The applicant must specifically reject this inflation protection if he or she does not want it. This provision does not apply to life insurance policies that provide accelerated LTC benefits.

Marketing

As briefly outlined in chapter 7, some of the provisions of the model legislation that pertain to marketing include an outline of coverage, a shopper's guide, a 30-day free look, standards for appropriateness of coverage, limitations on post-claims underwriting, third-party notification of pending policy lapse, and policy replacement.

Outline of Coverage—An outline of coverage must be delivered to a prospect at the time of initial application. This outline must contain

- a description of the principal benefits and coverage provided in the policy
- a statement of the policy's principal exclusions, reductions, and limitations
- a statement of the terms under which the policy may be continued in force or discontinued
- a statement that the outline of coverage is a summary only, not a contract of insurance, and that the policy contains governing contractual provisions
- a description of the terms under which the policy or certificate may be returned and premium refunded
- a brief description of the relationship of cost of care and benefits
- a statement if the policy is intended to be federally tax-qualified

Shopper's Guide—A shopper's guide must be delivered to all prospects. The guide must either be in the format developed by the NAIC or be a guide developed by the state insurance commissioner. The guide must be presented prior to completing the application or enrollment form. A few states also require that a guide explaining Medicare Supplement policies be provided to applicants over age 64. Shopper's guides are discussed in more detail in chapter 4.

30-day Free Look—The insurer must allow applicants 30 days to review the policy after delivery. During that time, an applicant may have the premium refunded if, after examining the policy, he or she is not satisfied for any reason. A notice of this privilege must be permanently displayed on the policy's first page or attached thereto.

Standards for Appropriateness of Coverage—Any entity marketing LTCI—excluding life insurance policies that accelerate benefits for LTC—must develop and use suitability standards to determine whether the purchase or replacement of coverage is appropriate for the applicant's needs, and advisors must be trained in the use of these standards. In addition, the advisor and insurer must develop procedures to determine the following:

- the applicant's ability to pay for the proposed coverage and other relevant financial information
- the applicant's goals or needs with respect to LTC and the advantages and disadvantages of insurance to meet these goals or needs
- the values, benefits, and costs of any existing insurance the applicant has when compared to the values, benefits, and costs of the recommended purchase or replacement

Limitations on Post-Claims Underwriting—Post-claims underwriting has been an issue of concern to regulators, consumers, and insurance professionals. This practice occurs when an insurer does little underwriting at the time of the initial application for coverage. Then, after a claim is filed, the insurer obtains medical information that could have been obtained earlier and may rescind the policy or deny the claim based on this new information.

To control post-claims underwriting, applications for insurance must be clear and unambiguous so that an applicant's health condition can be properly ascertained. Except for policies that are guaranteed issue, the application must also contain a conspicuous statement near the place for the applicant's signature that says the following: "If your answers to this application are incorrect or untrue, the company has the right to deny benefits or rescind your policy."

If an application contains a question about whether an applicant has had medication prescribed by a physician, the application must also ask the applicant to list the medications that have been prescribed. If the policy is issued and the medications listed in the application were known by the insurer at time of application, or should have been known, to be related to a condition for which coverage would normally denied, then the policy cannot be rescinded for that condition.

The insurer is also required to obtain additional information on applicants aged 80 or older. This includes at least one of the following: a report of a physical examination, an assessment of functional capacity, an attending physician's statement, or copies of medical records.

Finally, a copy of the completed application must be delivered to the insured no later than the time of the delivery of the policy unless it was retained by the insured at the time of the application.

Third-Party Notification of Pending Policy Lapse—No policy can be issued until the applicant has been given the option of electing a third party to be notified of any pending policy lapse because of nonpayment of premium. The purpose of this provision is to eliminate the problem of policy lapse because a senile or otherwise mentally impaired person fails to pay the premium.

Policy Replacement—If one LTCI policy replaces another, the new insurer must waive any time periods pertaining to preexisting conditions and probationary periods for comparable benefits to the extent that such periods were satisfied in the original policy. The Model Regulation also requires applications to contain questions as to whether the applicant has other LTCI in force and whether a LTCI policy is intended to replace any other medical expense policy or LTCI policy in force.

The questions include:

- Do you have another LTCI policy?
- Did you have another LTCI policy in force during the last 12 months? If so, with which insurer? If that policy lapsed, when did the lapse take place?
- Do you intend to replace any medical or health insurance coverage with this policy?
- Are you covered by Medicaid?

Advisors must also list any other health insurance policies they have sold to the applicant that are still in force, as well as any policies sold to the applicant in the past 5 years that are not in force.

If it is determined that a sale will involve a policy replacement, the insurer or its advisor must furnish the applicant with a notice regarding replacement of the LTCI coverage and its potential disadvantages for the policyowner. One copy of the notice is retained by the applicant; another copy, signed by the applicant, is retained by the insurer. In addition, the insurer replacing the coverage must notify the existing insurer of the proposed replacement within 5 days of the earlier of the date of application or the date the policy is issued.

State Regulation

The insurance industry in the United States is regulated primarily by the individual states, not by the federal government. Each state has its own laws and regulations that deal with insurance sales. Likewise, each state has its own rules for the approval and licensing of insurance products and advisors. For a particular product to be sold in a given state, both the company and the product must be approved.

Licensing—Each state is responsible for approving the advisors who are licensed to sell approved products. Generally, advisors must hold a resident license in the state in which they live and must hold a nonresident license in any other state in which they do business.

Licensing procedures vary from state to state, although all states require the successful passing of an examination before issuing a resident license. Nonresident licenses are often granted through reciprocal agreements between the states, without additional testing. Licenses are granted for a specific time period, and most states now require proof of continuing professional education before a license is renewed.

You have the responsibility to abide by the insurance regulatory laws of those jurisdictions in which you conduct business. You must also adhere to each state's continuing education requirements that are necessary to maintain your license to sell LTCI in those states where you work. There are some unique variations in these requirements in several jurisdictions. For example, in the states of Delaware and California, there are separate licensing and continuing education requirements that must be periodically maintained solely to be able to sell LTCI.

The licensing process is a state's way of providing some control over insurance advisors' activities. The state's insurance department also serves as a place for consumers to turn if they have a complaint or feel that an advisor has misrepresented the facts in making a sale. If an advisor fails to comply with the state's regulations, the state has the right to rescind the license and may take legal action against the advisor and possibly against his or her company.

While state laws regulating insurance vary, the state commissioners work together through the NAIC to identify the issues of greatest importance to consumers and to set legislative standards through model legislation. Because of their work, there is general agreement on some practices involved in insurance sales.

Misrepresentation—All states are concerned with the misrepresentation of insurance products and their benefits. Suggesting that a policy has certain features, benefits, values, or guarantees that are not specifically guaranteed in the written contract likewise is a misrepresentation. So is a failure to reveal limitations or exclusions of coverage. In the sale of LTCI you must provide a prospect with all the materials prescribed the

NAIC model legislation, as well as those disclosure forms required by your company.

Illustrations—One concern over misrepresentation comes from the use of illustrations in the sales process. Allowing misconceptions regarding benefits to exist, or fostering it through the sales presentation, is a serious form of misrepresentation. A complete illustration should clearly explain which values are guaranteed and which are not. The advisor should make sure that the prospect reads and understands the limitations of any projections that are made. A full illustration, including all footnotes and explanation pages, should be given to and reviewed with the prospect.

Replacement—Another major area of concern shared by the states is the unjustified replacement of existing policies in order to sell new policies. Unwarranted replacements can threaten the policyowner's benefits, undermine the insurer's underwriting practices, and damage your integrity.

There are circumstances when LTCI policy replacement is desirable. LTCI contract enhancements that have emerged in the last few years along with the advent of tax-qualified policies may warrant a person's review of their existing coverage. However, it is extremely important to adhere to the NAIC Model Regulation procedures discussed earlier in this chapter. You also should never encourage a prospect to lapse existing coverage until a new policy has passed through underwriting and been satisfactorily issued and put into force.

Advice—States are also concerned with what advisors call themselves and the kinds of advice they give their prospects and clients. Advisors who call themselves financial planners or financial consultants may be breaking state laws unless they have obtained special licenses. In many states, financial advisors, planners, and consultants are considered separate professional groups, and specific licenses are required.

Even in routine contacts, an insurance or financial advisor's discussions with a prospect or client may touch on legal or tax matters. Giving a client or prospect specific legal or tax advice can be construed as practicing law without a proper license, and that is illegal. While discussing legal or tax matters with clients in very general terms is allowed, an advisor cannot give specific advice in these areas. When specific advice is requested, you should always advise your prospects and clients to consult an attorney or tax advisor.

Ethical Considerations

Suitability—Your professional obligation to prospects is to help them determine and carry out the best solutions available to meet their financial needs. In identifying the need for insurance and by helping the prospect understand that need and seek protection, you have fulfilled your professional obligation.

If the prospect has medical or other problems that lead to the company offering a different policy than the one applied for, or a policy at a higher premium, then your responsibility is to help the prospect decide if the rated policy meets his or her needs and is the best solution to the problems it is meant to cover. If, for some reason, a prospect is not insurable, you are not at fault and have not failed to meet your professional duty.

Your obligation to both the prospect and to the company you represent is to provide the most accurate and complete information possible. Only then can the company decide if it is willing to offer a policy, and at what premium. You have a primary duty to the company to provide factual information that supersedes your responsibility to get coverage for the prospect.

The need to provide complete and accurate information about a prospect goes beyond the need to protect the company from inadvertently accepting extra risk. Failure to provide complete and accurate information, failure to record information provided by the prospect, or intentional misrepresentation of facts by the advisor or the prospect can void the insurance contract, leaving that person unknowingly unprotected.

In the case of a contested or denied claim, both the advisor and the company may be held accountable for the misinformation. If the client is responsible, his or her family may suffer. If the advisor is responsible, he or she can be held personally liable. The risk to all parties involved is substantial.

The conflict that may arise between the prospect's need for insurance and the company's underwriting rules and issuing standards spans both compliance and ethics. You may encounter situations when fair business practices, legal requirements, and company rules sometimes seem to conflict with your best efforts. How the apparent conflict is resolved is a matter of ethics, and it goes beyond compliance with the law.

> The conflict that may arise between the prospect's need for insurance and the company's underwriting rules and issuing standards spans both compliance and ethics.

Burke A. Christensen, JD, CLU, former vice president and general counsel of the American Society of CLU & ChFC, wrote the following in an article for the *Journal of the American Society of CLU & ChFC:*

> ...remember that there is sometimes a gap between what is legal and what is ethical. According to Potter Stewart, retired justice of the United States Supreme Court, that gap represents "the difference between what you have a right to do, and what is the right thing to do." To infuse your character with ethics, you must not be content to merely comply with the law. . .

Another way to say it is that ethical behavior is doing the right thing. Professional ethics can be defined as behaving according to the principles of right and wrong that are accepted by the profession. It is doing what is right and putting the prospect's best interest before your own. It is maintaining the highest possible standard of behavior in all your business dealings. It is continuing to develop your skills so you can provide the best possible service to those with whom you work. It is representing the industry, its companies, and its advisors, in the best possible light.

Professional Code of Conduct and Ethics

By adopting and practicing a professional code of ethics, you will achieve the high standard of professionalism that a career in financial services requires. The following examples of the codes of ethics of The American College and The National Association of Insurance and Financial Advisors (NAIFA) are standards of professional behavior to which you should constantly adhere.

The American College
Code of Ethics

To underscore the importance of ethical standards for Huebner School designations, the Board of Trustees of The American College adopted a Code of Ethics in 1984. Embodied in the Code is the Professional Pledge and eight Canons.

The Professional Pledge and the Canons

The Pledge to which all Huebner School designees subscribe is as follows:

"In all my professional relationships, I pledge myself to the following rule of ethical conduct: I shall, in light of all conditions surrounding those I serve, which I shall make every conscientious effort to ascertain and understand, render that service which, in the same circumstances, I would apply to myself."

The eight Canons are:

I. Conduct yourself at all times with honor and dignity.

II. Avoid practices that would bring dishonor upon your profession or The American College.

III. Publicize your achievement in ways that enhance the integrity of your profession.

IV. Continue your studies throughout your working life so as to maintain a high level of professional competence.

V. Do your utmost to attain a distinguished record of professional service.

VI. Support the established institutions and organizations concerned with the integrity of your profession.

VII. Participate in building your profession by encouraging and providing appropriate assistance to qualified persons pursuing professional studies.

VIII. Comply with all laws and regulations, particularly as they relate to professional and business activities.

N • A • I • F • A
The National Association
of Insurance and Financial Advisors
Code of Ethics

PREAMBLE: Those engaged in life underwriting occupy the unique position of liaison between the purchasers and the suppliers of life and health insurance and closely related financial products. Inherent in this role is the combination of professional duty to the client and to the company, as well. Ethical balance is required to avoid any conflict between these two obligations. Therefore,

I Believe It To Be My Responsibility

To hold my profession in high esteem and strive to enhance its prestige.

To fulfill the needs of my clients to the best of my ability.

To maintain my clients' confidences.

To render exemplary service to my clients and their beneficiaries.

To adhere to professional standards of conduct in helping my clients to protect insurable obligations and attain their financial security objectives.

To present accurately and honestly all facts essential to my clients' decisions.

To perfect my skills and increase my knowledge through continuing education.

To conduct my business in such a way that my example might help raise the professional standards of life underwriting.

To keep informed with respect to applicable laws and regulations and to observe them in the practice of my profession.

To cooperate with others whose services are constructively related to meeting the needs of my clients.

Adopted April, 1986
NAIFA Board of Trustees

Building Your Practice

Your Role as the Financial Service Professional

Your role in the financial planning process can be that of both catalyst and coordinator. First, through your work by locating qualified prospects, uncovering and quantifying their needs, developing suitable recommendations, and then by motivating them to take appropriate action, you play a unique role in the financial service arena. You are the one and only member of the financial planning team that both solicits prospective business from new prospects and insures them (and their family and heirs) from the detrimental effects of those risks that can threaten their financial well being. Finally, you monitor their financial plan and make recommendations as needed.

Coordinating the labors of other financial planning professionals can be a daunting task, which is one reason that many clients delay doing the financial and estate planning they need. The tasks involved in planning for the security of one's finances and the proper disposition of one's assets can seem overwhelming to many people. This feeling of confusion about where to begin the complex process of wealth management contributes to the tendency for procrastination in addressing these matters. Therefore, we often have to orchestrate a team effort to assist our prospects and clients in achieving their financial goals.

Professionalism

In order to work successfully with other professionals, you must be a professional. You must have the technical knowledge necessary to provide meaningful support and accurate advice to your prospects and clients. As a competent financial service professional, you must be fully conversant in the legal and tax ramifications of the recommendations you make. You must also be able to outline the positive and negative implications of the various LTCI options available, so that your prospects and clients can make informed purchasing decisions. You therefore must have a thorough understanding of your products, the

When one financial advisor was asked, "Why are you involved in the LTCI market?" she responded, "First of all, it's the right thing to do for your clients. If you're trying to fulfill the needs of your clients, obviously LTCI is one of the greatest needs that people have, whether they are trying to protect their estate or their peace of mind. When you consider the huge number of baby boomers who are all aging together, it's obvious that in the future there will be a strain on LTC resources and the funding for quality care…and the government has given us pretty clear signals that they are not prepared to handle this strain. Therefore, if you want to do the right thing for your clients now and in the future, LTCI is something you need to be selling to them."

problems that face your prospects and clients, and how your products can be used to provide solutions.

Client Focus—To be a professional, you also need to be client-centered. This means you have to put your clients' interests before your own. In financial, estate, and retirement planning, your job goes beyond simply making an insurance sale. Your professional responsibility is to help your prospects and clients identify and implement all the steps that will help them accomplish their financial planning goals.

Professionals also adhere to a code of ethics. You should endorse and follow the code of ethics of your chosen organizations. NAIFA, The American College, the Society of Financial Service Professionals, and the Million Dollar Round Table all provide professional codes of ethics.

Legal Requirements—Professionalism requires you to meet the legal and ethical standards of the insurance and financial services industry. You must, for example, be licensed to discuss the products you sell in all jurisdictions in which you work. Unless you are a licensed attorney, it is illegal for you to give legal advice. It is also illegal for you to give tax advice when acting in the role of insurance advisor. While you can discuss legal and tax considerations in general terms, you cannot provide specific legal or tax advice, nor draft legal documents.

Protect Yourself—In spite of all your professionalism, mistakes and misunderstandings do happen, therefore you need to protect yourself. Your exposure to the risk of lawsuits, like any other liability, can and should be insured with errors and omissions insurance.

Proper documentation helps you protect yourself. As you start making a complete assessment of your prospect's needs, consider all needs, not just the ones that may represent a sale for you. Make your recommendations in writing and keep copies that are signed or initialed by your prospect in respective files. Likewise, keep copies of all correspondence and records of all conversations.

Working with Other Professional/Financial Service Advisors

It is certainly inadvisable, not to mention being virtually impossible, to work in the LTCI market today without working with other professional advisors. Consequently, you will inevitably need to put your clients in touch with various members of a network of professional advisors that you will develop throughout your career. You must also learn effective techniques to work with their existing advisor(s). For example, in basic estate planning, a qualified attorney should be involved in preparing a will, a trust, a durable power of attorney, and an advance medical directive. As a person's estate becomes more complicated with the acquisition of more assets and various forms of property, accountants, trust officers, and securities brokers may also be needed.

Creating Relationships—Most advisors who have been in the financial services business for any length of time have at least one story of an accountant or attorney who squelched a big sale. This experience, which is common to many of you, can leave a bad impression regarding the effect that other professionals can have on your recommendations.

If prospects already have a relationship with a professional advisor, it is unrealistic to expect the prospect to make a decision without first consulting him or her. These advisors are important to the planning process, so try to involve them in your planning as it becomes apparent that they will influence the prospect's decision. Your relationship with the prospect's advisors should not be adversarial; instead it should be a cooperative one with all of you having the same objective, which is the best plan for your prospect.

Other Advisors—One of the first things you should determine as you develop your relationship with a prospect is whom he or she turns to for advice. This should be done early in your first fact-finding interview, as discussed in chapter 4. Find out if the advisors help in a professional or personal capacity. Also, try to ascertain the strength of the relationship with that advisor, so that you can determine how influential they will be in the final decision about LTCI.

The attitude of outside advisors, whether they are professional or personal, can make or break your LTCI proposal. Try to involve them in

> It is certainly inadvisable, not to mention being virtually impossible, to work in the LTCI market today without working with other professional advisors.

the sales process from the beginning. Make sure they understand your proposal and buy into it before you try to close the sale. Try to make them advocates for what you are proposing instead of adversaries.

Confidentiality—As a professional, you have an obligation to keep the prospect and client information you collect confidential. By the same token, you should not expect other professionals to share information or discuss your prospect's financial planning matters with you without the prospect's permission. When you begin working with new prospects, share with them your potential need to discuss their situation with their other advisors.

If there is an outside advisor with whom you find it necessary to make contact, you should never contact that person directly without first getting the prospect's permission to do so. Otherwise, you may find the advisor very unreceptive to your call. Like you, attorneys and accountants have a responsibility to keep confidential the information they possess about a client.

Getting Permission—The best way to get permission is to have your prospect contact his or her other advisors, alerting them to the fact that you are working together and authorizing the advisors to provide the information you need. If possible, it is best to have this done in writing so the other advisors have a copy for their files. You can provide the prospect with a letter or form to be used.

If any of the other advisors are family members, invite them to attend your next meeting with the prospect. This will avoid many misunderstandings of what is being discussed and demonstrate your willingness to work amicably with them through the planning process.

Follow Up—When you know that letters to the advisors have been sent, follow up with a phone call. You will want to introduce yourself, reference the prospect's letter, and then tell them briefly the area of planning you are doing for the prospect. If you agree that it is appropriate to meet with them, ask for an appointment.

In order to be effective, you will need to prepare carefully for a meeting with the prospect's other advisors. You want your discussion with them to be concise, so be prepared to explain what you are proposing and know what information you seek, if any. If the other advisors include an eldercare attorney, you may suggest that some planning documents such as a durable power of attorney be drafted or considered. You can also educate the attorney on the terms of the LTCI policy you are recommending. Remember, this may be an opportunity to develop an ongoing and mutually beneficial professional relationship with this person. It does not hurt to encourage teamwork on behalf of the prospect. Be sure to let the attorney know that both you and the prospect value his or her input.

Keeping it Positive—If the other advisors oppose your ideas or have a preferred approach, it is best to know this early in the process. Sometimes the first sale must be made to the advisors. Ask about their objections and tell them that you need their input to tailor the plan to the prospect's needs. Try to get the advisors' opinions on how to approach LTC planning. Listen closely and always try to find common ground.

If the other advisors disagree with each other, consider the validity of their opinions, explore additional options, and try to build a consensus. This is a useful strategy whether the advisors are the prospect's accountant and attorney, or his or her son and daughter.

Under no circumstances should you make negative comments about other advisors to your prospect. In addition to being unprofessional, it can cause the prospect to become confused about the merit of the options being proposed, which may in turn lead to his or her not taking any needed action at all. Instead, acknowledge different points of view and explain why you think yours is the best one. You can address the concerns or objections of the other advisors without attacking their credibility or expertise.

Professional Development Through Education

In order to educate your prospects, you must first become educated. Not only do you have to learn the basic concepts involved in financial planning, but you must keep studying in order to learn advanced concepts as well. You have to be prepared to address the exceptions and complications that are often part of the responsible planning process, as well as the routine situations that you most frequently encounter. You must stay abreast of new product innovations, legislative trends, and tax rulings that can impact your ability to provide the highest possible level of service.

By continually educating yourself, you will become a competent member of your prospects' and clients' financial planning teams. Additional knowledge and skill development can result from pursuing the recognized professional designations of the financial services industry. The LUTCF, CLU, ChFC, RHU, REBC, and CFP designations, which are all earned in part by the successful completion of a qualified course of study, indicate your ongoing commitment to professionalism.

Membership and participation in the industry's professional organizations such as NAIFA, the Society of Financial Service Professionals, and the National Association of Health Underwriters offer an opportunity for continuing education. You may also want to explore the various training and educational programs that are provided by insurance companies, universities, proprietary training organizations, and other professional organizations. *Advisor Today* (the magazine of NAIFA) and *Life Insurance Selling* are excellent magazine sources of insurance news and sales ideas. In addition, the quarterly publication of the American Association for Long-Term Care Insurance, titled *Long-Term Care Insurance Sales Strategies,* is worthwhile reading for advisors who want to focus on the LTCI market. Information about this publication and how to join the Association can be found at *www.LTCSales.com.*

Formal programs can supplement your self-training regimen of daily and weekly readings of financial literature. For more information on training resources, log onto the American College Web site at *www.amercoll.edu.*

A Concluding Thought—You have finished reading the last chapter of *Essentials of Long-Term Care Insurance.* Now it is time to assimilate the foregoing LTCI sales skills techniques, product essentials, and planning foundations into your marketing activities. As you develop your business and focus on your future, remember that one day you too may need LTC. At the very least, use what you have learned from reading this book to design your own LTCI plan.

Chapter Eight Review

Key Terms and Concepts are explained in the Glossary. Answers to the Review Questions and Self-Test Questions are found in the back of the book in the Answers to Questions section.

Key Terms and Concepts

Federal Long-Term Care Insurance
    Program (FLTCIP)
group LTCI
group underwriting
key employee LTCI plans
mass-marketed individual insurance
National Association of Insurance
    Commissioners (NAIC)

NAIC LTCI model legislation
    NAIC LTCI Model Act
    NAIC LTCI Model Regulation
partnership programs for LTC
professional ethics
professionalism
state regulations
types of groups
voluntary benefit plan

Review Questions

8-1. What two types of LTCI are marketed to employees at the worksite?

8-2. Explain the tax treatment of premiums paid by a C corporation employer for a tax-qualified LTCI contract.

8-3. What are the goals of state partnership programs for LTC?

8-4. Who is eligible for coverage under the FLTCIP?

8-5. What is the purpose of the NAIC's model legislation with regard to LTCI?

8-6.   Under what circumstances does the NAIC's Model Act exclude life insurance policies from the definition of LTCI?

8-7.   What are the NAIC Model Act's rules on incontestability for a LTCI policy?

8-8.   Explain what is meant by the apparent conflict between doing what is legal and doing what is ethical in dealing with prospects and clients.

Self-Test Questions

Instructions: Read chapter 8 first, then answer the following questions to test your knowledge. There are 10 questions; circle the correct answer, then check your answers with the answer key in the back of the book.

8-1.   For employer-sponsored groups, the least stringent and most liberal form of LTCI underwriting from the standpoint of employees is

(a) guaranteed issue
(b) modified guaranteed issue
(c) simplified issue
(d) full individual underwriting

8-2.   Under the federal long-term care insurance program (FLTCIP), children who are qualified relatives are eligible for coverage if they are at least age

(a) 16
(b) 18
(c) 21
(d) 30

8-3.   The NAIC LTCI model legislation focuses on

(a) rate making and underwriting
(b) policy provisions and marketing
(c) education and professionalism
(d) group and individual product comparisons

8-4. Purchasers of LTCI under employer-sponsored plans differ from purchasers of LTCI in the individual market in which of the following ways?

    I.   Purchasers of employer-sponsored coverage tend to be younger.
    II. Purchasers of employer-sponsored coverage tend to select higher benefits.

    (a) I only
    (b) II only
    (c) Both I and II
    (d) Neither I nor II

8-5. A LTC insurer will generally use guaranteed-issue underwriting for employees in an employer-sponsored group only if the group meets which of the following criteria?

    I.   The employer pays some or all of the premium costs.
    II. The employees have maximum choice in picking the level of benefits.

    (a) I only
    (b) II only
    (c) Both I and II
    (d) Neither I nor II

8-6. Under the federal long-term care insurance program (FLTCIP), the comprehensive option provides reimbursement for all of the following services at 100 percent of the MDB amount (up to any specified limits) **EXCEPT**

    (a) nursing home care
    (b) respite care
    (c) adult day care
    (d) hospice care at home

8-7. In your capacity as a financial services professional, you should do all of the following **EXCEPT**

(a) put your clients' interests before your own
(b) adhere to a professional code of ethics
(c) protect yourself with errors and omissions insurance
(d) draft legal documents for your clients

8-8. When working with other professional/financial service advisors, you should do all of the following **EXCEPT**

(a) involve the prospect's other advisors in the sales process from the beginning
(b) keep information you collect about the prospect confidential unless he or she authorizes you to share it with other advisors
(c) have the prospect contact his or her other advisors to let them know that you may contact them
(d) attack the credibility or expertise of the prospect's other advisors who disagree with you

8-9. All of the following are abbreviations for recognized professional designations in the financial services industry **EXCEPT**

(a) CLU
(b) CFP
(c) LTCI
(d) LUTCF

8-10. Partnership Programs for Long-Term Care are approved in all of the following states **EXCEPT**

(a) California
(b) Texas
(c) Indiana
(d) New York

Glossary

A-B trust—the grantor's will sets up two trusts. The marital A trust is designed to hold assets that qualify for the marital deduction. The nonmarital B trust is designed to preserve the full estate tax credit for the grantor spouse.

accelerated death benefit—a cash advance made from a life insurance policy's death benefit that goes to an insured who is terminally ill. A growing number of policies include chronic illnesses as a legitimate reason to apply for the cash advance.

active listening—a method of listening in which the advisor demonstrates his or her understanding of the prospect's perspective and can state in the prospect's own words what the prospect has said and meant to communicate

activities of daily living (ADLs)—those activities geared toward the care of bodily needs that enable an individual to live independently. They include bathing, dressing, using the toilet, eating, transferring, and continence.

acute care—health care needs in which a patient receives medical care in a hospital for a relatively brief period of time for a severe episode of illness, an accident or other trauma, or recovery from surgery

adult day care—a relatively new type of care that provides social, medical, and rehabilitative services to people with physical and mental limitations. Adult day care takes place at a center that is designed for the elderly who may be severely impaired but who live at home and whose family caregiver is unavailable to provide care during the day.

advance medical directive—either a durable power of attorney for health care or a living will is referred to as an advance medical directive. Preparing an advance medical directive lets the physician and other health care providers know the kind of medical care an individual wants, or does not want, if he or she becomes incapacitated.

adverse selection—the tendency for those with a higher than average probability of loss to seek or continue insurance to a greater extent than those with an average or below average probability of loss

age-based—an effective way to segment the LTCI market is by age

alternative funding sources—financing alternatives to LTCI that include personal savings and assets, relying on family members, reverse mortgages, and/or viatical settlements

alternative plans of care—a clause that serves as a "catch-all" provision to accommodate changes in LTC services and coverage that will most certainly occur in the future. Many policies provide benefits for alternative plans of care, even though the types of care might not be covered in the policy.

Alzheimer's disease—a form of dementia that results in the progressive deterioration of a person's mental faculties

approach—the step in the selling process that involves asking the prospect for an appointment. An approach can be done face-to-face or via the telephone.

assisted-living facility—a place that provides a supportive-living arrangement for elderly residents who, despite some degree of impairment, remain independent to a significant degree, but require continuing supervision and the availability of unscheduled assistance

APS (attending physician's statement)—typically the primary source of medical information for LTCI. The APS provides the underwriter with detailed information from any physician that has treated the applicant.

baby boomers—the name for the generation born between 1946 and 1964. Their name reflects the sheer size of this group. Boomers are characterized as spenders, inheriters, image-conscious, and youth-oriented.

bed reservation benefit—a benefit that continues policy payments to an LTC facility for a limited time (such as 20 days) if the insured temporarily leaves the facility for any reason. For example, the insured may need to be hospitalized for an acute condition or wish to take a personal leave from the nursing home to attend a family reunion or holiday activity. Without the continuation of payments to the facility, the bed may be rented to someone else and unavailable upon the insured's return.

benefit period—the maximum period for which benefits are paid. It begins when the elimination period is satisfied and benefits are payable. When the maximum benefit amount is paid, the policy terminates.

benefit triggers—the conditions specified by the insurance company that must be met in order for the policy to pay benefits

building prestige—a preapproach strategy in which an advisor implements a personal public relations campaign designed to build and maintain a good reputation within a target market and the community-at-large

buying signals—obvious verbal and nonverbal signals that indicate acceptance or rejection of what an advisor is selling

care coordinator—a person who assesses a LTC patient who shows some degree of impairment to determine the care needs and the development of a care plan to meet those needs

caregiver training—a benefit that provides the training of a family member or friend to provide care so that a person requiring LTC services can remain at home. The caregiver may need training in how to give safe and effective care. The amount payable is limited and will typically pay up to a maximum of three to five times the maximum daily benefit (MDB).

care setting—the places where LTC services can be provided including skilled nursing facilities, residential communities, community-based facilities, or a care recipient's home

center of influence—an influential person who knows an advisor favorably and agrees to introduce or recommend him or her to others

chronic care—health care needs that represent the broad range of medical, custodial, social, and other care services to assist people who have an impaired ability to live independently for an extended period of time. Chronic care needs are the needs that LTCI addresses and that are provided by nursing homes, assisted-living facilities, and home health care agencies.

circle of health protection—a graphic circle that is made up of two halves, each with three sections. The left half of the circle represents protection for acute health care needs; the right half of the circle represents protection for chronic health care needs.

classification—classification recognizes the differences in the applicants who are accepted. It involves determining which rate category is appropriate for an applicant once he or she is accepted.

client-focused selling—a selling philosophy based on principles of effective communication such as asking good questions and listening carefully in order to cultivate a long-term, mutually beneficial relationship with a client.

cognitive impairment—any deficiency of a person's mental faculties such as short- or long-term memory, deductive or abstract reasoning, or judgment

cold calling—using the telephone to arrange appointments with prospects who are total strangers

combination products—products that package other insurance coverages with LTCI. Under these package products, either life insurance, disability income insurance, or an annuity is combined with LTCI to provide customized solutions to a variety of prospect needs and goals. These combination products have also been referred to as hybrid products, linked policies, blended polices, or packaged policies.

community spouse—the spouse of a Medicaid beneficiary who does not require Medicaid assistance himself or herself

comprehensive policy—a type of policy that combines benefits for facility care and home health care into a single contract. Variations exist within this type of policy with respect to what is covered as part of the standard policy and what is an optional benefit that the prospect may select. It is sometimes referred to as an integrated policy.

contingent benefit upon lapse—a benefit that allows the policyowner to select certain options each time the insurer increases the premium rate to a level that results in a cumulative increase of the annual premium equal to or exceeding a specified percentage of the premium at the time of policy issue

continuing care retirement community (CCRC)—a care setting, also known as a *life-care facility*, that provides the full continuum of supportive-living arrangements and is obligated to provide the housing and defined LTC services at each level of care for the life of the resident

countable assets—the assets that a person must exhaust before he or she can qualify for Medicaid benefits. These assets include: cash, checking and savings accounts; bonds and CDs; investment property; vacation property; second vehicles; deferred annuities; all general investments; all accessible qualified plans (if the person can liquidate the account); life insurance cash surrender values if the face amount exceeds $1,500; and every other item not specifically listed as exempt by Medicaid. Asset exceptions vary by state.

couples versus singles—couples and singles buy LTCI for different reasons. For couples, the desire to protect their standard of living is paramount. For singles, there is no one there to care for them should they need it.

custodial care—care services that include assistance with the activities of daily living (ADLs) or instrumental activities of daily living (IADLs)

deductive approach—an approach to the personal information-gathering process that is characterized by starting with a thorough and lengthy fact-finding form that broadly covers all the prospect's financial needs. The process requires quantifying a prospect's financial planning needs, prioritizing them, and then selling the prospect the appropriate product or products that address the highest priority of need.

depleting assets—some people who are not poor become poor by spending nearly all their income and assets on care. Generally, a person can have no more than $2,000 of assets to qualify for Medicaid.

direct mail—a preapproach strategy that involves sending a letter or postcard to a prospect. Some direct mail strategies involve a giveaway (or premium offer).

discovery agreement—a verbal or written mutual agreement between the advisor and the prospect to work together to address the expressed financial goals of the prospect. It is formulated at or after the conclusion of the initial fact-finding interview.

durable power of attorney—a document signed by one person (the principal) authorizing another person (the attorney-in-fact) to act on behalf of the signer. The word *durable* indicates that the power stays in effect in the event that the signer becomes incapacitated.

durable power of attorney for health care—a durable power of attorney limited to health care issues. It permits a designated family member or decision maker to make health care decisions on behalf of an individual who cannot make his or her own health care decisions.

effective communication—important interviewing skills such as knowing how and when to ask appropriate types of questions, being an active and empathetic listener, and being able to explain financial needs and insurance products to prospects

elimination period—the period of time between the start of LTC services and the start of benefit payments (also called a waiting or deductible period). Elimination periods may range from 0 to 365 days and will stipulate that LTC services must be necessary for either a consecutive or total number of days in order for it to be satisfied.

face-to-face assessment interview—a personal interview at the underwriter's discretion or because underwriting guidelines call for such an assessment if a certain age or certain medical condition is present. It may be used to determine an applicant's medical history, ability to perform activities of daily living (ADLs) or instrumental activities of daily living (IADLs), or to evaluate an applicant's cognitive ability.

facility-only policy—a policy that is designed to provide benefits only if the insured is in a nursing home (referred to as a nursing home policy) or in another care setting, such as an assisted-living facility or hospice

features and benefits—a characteristic (feature) explaining what a product is and what it does. A *benefit* is what the prospect gets as a result of the feature. It is what the product does for the prospect and usually why he or she wants it.

Federal LTCI program (FLTCIP)—a government-sponsored LTCI program that provides coverage on a voluntary basis with participants paying 100 percent of the premium. Those eligible for coverage include federal and postal employees and retirees, military personnel and retirees, and qualified relatives.

field underwriting—the process of an advisor selecting a prospect and fully completing an application that accurately reflects the applicant's medical condition and current situation. It is the advisor's responsibility to communicate all relevant facts about the applicant and identify special circumstances and clarify questionable situations.

financial and emotional needs—the motivations for purchasing LTCI

financial and personal resources review—a short fact finder designed to uncover basic prospect information and potential objections to purchasing LTCI

formal caregiver—an individual who provides care and services as a profession or occupation to LTC recipients. Formal caregivers include physicians, nurses, other licensed medical personnel, and nonmedical personnel.

general power of attorney—a document signed by one person (the principal) authorizing another person (the attorney-in-fact) to act on behalf of the signer. A general power is effective as long as the person granting the power remains in good health, but it becomes legally ineffective in cases of mental incompetence or medical incapacity.

generation—an age-based segmentation of the general population developed by demographers. It is based on the theory that the general population's psyche and behavior are shaped by significant life experiences, such as the way people are raised, national and world events, wars, the social and economic climate of the times, and so forth.

generation X—the name for the generation born between 1965 and 1980. They are considered to be risk takers, skeptical, self-oriented, practical, and work-life balance oriented. They are also referred to as *Xers* or *baby busters*.

grace period—the period of time between the date the policy's premium is due and the date the policy will lapse. Most policies have a 31-day grace period. This means that the premium can be paid any time within the 31-day period after it is due, and during this period the policy will remain in force.

group LTCI—LTCI products marketed at the worksite include two types of group products—group insurance and mass-marketed policies of individual insurance

group underwriting—several levels of underwriting that may apply to employees of employer-sponsored groups. These include guaranteed issue, modified guaranteed issue, simplified issue, and full underwriting. Large groups typically are accompanied by some degree of underwriting of the groups themselves.

guaranteed renewable—a type of policy in which the policy will be renewed as long as the premium is paid. In addition, premiums cannot be raised for a particular insured. However, premiums can and often are raised for the whole underwriting class to which the insured belongs. LTCI policies currently being sold are almost always guaranteed renewable.

Health Insurance Portability and Accountability Act (HIPAA)—legislation passed in 1996 that established standards for LTCI and made the tax treatment of LTCI policies more favorable if they met the prescribed standards. Policies issued on or after January 1, 1997, generally must meet the federal standards to be considered tax qualified, while policies in force before January 1, 1997, generally are grandfathered and automatically qualify for tax benefits.

HIPAA chronic illness certification—a HIPAA requirement that a licensed health care practitioner must at least annually certify that the insured remains chronically ill

HIPAA chronic illness definition—a HIPAA requirement that the insured must require substantial assistance with at least 2 of 6 ADLs or be cognitively impaired for a tax-qualified policy to pay benefits

home health care—care that takes place where the care recipient resides and encompasses virtually any home environment outside of a nursing home

home health care only policy—a policy that is designed to provide benefits for care outside an institutional setting. Some home health care policies also provide benefits for care in assisted-living facilities, one area in which they often overlap with facility-only policies.

homemaker companion—a person, normally an employee of a home health care agency, who assists with homemaker services such as cooking, laundry, shopping, cleaning, bill paying, or other household chores (also referred to as a home health aide). Homemaker companion also refers to a LTCI policy benefit that provides these and other personal care services assisting with daily living, such as grooming, personal hygiene, and taking medications.

hospice—a place that treats terminally ill persons. Hospice care also offers help with the physical, psychological, social, and spiritual needs of those experiencing the loss, grief, and bereavement that come with a terminal illness.

hospice care—a system of treatment designed to relieve the discomfort of a terminally ill individual and to maintain quality of life to the extent possible throughout the phases of dying

indemnity or per diem basis—a method of paying LTCI benefits in which the MDB amount is paid regardless of the actual cost of care. For example, if the cost of a nursing home under an indemnity (per diem) policy is $150 and the insured has a MDB amount of $200, then the full $200 will be paid. Benefits typically range from $50 to $500 per day.

inductive approach—the converse of the deductive approach to information gathering. It starts with a dominant or single need, then broadens into a full-blown comprehensive financial need analysis where several financial planning needs are identified and prioritized.

inflation protection—an optional LTCI policy rider that increases the maximum daily benefit (MDB) to keep pace with inflation. The amount of the increase is either specified as a percentage or tied to an inflation index, such as the consumer price index (CPI). If the policy specifies a percentage, that percentage may either be compounded annually or be a flat percentage (simple interest) of the initial MDB. The cost of an automatic increase in benefits option is usually built into the initial annual premium, or the premium will increase each year in a step-rate fashion to reflect the automatic increase in benefit amount.

informal caregiver—an individual who voluntarily cares for a LTC recipient without pay and without formal education and training in LTC. Informal caregivers include immediate family members and others related to the care recipient by blood or marriage or friends, neighbors, and volunteers.

instrumental activities of daily living (IADLs)—activities that deal with one's ability to function cognitively such as preparing meals, shopping, cleaning, managing money, taking medications, and so forth

irrevocable life insurance trust (ILIT)—In an ILIT, a life insurance policy covering the grantor spouse's life is purchased and owned by the irrevocable trust. It allows the grantor spouse to provide support benefits for the surviving spouse, while avoiding inclusion of the proceeds in the estate of either spouse.

key employee LTCI plans—a recent phenomenon in the worksite marketing of LTCI where employers selectively provide individual policies to their key employees and executives and pay for their coverage using the company's funds.

lapse—the termination of coverage in a policy when the renewal premium is not received by the insurance company within the grace period

living will—a legal document that describes the types of medical treatment an individual chooses to accept or reject. The purpose of a living will is to let others know a person's medical wishes when he or she is terminally ill or in a vegetative state and unable to communicate.

long-term care (LTC)—the broad range of medical, custodial, and other care services provided over an extended period of time in various settings due to chronic illness, physical disability, or cognitive impairment

LTC fact finder—a comprehensive questionnaire that is designed for the discovery of factual, quantitative, and attitudinal information about a LTCI prospect

long-term care insurance (LTCI)—the insurance product designed to cover long-term care expenses

LTCINS Links—an acronym (which stands for LTC insurance) for key information that an advisor obtains from asking a series of questions. When the information is linked together, the advisor can make a relatively quick judgment about whether it is possible to underwrite a prospect.

market segment—an identifiable group of people with common characteristics and needs

mass-marketed individual insurance—individual polices of insurance sold through a sponsoring organization, such as an employer or association

maximum dollar amount—the total dollar amount of benefits the insurance company will pay under the policy. Typically, the maximum dollar amount is calculated by multiplying the MDB by the benefit period in years and then by 365. If the policy has a lifetime benefit, then there is no limit on the total dollar amount for which the insurance company is responsible.

maximum daily benefit (MDB)—the maximum level of benefits per day that the prospect purchases up to the maximum amount the company provides. Typically, benefits are sold in increments of $10 per day up to $200 or $250 or, in a few cases, up to as much as $400 or $500 per day.

Medicaid—a joint federal and state program to provide medical assistance to the poor. If an individual meets certain income and resource tests, the state of residence may consider an individual a qualified Medicaid beneficiary.

Medicaid asset rules—rules that classify a Medicaid beneficiary's assets and determine which ones need to be used before Medicaid will provide assistance. There are two main asset classifications: countable and noncountable (see definitions for these terms). Such rules take into consideration the presence of a community spouse who is not a Medicaid beneficiary.

Medicaid eligibility—a state-determined set of qualifications for Medicaid that meet federal guidelines. Typically, a recipient cannot have access to any financial resources, such as bank accounts, stock and bond accounts, or mutual funds.

Medicaid estate recovery rules—rules that allow the government to recover from the estate of a Medicaid recipient an amount equal to the cost of care

Medicaid income rules—rules that govern how much of a Medicaid beneficiary's income must be applied to the cost of care. Such rules take into consideration the presence of a community spouse who is not a Medicaid beneficiary.

Medicaid look-back rules—a set of rules that attempt to close the loophole of transferring assets to qualify for benefits by creating a period of ineligibility for Medicaid. If assets are transferred for less than their market value during a specified period before receiving benefits for nursing home, home, or community-based services, ineligibility results. The "look-back" period is 3 years (36 months) for outright transfers and 5 years (60 months) for transfers into trusts. This period of time is measured from the date of the application for benefits.

Medicare—a federal health insurance program primarily for people aged 65 and older. There are two parts to the original Medicare program: Part A provides hospital insurance and Part B provides medical insurance. (The third part, Part C, is simply an indirect way to access the original Medicare coverage of Parts A and B through insurance companies rather than directly through the federal government.)

Medicare Part A: Hospital Insurance—Part A helps pay the expense of inpatient hospital care and provides limited benefits for skilled-nursing home care, home health care, hospice care, and psychiatric hospital care. There are no monthly premiums.

Medicare Part B: Medical Insurance—Part B helps pay for doctors' services, medically necessary outpatient hospital services, x-rays, and other diagnostic services, durable medical equipment, and some other services and supplies. There are monthly premiums required and therefore a person may opt out.

medigap policy—a policy usually designed specifically to cover deductibles and any coinsurance required by Medicare coverage. Medigap policies are also known as *Medicare supplement* policies.

MIB, Inc.—a not-for-profit association of insurance companies that exchanges information among its members relevant to the underwriting of life, health, disability income, and LTCI. Its purpose is to protect insurers, and ultimately their policyowners, from losses by facilitating the detection and deterrence of fraud by those who may omit or try to conceal facts essential to proper classification and selection of insurance applicants.

National Association of Insurance Commissioners (NAIC)—membership organization of insurance commissioners whose goal is to promote uniformity of state regulation and legislation as it relates to insurance. The NAIC often drafts model legislation that is eventually adopted by individual states.

NAIC LTCI Model Act—the NAIC promulgated the Model Act in 1987. It is designed to be incorporated into a state's insurance law.

NAIC LTCI model legislation—important legislation adopted by the National Association of Insurance Commissioners in 1987 and in 1988 that established guidelines for insurance companies to follow regarding LTCI policy design, policy definitions, and policy provisions. This legislation also specified marketing procedures and important notifications that must be provided to an insured or prospective insured, before taking the application, during the underwriting process, and after the coverage takes effect.

NAIC LTCI Model Regulation—the NAIC issued the Model Regulation in 1988. It is designed to be adopted for use in implementing the Model Act.

NAIC Shopper's Guide—a piece that explains important aspects of LTCI and the need for it and serves as a *neutral* source of information from a third party. It helps guide prospects to understand LTCI and to decide which policy to buy.

networking—the process of continuous communication and the sharing of ideas and prospects with others whose work does not compete with yours as an advisor

noncancelable—a provision that offers the highest level of protection for the policyowner, since the premiums are guaranteed and the contract cannot be changed. The insurer assumes all the risk concerning the actuarial assumptions used in underwriting the policy, no matter what changes subsequently take place. The NAIC LTCI Model Regulation allows only noncancelable policies to use the term "level premium".

noncountable (exempt) assets—certain assets that are not counted toward Medicaid eligibility a person may keep regardless of worth and still be eligible for benefits. They include items like: a small sum of money (usually $2,000–$3,000); a primary residence and household furnishings; a prepaid funeral and burial plot worth up to $1,500; term life insurance; business assets and real property, if one earns a livelihood from them; all personal property; one engagement and one wedding ring, regardless of value; and one automobile limited to $4,500 in value, unless medically equipped (then there is no limit).

nonforfeiture benefit—a benefit in which the policyowner will receive some value for the policy if the policy lapses because the required premium is not paid. The most common type of nonforfeiture option is a *shortened benefit period*. With this option, coverage is continued as a paid-up policy, but the length of the benefit period (or the amount of the benefit if stated as a maximum dollar amount) is reduced.

nonqualified LTCI policy (contract)—a term that refers to all LTCI policies being sold that do not meet the requirements of HIPAA. They are believed to not be eligible for the tax benefits provided under tax-qualified policies as defined by HIPAA.

nonverbal signals—gestures, bodily movements, or facial expressions, such as leaning forward, listening attentively, making eye contact, nodding, showing appreciation, or participating that indicate acceptance or rejection of a person or an idea

nursing home (care)—a state-licensed facility that provides skilled, intermediate, and custodial care services with the care recipient's condition determining the combination and extent of services provided

objections: four categories—resistance to purchasing LTCI that fall into one of four general categories: no need, no money, no hurry, and no confidence

other care services—the realm of services provided under the auspices of LTC has broadened beyond physical and medical needs. One example is social care, aimed at preventing the loneliness and isolation that a person requiring LTC often experiences. Also included are the services that are required in order to adapt the home to the care recipient's needs.

outline of coverage—a clear and simple description of the policy's most important features. It is an important tool for explaining the policy features to the prospect or applicant.

partnership programs for LTC—alliances between state governments and insurance companies to encourage the sale of approved LTCI policies in order to protect people from being impoverished by LTC expenses and to prevent them from becoming immediately dependent on Medicaid

personal history interview—a telephone interview that is conducted after the application is received and provides an independent verification of information on the application. It also affords an opportunity to clarify responses, ask additional questions, and assess cognitive ability. Some interviews are conducted by specialized agencies under contract; while others may be conducted by company personnel specially trained to do this.

pivot approach—transitioning from a successful or unsuccessful sale or discussion of one product and asking for an appointment to discuss another financial or insurance need and product

pivoting—a suggestion to the prospect that he or she consider alternative products for financing his or her LTC needs when that prospect does not qualify for LTCI

pool of money—a method introduced to determine total plan benefits regardless of where the services were provided. The pool of money is calculated by multiplying the number of days of coverage times the MDB amount. As benefits are paid for the actual charges incurred up to the MDB, the pool of money is reduced by the actual dollar amount of benefits paid.

post-claims underwriting—it occurs when an insurer does little underwriting at the time of initial application. Then, after a claim is filed, the insurer obtains medical information that could have been obtained earlier. Based on this new information, the insurer either rescinds the policy of denies the claim.

preapproach—any method or strategy used to create awareness of who an advisor is and interest in his or her products so that prospects are preconditioned to meet with the advisor and buy his or her products. Examples of methods include direct mail, building prestige, a ten-second commercial, and a résumé.

preexisting condition—some illness or disability for which the applicant was treated or advised within a time period prior to the issuance of an insurance contract that might affect underwriting and/or limit the payment of a claim

professional ethics—code of ethics mandating high standards of behavior to which those professionals in a chosen career (such as financial services) should constantly adhere

professionalism—participation in a chosen career that is characterized by peer acceptance, certifications or designations, technical knowledge, expertise, dedication, ethical behavior, and integrity

prospect—the potential buyer who has been identified by an advisor

prospecting—the continuous activity of identifying new candidates for the products and services an advisor provides

QTIP trust—It permits a spouse to provide for a surviving spouse by transferring assets to a trust that qualifies for the marital deduction and yet permits the transferor spouse to retain control over the ultimate disposition of the assets.

qualified prospect—A person who needs and values an advisor's products and services, can afford them, is insurable, and is approachable

referral—a person who has been suggested by another person as a prospect who may be interested in the products and services an advisor provides. Referrals are also known as referred leads and can come from clients, prospects, centers of influence, and even nonprospects.

reimbursement basis—the method of paying LTCI policy benefits in which the insured is reimbursed for actual expenses up to the specified policy limit. For example, if the insured has a reimbursement policy and has a MDB of $200 but has claims of $150 per day, only $150 would be paid. In contrast, an indemnity (per diem) policy would pay the full MDB of $200.

reinstatement—a provision that requires the insurer to restore coverage to its original premium-paying status. Usually it requires evidence of good health and payment of past-due premiums. This provision requires the insurer to reinstate the policy if the policyowner provides proof that the insured was cognitively impaired at the time the premium was due and the policy lapsed within 6 months of the due date.

rescind—the action an insurance company takes to void a policy

respite care—a LTC service that relieves a primary caregiver from the physical and emotional stress of providing care over a long period of time and/or to allow some period of personal time

restoration of benefits—under this provision insureds can have their full complement of benefits restored if they previously received less than full policy benefits and have not received any policy benefits for a certain time period, often 180 days

résumé—a preapproach method consisting of a professional, one-page promotion piece that contains information about the advisor and his or her professional qualifications and expertise

return of premium rider—a nonforfeiture benefit offered by some policies in which a portion of the premium is returned if the policy lapses. For example, the policy of one insurer pays nothing if the policy lapses before it has been in force for 5 full years and increasing percentages of the premiums are paid the longer the policy was in force (when it lapsed). Depending on the insurer, any benefits paid while coverage was in force may or may not be deducted from the refund.

reverse mortgage—a special type of housing loan that allows homeowners age 62 and over to convert the equity in their houses into cash. Payments can be in the form of a single lump sum, regular monthly advances, a line of credit, or a combination of these. There are no payments by homeowners or any obligations to make repayments as long as they remain in the house.

revocable living trust—a generally established way to avoid both the cost and the public nature of probate. By transferring ownership of all you own to the living trust, you avoid the costs, the time lag, and the public record aspects of probate. The living trust focuses on the management and distribution of assets during both life and death. The owner retains full control and the agreement is revocable and amendable at any time while the owner is alive. Trust assets are fully includable in the estate at the owner's death. Property that passes through the living trust has its ownership transferred to the trust.

selection—the underwriter must select those applicants who are within the insurer's range of acceptability. Selection implies there are both acceptances and rejections, since not all applicants are accepted for insurance.

selling process—the name given for the 10 steps involved in successfully making a sale, beginning with selecting a prospect and ending with providing ongoing service. It is also referred to as the sales cycle.

seminars—seminars are an extremely effective way to prospect, especially in the senior market. They are live infomercials that both educate and motivate a large number of people simultaneously. They are a form of mass marketing.

shared benefit—a benefit offered by some insurers when both a husband and wife are insured with them. It allows each spouse to access the benefits of the other spouse. For example, if each spouse has a 4-year benefit period and one spouse has exhausted his or her benefits, benefit payments can continue by drawing on any unused benefits under the other spouse's policy. An insurer may allow the transfer of any unused benefits to a surviving spouse's benefits or allow the spouses to purchase an extra benefit, equal to the separate benefit on each spouse.

silent generation—the name given to the generation born between 1925 to 1945. They are marked as people who are private, cautious, self-reliant, hardworking, and frugal. They are also referred to as *the Silents*.

skilled nursing facility—nursing homes that meet the accreditation criteria required for reimbursement of services provided to Medicare and Medicaid patients

social care—care that is aimed at preventing the loneliness and isolation that a person requiring LTC often experiences

social style—predictable patterns of behavior that people display in assertive/responsive situations. Appropriate responses to the characteristics of each social style indicate how you can best establish rapport with a prospect who has that style.

spousal discounts—policies that offer some type of married couple or (partner) reductions. The discounts vary depending on whether both spouses apply for and are accepted by the same company; or whether both spouses apply for but only one spouse is accepted. Some states require that a married person be given the discount whether or not the spouse applies for or is even insurable for LTCI. Some companies offer the discount to unmarried couples or same sex partners. The two adults typically must be from the same generation and live in the same household. Some newer policies cover several members of the same family who are from different generations. Living with another person tends to lower the need for LTC, so companies are gradually becoming more favorably disposed to offering these types of discounts.

springing durable power of attorney—a document signed by one person (the principal) authorizing another person (the attorney-in-fact) to act on behalf of the signer. A springing durable power becomes operative only when a specified event occurs, such as the physical or mental incapacity of the principal.

state regulations—state laws that deal with insurance companies, insurance products, and that establish rules for advisors regarding licensing and sales practices

substantial assistance—involves the physical assistance of a person to help him or her perform ADLs or the necessary presence of another person within arm's reach to prevent, by physical intervention, injury to the individual while performing ADLs

suitability—means determining whether LTCI is appropriate for meeting an applicant's needs. Suitability standards must take the applicant's ability to pay, his or her goals or needs, and his or her values, benefits, and costs of coverage into account.

survivorship benefit—a typical provision that states that if the coverage remains in force for a specified number of years and one spouse dies without having received any benefits, the surviving spouse would then have a paid-up policy. Different policies require different in-force time durations, as well as consideration of whether or not the payment of a claim would terminate the benefit.

target market—an identifiable group of people with common characteristics and needs (a market segment) that is accessible and has a communication or networking system

tax-qualified LTCI policy (contract)—LTCI policies that meet the requirements of HIPAA and therefore are eligible for favorable tax treatment

telephone approach—using the telephone to set an appointment with a prospect

ten-second commercial—a preapproach strategy that involves having several creative, well-thought-out, customized responses to the question, "What do you do for a living?"

third-party notification—a method of preventing the inadvertent lapse of a policy, particularly by a person with physical or cognitive impairment, whereby the policyowner must be given the option of naming another person to receive notification of the cancellation of a LTCI policy for nonpayment of premium. This provision requires the insurer, after the premium is overdue by at least 30 days, to notify both the policyowner and the alternative premium payor that (1) the premium is overdue and (2) the policy will lapse 30 days after the notice is mailed unless the premium is paid prior to that time.

30-day free look—a policy provision that gives the policyowner the opportunity to return the policy for a full refund of premium without explanation. The policyowner has 30 days from the day he or she receives the policy.

trust—the trust agreement contains the provisions that act as the instructions to the trustee from the grantor regarding what can and cannot be done with the trust property. The four components of a trust are the corpus, grantor, trustee, and beneficiary.

types of groups—the name given for basically two types: Employer-sponsored plans and affinity groups or associations that make coverage available as a member benefit

underwriting—the insurer's process for selecting and classifying insurance applicants. It is a critical component of the insurance equation. Determining who qualifies for coverage (selection) and on what terms and conditions and at what price (classification) is what underwriting is all about.

viatical settlement—a method used by terminally ill insureds that leverages the death benefit of life insurance policies while the insured is still living. It involves a third party, typically a viatical settlement company, that pays a percentage of the policy's face amount in a lump sum. The third party assumes ownership of the policy and is responsible for the premium payment and, in return, receives the death proceeds and any dividends.

voluntary benefit plan—the term that is often used to refer to worksite-marketing situations in which LTCI coverage is made available as part of an employee-employer relationship and the insured pays the entire premium

waiver-of-premium—a benefit in which the policyowner does not have to pay premiums after the insured has begun to receive benefit payments or has received them for a period of time. While the premiums are being waived, the policy remains fully in force. Unlike comparable provisions in life insurance and many other types of health insurance, there are a variety of circumstances that might apply to the waiver-of-premium provision for LTCI.

women—as a market segment, women have a greater exposure to LTC than men. They have a much higher probability of caring for an elderly parent or relative than men, and they typically purchase LTCI because they do not want to be a burden to their loved ones. Men typically purchase LTCI to preserve assets.

Answers to Questions

Chapter 1

Answers to Review Questions

1-1. The 10 steps in the selling process are:

1. Select the Prospect—This involves picking prospects that have a high probability of needing, wanting, and affording LTCI as well as qualifying for it.

2. Approach the Prospect—This involves getting appointments, and it can be done either by telephone or face to face.

3. Meet the Prospect—This involves establishing rapport, explaining your business purpose, asking thought-provoking questions, and listening.

4. Gather Information—This involves conducting a fact-finding interview to uncover the prospects needs, goals, priorities, attitudes, and financial situation.

5. Analyze the Situation—This involves analyzing the products you have to see how they might best fit into a plan that meets the prospect's situation.

6. Present Solutions—This involves positioning your plan to meet the prospect's situation as detemined by the fact-finding interview.

7. Implement the Solution—This involves helping the prospect acquire the products and services required to put the plan into action.

8. Underwrite—This involves completing the application, performing all necessary field underwriting, and submitting the case to the company.

9. Deliver the Contract—This involves delivering the policy, reviewing the policy's benefits with the insured, explaining how the benefits resolve the insured's situation, and setting the stage for monitoring the situation through a plan of periodic review.

10. Service the Plan—This involves servicing the policy during the claims process and setting the stage for obtaining quality referrals.

1-2. The four major factors involved with the impending LTC crisis are the

- increasing need for LTC services
- decreasing ability of families to provide care
- high cost of care
- lack of viable options to pay for care

1-3. LTC can best be defined as the broad range of medical, custodial, and other care services provided over an extended period of time in various care settings due to a chronic illness, physical disability, or cognitive impairment.

1-4. Emotional reasons why people buy LTCI are to
- be independent and not have to depend on anyone else for their care
- avoid being a burden on family and/or friends
- have a choice of care providers and care settings
- protect assets and be able to leave a legacy for their children

1-5. The three age-based market segments described in the text are
- under age 50
- ages 50 to 65
- over age 65

Answers to Self-Test Questions

1-1.   c
1-2.   e
1-3.   b
1-4.   d
1-5.   b
1-6.   a
1-7.   d
1-8.   c
1-9.   d
1-10. a

Chapter 2

Answers to Review Questions

2-1. A qualified prospect is a person who
- needs and values your products and services
- can afford to pay for your products and services
- is insurable
- can be approached by you on a favorable basis

2-2. Ways in which prospects in the under age 50 market segment can be approached to buy LTCI are to
- buy LTCI for themselves
- buy or facilitate the buying of LTCI for their parents or other relatives for whom they feel responsible

2-3. Reasons why the ages 50 to 65 market segment will be the bread and butter market for LTCI for the next several years are:

- Over the next several years, the Baby Boomer population bulge will dominate the ages 50 to 65 market segment, making it the market segment with the most prospects by sheer numbers alone.
- People in this market segment typically are at their peak income levels and LTCI premiums are relatively low for the younger ages in the segment.
- People generally view LTC as a retirement planning issue and ages 50 to 65 are when planning for retirement becomes a front-burner issue.
- People in this market segment have a greater likelihood of experiencing a parent or other elderly relative needing LTC, and people who have had this type of experience are more receptive to buying LTCI.

2-4. You have a target market if you can find a market segment that has a communication or network system. The communication system or network provides the means by which your reputation as a professional advisor can precede you. Market segmentation is a powerful marketing strategy that allows you to customize your approach and presentations based on the common needs and characteristics of the prospects in the segmented market.

2-5. Prospecting methods include
   a. referrals: These are people to whom you are introduced by someone who knows and values your work.
   b. centers of influence: These are influential people who know you favorably and agree to introduce or recommend you to others.
   c. networking: This is the process of continuous communication and the sharing of ideas and prospects with others whose work does not compete with yours.
   d. seminars: These are a means to present LTCI to several prospects at one time, resulting in less time needed to conduct one-on-one interviews.
   e. cold calling: This involves contacting strangers by telephone, typically from a list purchased from a reputable vendor.

2-6. Ways to preapproach a prospect include
   - direct mail: a letter or postcard that preconditions prospects to be receptive when you call them
   - building prestige: build a reputation that allows you to approach prospects on a favorable basis
   - a ten-second commercial: a short response to the question, "What do you do for a living?" that is relevant and interesting to the person asking the question
   - a résumé: a one-page self promotional piece that introduces you

2-7. A good approach script should
   - have a greeting: you want to make a good first impression
   - create interest: you are trying to motivate prospects to see you

- ask for an appointment: you are calling to get this
- have a closing: you need to reconfirm the appointment and affirm your desire to meet

2-8.   Four advantages of seminars are
- they enable you to use time efficiently: Seminars enable you to present yourself and your products to a large number of prospects at one time.
- they enable you to meet prospects in a nonthreatening way: Seminars allow prospects to warm up to you because they do not have to share any financial and health information at this time.
- they enable you to maximize your public speaking ability: Some advisors are natural-born public speakers, making seminars an extremely enjoyable and effective form of marketing.
- they enable you to prequalify prospects: Although you initiate the seminar by inviting the prospects, they confirm their interest by attending and represent a much better prospect pool than a cold call list.

Answers to Self-Test Questions

2-1.   c
2-2.   d
2-3.   a
2-4.   c
2-5.   d
2-6.   b
2-7.   c
2-8.   d
2-9.   a
2-10.   d

Chapter 3

Answers to Review Questions

3-1.   a. An informal caregiver is an individual who voluntarily cares for a LTC recipient without pay and without formal education or training in LTC.
        b. A formal caregiver is an individual who provides care and services as a profession or occupation to LTC recipients.

c. A respite caregiver is an alternate caregiver who provides services to relieve a primary caregiver from the physical and emotional stress of providing care or to allow some period of personal time.

d. A care coordinator is also known as a care planner or care manager. This person assesses an elderly person who shows some degree of physical or cognitive impairment to determine his or her care needs and then develops a care plan to meet those needs.

3-2. a. Home health care encompasses care provided in the care recipient's home, his or her child's home, or even in an independent living or assisted living facility.

b. An adult day care center is a place that provides social, medical, and rehabilitative services to people with physical and cognitive impairments. It provides a place for such people to go while their primary caregiver works.

c. Independent housing encompasses a wide range of housing arrangements for seniors who require little or no assistance. It includes senior apartments, home sharing, and accessory apartments.

d. An assisted-living facility is a place for elderly residents who remain significantly independent but have some impairment and require some degree of supervision or help.

e. A nursing home is a facility that provides skilled, intermediate, and custodial care services with the care recipient's condition determining the combination and extent of services provided.

f. A combined facility offers two or more shared-living arrangements that provide the same housing and services as provided under a separate supportive living arrangement.

g. Hospice care is a system of treatment designed to relieve the discomfort of a terminally ill individual and to maintain quality of life to the extent possible throughout the phases of dying.

3-3. The four sources used to pay for LTC are
- self-funding
- government programs
- LTCI
- charity

3-4. There are a couple of ways to use life insurance to pay for LTC.
- Accelerated death benefits: Many policies make cash advances to terminally ill insureds, while some policies also include chronic illnesses as a legitimate reason for making cash advances.
- Viatical settlements: A terminally ill insured sells his or her policy to a viatical company for a lump-sum payment. When the insured dies, the viatical company receives the proceeds.

3-5.   Yes, Medicare will cover Jane's nursing home care for up to 100 days. A copayment will be charged for days 21 to 100 of care.

3-6.   • Jack: No, Jack is not eligible for Medicare benefits because Medicare does not cover custodial care. To receive care, Jack would have to have received care in a hospital for at least 3 consecutive days before being transferred to a skilled-nursing facility. The facts give no indication of Jack needing acute care in a hospital.

   • Jill: Possibly, if Jill had a 3-day hospital stay, she would be eligible for skilled-nursing facility care. However, without the hospital stay, Jill is not eligible for benefits to rehabilitate her broken leg.

   • June: No, June is not eligible for Medicare benefits because cognitive impairments are not covered.

3-7.   a. Joe would have to spend all but $30 to $50 per month of his income on care. This amount is known as a personal needs allowance and is designed to cover a Medicaid recipient's personal expenses. There is no specific income limit in medically needy states.

   b. Joe would have to spend all of his income on care because he does not qualify for Medicaid since his monthly income of $3,288 is not less than 3 times the SSI benefit level of $1,656 (in 2003).

3-8.   a. The $80,000 in stocks and bonds are countable assets that Joe must exhaust before he can qualify for Medicaid benefits.

   b. The residence, household furnishing and personal effects, car (limited to $4,500 in value), and cash (usually no more than $2,000 to $3,000) are noncountable assets and do not count toward Medicaid eligibility. Joe may keep these assets and still be eligible for benefits.

Answers to Self-Test Questions

3-1.   a
3-2.   c
3-3.   b
3-4.   d
3-5.   b
3-6.   b
3-7.   c
3-8.   a
3-9.   d
3-10. c

Chapter 4

Answers to Review Questions

4-1. The main purpose of the initial interview in a two-interview sales approach is to build the foundation for a collaborative relationship with the prospect, not to make a sale.

4-2. The four social styles and the characteristic that best explains what a prospect with a particular style wants are:
- Driver: a prospect who wants to be in control
- Expressive: a prospect who wants to be recognized
- Amiable: a prospect who wants to be accepted
- Analytical: a prospect who wants to be accurate

4-3. The steps involved in the LTC planning process are to
1. assist the prospect in forming goals and objectives
2. help the prospect identify existing resources for meeting the goals and objectives
3. analyze the gap between the goals and objectives and the existing resources
4. devise a plan for bridging the resource gap
5. implement the plan
6. monitor the plan

4-4. Sales presentation tools and techniques that can be used by an advisor to help explain the need for LTCI are
- visual materials to help focus attention
- third-party substantiation brochures, fact sheets, and testimonials
- statistical evidence using charts and graphs to show the cost of LTC and its trend
- real-life stories and case histories of people needing LTC
- a shoppers guide that can assist people in determining whether LTCI is appropriate for them

4-5. The initials LTCINS stand for Long-Term Care Insurance. It is an acronym for key information that an advisor needs to obtain from a prospect. With the information linked together, the advisor can make a relatively quick judgment about whether the prospect is insurable. The acronym's letters stand for a series of questions that the advisor needs to ask the prospect.
- L is Life Span and the questions relate to date of birth.
- T is Time in Hospital and the questions relate to health.
- C is Children and the questions relate to family.
- I is Insurance Proposals and the questions relate to potential competition.
- N is Nursing Home Experience and the questions relate to exposure to nursing homes.
- S is Savings Level and the questions relate to ability to pay for the coverage.

4-6. The four characteristics of qualified prospects for LTCI are:
- They need and value your products and services.

- They can afford to pay for LTCI.
- They are insurable for LTCI.
- They can be approached by you on a favorable basis.

4-7.   Some prospects fail to qualify for LTCI during the fact-finding interview because they
- are hostile or uncooperative
- are uninsurable for LTCI
- have insufficient funds to purchase LTCI
- are shopping for a better deal

4-8.   The three distinct discovery components of a formal LTC fact-finding form are the
- factual component
- quantitative component
- attitudinal component

4-9.   The name of the implied contract that represents mutual consent between the prospect and you to continue working together is the discovery agreement.

4-10. Two three-step techniques for responding to prospect resistance are
- *acknowledge* a concern, *clarify* it, and then *resolve* it
- to use the words *feel, felt,* and *found* in three successive sentences as demonstrated below:
  - I understand how you *feel.*
  - Many of my prospects have *felt* the same way.
  - Until they *found* that . . . (state a benefit or explain how the plan was a good solution for their situation.)

4-11. The four general categories of objections to purchasing LTCI are
- no need
- no money
- no hurry
- no confidence

Answers to Self-Test Questions

4-1.   b
4-2.   a
4-3.   b
4-4.   c
4-5.   a
4-6.   b
4-7.   d
4-8.   b
4-9.   d
4-10. c

Chapter 5

Answers to Review Questions

5-1. It is advisable not to emphasize price when selling LTCI because price is usually a function of the benefits a policy has to offer. Typically, if a policy is inexpensive, it probably is so because its benefits are not as generous as those in higher-priced policies. Significant variations in policy benefits exist from one insurance company to another, and these variations can usually be tied to price. Consequently, when selling LTCI, focus on a policy's benefits because they usually account for the price being charged. In this regard, however, it should be noted just how difficult it is to compare the benefits of any two LTCI policies because of the wide variations that often exist between policies.

5-2. The following pertain to LTCI as follows:

    a. Respite care provides for temporary institutional or home care for an insured whose informal caregiver takes vacation or break time.

    b. Caregiver training provides training for a family member or friend in how to give safe and effective care, so that an insured in need of care can remain at home.

    c. A pool of money is a method for measuring the maximum dollar amount that can be paid under certain LTCI policies. The pool of money can be calculated by multiplying the number of days (years) of coverage times the MDB amount.

    d. A bed reservation benefit continues policy payments to a LTC facility for a limited time (such as 20 days) if the insured temporarily leaves the facility for any reason.

5-3. The pool of money available for Matthew's reimbursement type of LTCI policy with a 4-year benefit period and a MDB amount of $200 is calculated by multiplying the benefit period by the MDB amount. Thus, 4 years or 1,460 days is multiplied by $200 and equals $292,000.

5-4. Home health care services can be counted toward the elimination period in several different ways.

    • Under the days-of-service method, only those days when actual services are received are counted.

    • Under the calendar-days method, once the insured qualifies for benefits and begins to receive services, only a specific number of calendar days must pass before the policy would actually pay benefits.

    • Under a blended variation of the days-of-service and calendar-days approaches, each week is counted as seven days toward the satisfaction of the elimination period if services were received on at least one day of the week.

    • Another variation of the elimination period found in reimbursement policies is for the insurer to start counting days toward the satisfaction of the period as soon as a physician certifies that LTC is necessary.

5-5. Most insurers offer spousal or partner discounts for LTCI policies because living with another person tends to lower the need for LTC. Spouses or partners can assist with and/or supervise the caregiving process and provide for companionship and support. Consequently, individual people are more likely to go on claim than are people with spouses or partners.

5-6. Other insurance coverages that have been packaged with LTCI in combination products are
- life insurance
- disability income insurance
- annuities

5-7. Under HIPAA, a person is defined as being chronically ill if he or she requires substantial assistance with at least 2 of 6 ADLs for a period of at least 90 days due to a loss of functional capacity or requires substantial services to protect him or her from threats to health and safety due to substantial cognitive impairment.

5-8. The tax treatment of nonqualified LTCI policy benefits has been the subject of controversy and uncertainty because HIPAA provides no clear statement regarding their taxation. Nevertheless, there is a growing consensus that such policies are in fact taxable because they are not listed by HIPAA as tax-free. On the other hand, some experts have concluded that the benefits of nonqualified policies are not taxable income because they should be treated for tax purposes like any other accident and sickness insurance benefits. Adding to the uncertainty is the fact that the IRS has thus far not issued a ruling on this matter.

Answers to Self-Test Questions

5-1. c
5-2. c
5-3. a
5-4. a
5-5. b
5-6. b
5-7. c
5-8. a
5-9. d
5-10. c

Chapter 6

Answers to Review Questions

6-1. The three things that must happen before LTCI policy benefits can be paid are
   1. an impairment must exist, as assessed by a health care professional
   2. services must be received for the impairment
   3. the elimination (waiting) period must be satisfied

6-2. The steps in calculating the MDB amount to include in a LTCI policy are
   1. determine the daily cost of nursing home care in the area
   2. subtract the daily amount of care that can be paid from income
   3. subtract the daily amount of care that can be paid from assets
   4. the difference represents the MDB to include in the policy

6-3. Key areas to evaluate when comparing the competition with your company and its products are
   - financial strength and claims-paying ability
   - reputation
   - product price
   - rate stability over time
   - company and advisor service
   - differences in the policies

6-4. Possible funding alternatives for LTC services other than LTCI are
   - savings and investments
   - annuity cash values and income payments
   - life insurance cash values and accelerated death benefits
   - life insurance viatical settlements
   - reverse mortgages
   - family members
   - Medicare and Medicaid

6-5. The difference between a policy feature and a policy benefit is that a feature is a characteristic of the policy itself—what it is and what it does. A feature is a fact about the policy. On the other hand, a benefit is what the insured gets as a result of the feature. It is what the policy does for the insured and usually why he or she wants it. Features produce benefits.

6-6. It is important to have the prospect's participation and involvement in the sales process for several reasons:
   - It helps the prospect feel responsible for solving his or her own problems.
   - It helps the advisor know whether he or she is on target with the presentation.
   - It builds agreement one step at a time.
   - It helps to clarify any misunderstandings by either party.

- It helps lead to a logical and successful close—a conclusion to buy.
- It provides opportunities to deal with objections before asking the prospect to buy.

6-7.   Examples of nonverbal buying signals are
- leaning forward
- listening attentively
- good eye contact
- nodding, showing appreciation
- speaking up, participating

6-8.   The three things that should be put in focus when taking a problem-solving approach to handling a prospect's objections to buying LTCI are
- building trust and rapport with the prospect
- dealing with the prospect's needs rather than his or her personality
- instilling a sense of urgency to act now and buy LTCI

Answers to Self-Test Questions

6-1.   c
6-2.   d
6-3.   g
6-4.   f
6-5.   e
6-6.   a
6-7.   b
6-8.   b
6-9.   d
6-10.   a

Chapter 7

Answers to Review Questions

7-1.   Steps the advisor must take in completing the application are to
- obtain all the information requested
- complete the application in the applicant's presence
- record accurately all information provided by the applicant
- obtain the necessary signatures
- complete a suitability statement
- provide the applicant with an outline of coverage; a shopper's guide; and all required receipts, documents, and disclosure information

7-2. Suitability standards must take into account the
- applicant's ability to pay for the coverage and other financial information appropriate to its purchase
- applicant's goals or needs with respect to LTCI and the advantages and disadvantages of LTCI in meeting those goals or needs
- values, benefits, and costs of any of the applicant's existing LTCI compared to the values, benefits, and costs of the recommended purchase or replacement

7-3. The sources of information used by an underwriter are
- the application
- attending physicians' statements
- the MIB
- a personal history telephone interview
- a face-to-face assessment interview

7-4. Factors used to classify LTCI applicants into rate categories are
- age
- medical condition
- marital status
- tobacco use

7-5. The objectives of the delivery interview are to
- reinforce the buying decision
- review the policy
- build the advisor-client relationship
- obtain required forms
- develop other sales opportunities

7-6. a. The tremendous financial and personal risk exposure that LTC poses must be a serious consideration in every retirement plan. A retirement plan that does not address this issue would have to be considered incomplete. A secure retirement depends not only on accumulating sufficient assets, but also on protecting those assets from the potentially devastating effects of LTC.

b. LTC and estate concerns are inextricably intertwined, as both are concerned with the preservation of assets. Because of the enormous potential costs of LTC, everything a person owns may be lost. The ultimate goal of estate planning is to fulfill the wishes of the individual regarding the disposition of his or her property at death. LTC planning is an important part of this process, because one can protect assets that might otherwise be used to pay for LTC.

Answers to Self-Test Questions

7-1. b
7-2. b

7-3.   a
7-4.   c
7-5.   a
7-6.   d
7-7.   a
7-8.   c
7-9.   d
7-10.   b

Chapter 8

Answers to Review Questions

8-1.   The two types of LTCI marketed to employees at the worksite are
  • traditional group insurance: This type of worksite coverage is characterized by a master group contract with individual certificates, group underwriting, and possibly experience rating.
  • mass-marketed individual insurance: This type of worksite coverage is not true group insurance but individual policies.

8-2.   The tax treatment of premiums paid by a C corporation employer for tax-qualified LTCI contracts is
  • income tax deductible by the employer as a legitimate business expense because LTCI is regarded as accident and health insurance
  • to not include them in the gross income of covered employees

8-3.   The goals of state partnership programs for LTC are to
  • protect people from being impoverished by LTC expenses
  • prevent people from becoming immediately dependent on Medicaid

8-4.   Those eligible for coverage under FLTCIP include federal and postal employees and annuitants, members and retired members of the uniformed services, and qualified relatives. Qualified relatives include spouses, children (at least 18 years old), parents, parents-in-law, and stepparents.

8-5.   The purpose of the NAIC's model legislation with regard to LTCI was to establish guidelines for insurance companies to follow regarding policy design, policy definitions, and provisions that should be offered in policies, as well as marketing procedures and important notifications that should be provided to prospects before taking their applications and to insureds after their coverage takes effect. The legislation consists of a Model Act that is designed to be incorporated into a state's insurance law and a Model Regulation that is designed to be adopted for use in implementing the law.

8-6.   The NAIC's Model Act excludes life insurance policies from the definition of LTCI if the life insurance policies
   - accelerate the death benefit specifically for one or more of the qualifying events of terminal illness, medical conditions requiring extraordinary medical intervention, or permanent institutional confinement
   - provide the option of a lump-sum payment for the previous benefits if neither the benefits nor the eligibility for benefits is conditional upon the receipt of LTC

8-7.   The NAIC Model Act's rules on incontestability for a LTCI policy depend on how long the policy has been in force.
   - If the policy has been in force for less than 6 months, the insurer can rescind the policy or deny an otherwise valid claim upon showing that a misrepresentation was material to the acceptance of coverage.
   - If the policy has been in force for at least 6 months but less than 2 years, the insurer can rescind the policy or deny an otherwise valid claim upon showing that a misrepresentation was both material to the acceptance of coverage and pertains to the condition for which benefits are sought.
   - The policy must contain a provision that makes it incontestable after 2 years on the grounds of misrepresentation alone. However, the insurer can still contest the policy on the basis that the applicant knowingly and intentionally misrepresented relevant facts pertaining to the insured's health.

8-8.   The apparent conflict between doing what is legal and doing what is ethical in dealing with prospects and clients involves situations when fair business practices, legal requirements, and company rules seem to conflict with your best efforts. How this apparent conflict is resolved is a matter of ehtics, and it goes beyond compliance with the laws. Sometimes there is a gap between what is legal and what is ethical. The gap represents the difference between what you have a right to do, and what is the right thing to do. To infuse your character with ethics, you must not be content to merely comply with the law. Ethical behavior is doing the right thing. It is doing what is right and putting the prospect's or client's best interest before your own.

Answers to Self-Test Questions

8-1.   a
8-2.   b
8-3.   b
8-4.   c
8-5.   a
8-6.   c
8-7.   d
8-8.   d

8-9.   c
8-10.   b

Index